YANKEY

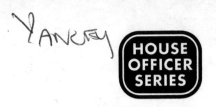

Orthopaedics

SECOND EDITION

D1435266

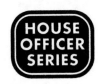

Orthopaedics

SECOND EDITION

Frank V. Aluisio, MD
Christian P. Christensen, MD
James R. Urbaniak, MD

Division of Orthopaedic Surgery
Department of Surgery
Duke University Medical Center
Durham, North Carolina

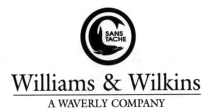

Williams & Wilkins

A WAVERLY COMPANY

BALTIMORE • PHILADELPHIA • LONDON • PARIS • BANGKOK
HONG KONG • MUNICH • SYDNEY • TOKYO • WROCLAW

Editor: Charles W. Mitchell
Managing Editor: Grace E. Miller
Marketing Manager: Rebecca Himmelheber
Production Coordinator: Felecia R. Weber
Project Editor: Jennifer D. Weir
Designer: Dan Pfisterer
Illustration Planner: Ray Lowman
Cover Designer: Graphic World
Typesetter: Bi-Comp, Inc.
Printer/Binder: Vicks Lithograph & Printing

Copyright © 1998 Williams & Wilkins

351 West Camden Street
Baltimore, Maryland 21201-2436 USA

Rose Tree Corporate Center
1400 North Providence Road
Building II, Suite 5025
Media, Pennsylvania 19063-2043 USA

Accurate indications, adverse reactions, and dosage schedules for drugs are provided in this book, but it is possible that they may change. The reader is urged to review the package information data of the manufacturers of the medications mentioned.

Printed in the United States of America

First Edition, 1990

Library of Congress Cataloging-in-Publication Data

Aluisio, Frank V.
Orthopaedics / Frank V. Aluisio, Christian P. Christensen, James
    R. Urbaniak.—2nd ed.
    p.   cm.—(The House officer series)
    Rev. ed. of: Orthopaedics for the house officer / William J.
    Mallon, Michael J. McNamara, James R. Urbaniak. c1990.
Includes bibliographical references and index.
ISBN 0-683-18213-7
1. Orthopedics.   I. Christensen, Christian P.   II. Urbaniak,
  James R.   III. Mallon, Bill.   Orthopaedics for the house officer.
  IV. Title.   V. Series.
[DNLM: 1. Orthopedics—methods.   2. Wounds and Injuries—therapy.
WE 168 A471o 1998]
RD731.A553   1998
616.7—dc21
DNLM/DLC
for Library of Congress   97-41655
                                                                                  CIP

The publishers have made every effort to trace the copyright holders for borrowed material. If they have inadvertently overlooked any, they will be pleased to make the necessary arrangements at the first opportunity.

To purchase additional copies of this book, call our customer service department at **(800) 638-0672** or fax orders to **(800) 447-8438.** For other book services, including chapter reprints and large quantity sales, ask for the Special Sales department.

Canadian customers should call **(800) 665-1148,** or fax **(800) 665-0103.** For all other calls originating outside of the United States, please call **(410) 528-4223** or fax us at **(410) 528-8550.**

Visit Williams & Wilkins on the Internet: http://www.wwilkins.com or contact our customer service department at **custserv@wwilkins.com.** Williams & Wilkins customer service representatives are available from 8:30 am to 6:00 pm, EST, Monday through Friday, for telephone access.

                                                                    98 99 00 01 02
                                                            1   2   3   4   5   6   7   8   9   10

We take great pride in dedicating this book to the following people:

To my wife, Karen, and children, Nicolette, Matthew, and Tyler; to our families for their tremendous loyalty, and to the memory of my brother, Jeff, and grandfather, Frank.

—Frank V. Aluisio

To my wife, Emily, and in the memory of my father, Bent V. Christensen.

—Christian P. Christensen

To my wife, Muff, and children, Kathi and Michael, who have all helped me in working and learning with residents, fellows, and students.

—James R. Urbaniak

We also dedicate this book to the residents, fellows, and students whom we have had an opportunity to work with and learn from over the past several years at Duke University Medical Center.

Foreword

The training years of an orthopaedic resident can be grueling. The hours spent on call and in the emergency room are far too long; the hours spent at home with family and friends are far too short; and the amount of reading and studying necessary to learn the trade seems endless at times.

In 1980, Mike McNamara and I began medical school together at Duke University and quickly became close friends. This continued through our years at Duke as orthopaedic residents, until we finished there a decade later. While serving our orthopaedic residency, we realized that no small pocket reference book for orthopaedic residents was available for reference in the emergency room or on call. This eventually led to our writing the first edition of *Orthopaedics for the House Officer,* with the assistance of Dr. James R. Urbaniak.

There are many books available from which orthopaedic residents may learn the craft. But late at night, when time is short and the patients are many, trying to read through a 75-page section on a certain type of fracture is difficult, if not impossible. Our goal with the first edition of this book was to provide orthopaedic residents a short reference that would enable them to have some knowledge of what to do, and teach them briefly how to handle the problem. The book is not intended to replace more encyclopedic texts. To fully understand orthopaedics, and become proficient and knowledgeable, all orthopaedic residents must still study and learn from those larger books.

But we hope that our small resident's handbook has served a purpose, and judging from the response to it over the last few years, we think that it has. We originally wrote the first volume in the years 1988–1989, but in this era of rapidly increasing medical technology, a decade is all but an eternity. Thus, it is certainly time for a new edition. Dr. McNamara and myself have both now moved on, having been in practice for seven years, and both of us subspecialize and no longer have the perspective of a House Officer. Thus, we thought it was natural to pass on the writing of a second edition to current orthopaedic residents.

Although I am no longer at Duke, I still work at a hospital across town, and the Duke orthopaedic residents rotate through our service. When I first worked with Frank Aluisio and Chris Christensen, I realized that these were two exceptional residents who would be both capable and willing to maintain, and probably even raise, the standards that we set with the first edition. They have added a lot to our original book, and I think have improved and upgraded it a great deal.

Dr. McNamara and I would both like to acknowledge our debt to Jim Urbaniak. He has served as a mentor to many orthopaedic residents at Duke since he began his practice there in the later '60s and especially so since he became Chief in 1984. This is certainly true in my case, as he provided assistance in my obtaining an orthopaedic residency above that which is normally called for. We would both like to thank him a great deal, not just for helping us with the first edition of this book, but for being our teacher and friend.

William J. Mallon, MD

Preface

When asked to write the second edition of *Orthopaedics for the House Officer*, Chris and I jumped at the opportunity. We soon realized that it would be a monumental task to create a book as informative and successful as the first edition. The goal of this edition is to provide a framework of orthopaedic knowledge applicable to commonly encountered situations involving musculoskeletal disorders. It is, by no means, meant to be an encyclopedic treatise on orthopaedic surgery.

This book serves as an accessible reference that can be carried in a lab coat for use in everyday situations. It was initially designed for use by junior residents in orthopaedics; general surgery and medical residents while on orthopaedic or emergency room rotations; emergency room and primary care physicians; physicians' assistants; and medical students. This edition, with its additional chapters, should also provide useful information for those near or beyond completion of their orthopaedic training.

With the assistance of Dr. Urbaniak, Chris and I have updated the chapters present in the first edition using the most current knowledge available in the orthopaedic literature. Several new chapters have been added to expand the scope of the book. These include chapters on pediatric orthopaedics, arthroplasty, commonly encountered rheumatologic conditions (the arthritides), and commonly used medications in orthopaedics. We hope that this additional information will be useful to those involved in the care of orthopaedic patients.

We give tremendous thanks to Bill Mallon, Mike McNamara and James R. Urbaniak, for their exceptional job in developing the first edition of this book. They provided an outstanding framework to expand upon with this edition. Dr. Urbaniak also utilized his vast experience and expertise in orthopaedics to make significant contributions to this edition. We also gratefully acknowledge the assistance and expert advice of our publishers and editors at Williams & Wilkins.

Frank V. Aluisio

Christian P. Christensen

Contents

Chapter 1

The Language of Orthopaedics

Orthopaedic surgery is a specialty that involves all facets of diagnosis and treatment of disorders of the musculoskeletal system. These range from primary diagnosis and treatment of soft tissue strains to complex surgical reconstruction for fractures, arthritic joints, and other musculoskeletal afflictions. The realm of orthopaedics includes musculoskeletal manifestations of congenital and developmental disorders (cerebral palsy, skeletal dysplasias), systemic diseases (arthritides), occupational or recreational injuries, degenerative conditions (osteoarthritis, tendinopathies), malignancies (primary bone and soft tissue tumors, metastatic lesions), endocrinopathies (hyperparathyroidism, Cushing's), and infectious diseases (osteomyelitis, septic arthritis). This book is intended to be a reference guide for recognizing and providing primary and emergency treatment of common orthopaedic problems and is, by no means, a comprehensive text on diseases and injuries of the musculoskeletal system.

A basic understanding of musculoskeletal anatomy is of tremendous assistance in diagnosing and treating these disorders. The bony skeleton provides structural support and protection for internal organs, has hematopoietic and metabolic functions, and provides a framework for muscular activity to allow for motion and locomotion. Afflictions of bone and joints represent the majority of musculoskeletal disorders treated by orthopaedists. Ligaments, tendons, muscles, and neurovascular structures of the spine and extremities are also essential elements of the musculoskeletal system, with their disorders also commonly treated by orthopaedic surgeons.

The essential component of a knowledge base for anyone interested in pursuing a career in orthopaedics, or for anyone frequently involved in the diagnosis and triage of musculoskeletal disorders, is an accurate history and musculoskeletal exam. This will allow for initial treatment in the emergency situation and also allow for generation of a differential diagnosis in the primary care setting for atraumatic and nonacute disorders. This book will focus on providing a knowledge base for an accurate physical exam, basic diagnostic techniques, and emergency treatment of common musculoskeletal conditions. An accurate initial assessment is of tremendous benefit to the orthopaedic surgeon for providing prompt, efficient, and cost-effective definitive treatment.

The remainder of this chapter will focus on common methods and terms used to describe orthopaedic disorders. Common abbreviations are also included since they are frequently used and can be confusing for those not familiar with them. An overview of bone formation and fracture healing is also included, as it assists in the understanding of fracture patterns and fracture description.

BONE[1,2,3]

Bone formation, or osteogenesis, occurs through one of two distinct mechanisms. The flat bones (skull, clavicle, pelvis) undergo mostly intramembranous ossification, while the remainder of the axial skeleton forms from endochondral ossification through a cartilaginous precursor.

The clavicle begins ossification in the seventh embryonic week and is the first bone to undergo this process. Intramembranous ossification initiates when osteoblasts (bone-forming cells) differentiate from fibrous mesenchymal cells to secrete osteoid, which represents the organic matrix of bone. The osteoid becomes calcified and organizes into a trabecular matrix known as the primary spongiosa. Remodeling then occurs through osteoblastic deposition of new osteoid and osteoclastic resorption of new bone from other sites within the structure. Eventually, growth occurs through the peripheral periosteum.

Endochondral ossification involves bone formation from a cartilaginous precursor. This precursor develops and elongates through chondrocyte growth and synthesis of a hyaline matrix, which becomes calcified. The chondrocytes eventually degenerate, and capillary invasion occurs with the subsequent arrival of osteoblasts, which secrete osteoid onto the calcified matrix to form bone. This represents the primary ossification center. Peripherally, osteoblasts secrete osteoid to form the periosteum.

Long bone elongation occurs through the physis or growth plate. The epiphysis is in the region of bone on the articular side of the physis, while the metaphysis is on the nonarticular side of the physis. In the physeal plate, several histologic zones exist (resting, proliferating, hypertrophic, calcifying) with distinct functions that overall serve to provide a matrix for further bone formation. Long bones increase in width through intramembranous bone formation via cells derived from the periosteum. This process is termed appositional bone growth.

Bone is constantly remodeling throughout life via the processes of osteoblastic deposition and osteoclastic resorption. Developmentally long bones obtain their mature shapes through the processes of elongation, funnelization, hemispherization, and cylinderization.

Figure 1.1 demonstrates the sections of immature long bones. These include the epiphysis, physis, and metaphysis, which have already been described. The diaphysis is the shaft of the long bone.

A basic understanding of bone formation is useful in understanding how they heal after injury. Bones heal by one of two general mechanisms: direct or indirect healing. The type of healing is generally dictated by the fracture pattern and the accuracy and stability of the fracture reduction[4].

Direct, or primary, healing occurs when a stable anatomic reduction has been performed. Prerequisites for direct healing are stable fixation without motion at the fracture site, anatomic reduction, and sufficient blood supply. Bone healing occurs in the initial phase through contact healing in areas of direct contact and gap healing in areas without direct contact. The gap ideally should be less than 1 mm to allow for rapid filling with lamellar bone. Gaps greater than 1 mm will initially fill with woven bone. Haversian remodeling is the second phase of direct bone healing and involves osteoblastic deposition and osteoclastic resorption to reconstitute the bone. Sufficient blood supply is essential for direct healing; thus, excessive soft tissue stripping for fracture reduction and fixation is not encouraged, as it disrupts blood supply. Callus formation is not involved in primary bone healing.

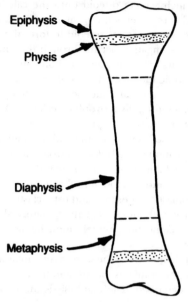

Figure 1.1. The four main parts of a long bone.

Indirect bone healing occurs through formation of callus and differentiation of interfragmentary tissue into bone. This type of healing occurs when the reduction is not anatomic, not stable, or in comminuted fractures with associated bone loss. Even an anatomic reduction will undergo healing through callus if motion occurs at the fracture site. Callus is formed by osteoprogenitor cells in periosteum and endosteum in response to activating factors released from freshly injured bone. The callus provides temporary stabilization and then differentiates in a process similar to endochondral ossification to form new bone, which undergoes remodeling to restore continuity and stability across the fracture site. Delayed unions and nonunions occur when there is a disturbance in the differentiation process of callus into bone (hypertrophic) or secondary to inadequate production of callus (atrophic).

MEASUREMENTS AND TERMS[5]

In diagnosing and treating musculoskeletal injuries and disorders, one will use terminology not commonly heard in other medical specialties. The following section will provide a partial list of basic descriptive terms frequently used by orthopaedic surgeons:

Proximal/Distal: These terms describe the relationship between two points on an extremity. The **proximal** portion will be that portion of the extremity closest to the axial skeleton, while the **distal** portion will be farther away. This relationship can be described for the entire extremity (femur is proximal to tibia, radius/ulna are distal to humerus) or for a single structure of the extremity (femoral head is proximal femur, femoral condyles are distal femur). These are important terms to understand when describing injuries.

Medial/Lateral: These terms describe the relationship to the midline, with medial being closer to the midline and lateral farther away.

Caudad/Cephalad: These terms refer to the orientation of a point with reference to the long axis of the body. **Caudad** refers to an orientation toward the feet and **cephalad** refers to an orientation toward the head from a given reference point. These are not commonly used to describe injuries but can be seen in radiographic descriptions.

Anterior/Posterior: Anterior refers to a structure pointing toward the front of the body, while **posterior** is toward the back of the body.

Prone/Supine: These terms refer to the position of the patient lying down on the operating or examination table. In the **supine** position, the patient is on his/her back, and in the **prone** position, the patient is lying face down.

Sagittal/Coronal/Axial: These terms are frequently used in computerized tomography (CT) and magnetic resonance imaging (MRI) to describe the orientation of the imaged slices in the study. **Sagittal** images are those oriented in the long axis of the body parallel to the midline in an anteroposterior direction. **Coronal** or **frontal** images are those oriented in the long axis of the body parallel to the midline in a mediolateral diection. **Axial** images are essentially cross-sectional anatomic images in a plane perpendicular to the long axis of the body.

Abduction/Adduction: These terms describe motion in the plane of the body toward (**AD**-duction) or away (**AB**-duction) from the midline of the body or limb. An easy way to remember this is that when someone abducts a body part, they are taking it away from the midline. In the distal appendages (hand/foot), these terms can be confusing, as abduction of the great toe is moving it toward the midline of the body; however, it is being moved away from the midline of the limb and is thus termed abduction.

Pronation/Supination: These terms describe the inward and outward rotation of the forearm and foot. In the **pronated** position, the **palm** of the hand is **down,** while in the **supinated** position, the **palm** is facing **upward.** This is best remembered by the mnemonic "Pick the *soup up* and *pro it away.*" Pronation can also be remembered by pouring a drink. In pronation of the foot, the plantar surface of the foot is turned outward laterally, while in supination, it is turned inward laterally. In runners, pronators will run on the inner border of their shoes while supinators will do the opposite.

Volar-flexion and Dorsiflexion: These terms refer to motion at the wrist. The volar or palmar surface of the hand and forearm is the flexor surface. The extensor surface of the forearm and hand is also known as the dorsal surface. Extension of the wrist is also termed dorsiflexion, while flexion is also termed volar flexion. This is similar to motion at the ankle, where extension is known as dorsiflexion and flexion is known as plantar flexion. The flexor surface or sole of the foot is also known as the plantar surface.

Radial/Ulnar Deviation: Because the forearm bones shift their orientation during pronation and supination, confusion can occur over what is medial or lateral. Motion in this plane is thus described in relation to the forearm bones. Radial or ulnar deviation implies an angulation toward the corresponding bone. For example, patients with rheumatoid arthritis commonly present with ulnar deviation of their fingers at the MCP joints.

Varus/Valgus: These terms refer to the angular relationship between the distal and proximal parts around a known axis. **Varus** means that the distal part is angled medially relative to the proximal part, and **valgus** (note the letter **L**) means the distal part is angled laterally.

Subluxation/Dislocation: Subluxation refers to an episode of instability in which two surfaces of a joint become partially separated and spontaneously reduce, while **dislocation** refers to complete separation of the two surfaces of a joint without spontaneous reduction. Dislocations generally need to be reduced by another individual depending on the involved joint. An example is the glenohumeral joint, in which a subluxation episode will give the feeling of the humeral head sliding along the glenoid with spontaneous reduction, while a dislocation will involve the humeral head lying completely out of the glenoid cavity, requiring reduction maneuvers to relocate it.

Ipselateral/Contralateral: Ipselateral refers to a point on the same side as a fixed orientation point, while contralateral refers to the opposite side.

COMMONLY USED ABBREVIATIONS

AAI, Atlanto-axial instability

AAOS, American Academy of Orthopaedic Surgeons

AAROM, Active Assisted Range of Motion

AC joint, Acromioclavicular joint

ACDF, Anterior cervical discectomy and fusion

ACL, Anterior cruciate ligament

AFO, Ankle-foot orthosis

AKA, Above knee amputation

AO, Arbeitsgemeinschaft für Osteosynthesfragen. This is a Swiss-based group that studies internal fixation of fractures.

AOA, American Orthopaedic Association

APB, Abductor pollicis brevis

APL, Abductor pollicis longus

AROM, Active Range of Motion

AS, Ankylosing spondylitis

ASIF, Association for the Study of Internal Fixation. This is the American counterpart of the AO group.

ATFL, Anterior talo-fibular ligament

AVN, Avascular necrosis

BKA, Below knee amputation

BR, Brachioradialis

BR, Bed Rest

BST, Balanced Skeletal Traction

CDH, Congenital Dislocation of the Hip

CFL, Calcaneo-fibular ligament
CMC, Carpo-metacarpal joint
CPM, Continuous Passive Motion
CRP, C-reactive protein
CTLS, Cervico-thoracic-lumbo-sacral (as in CTLS brace)
CTR, Carpal tunnel release
CTS, Carpal tunnel syndrome
DDH, Developmental Dysplasia of the Hip
DIP, Distal interphalangeal joint
DJD, Degenerative joint disease
ECRB, Extensor carpi radialis brevis
ECRL, Extensor carpi radialis longus
ECU, Extensor carpi ulnaris
EDB, Extensor digitorum brevis
EDC, Extensor digitorum comminus
EDL, Extensor digitorum longus
EDQ, Extensor digiti quinti
EHL, Extensor hallucis longus
EIP, Extensor indicis proprius
EPB, Extensor pollicis brevis
EPL, Extensor pollicis longus
FCR, Flexor carpi radialis
FCU, Flexor carpi ulnaris
FDB, Flexor digitorum brevis
FDL, Flexor digitorum longus
FDP, Flexor digitorum profundus
FDS, Flexor digitorum superficialis (sublimus)
FHL, Flexor hallucis longus
FPL, Flexor pollicis longus
FROM, Full Range of Motion
FWB, Full Weight Bearing
FX, Fracture
GH, Glenohumeral joint
HKAFO, Hip-Knee-Ankle-Foot orthosis
HMO, Health Maintenance Organization
HNP, Herniated nucleus pulposis
HOB, Head of Bed
HTO, High tibial osteotomy
ICBG, Iliac crest bone graft
IGHE, Isolated glenohumeral elevation
ITB, Ilio-tibial band

KAFO, Knee-Ankle-Foot orthosis
LAC, Long arm cast
LAS, Long arm splint
LCL, Lateral collateral ligament
LLC, Long leg cast
LLS, Long leg splint
LMT, Lateral meniscus tear
LS, Lumbosacral (as in LS corset)
MCL, Medial collateral ligament
MCP, Metacarpophalangeal joint
MMT, Medial meniscus tear
MTP, Metatarsophalangeal joint
NHP, Nursing Home Placement
N/V, Neurovascular
NWB, Nonweight Bearing
NSAID, Nonsteroidal anti–inflammatory drug
OA, Osteoarthritis
ON, Osteonecrosis
ORIF, Open Reduction and Internal Fixation
PCL, Posterior cruciate ligament
PF, Patellofemoral
PIP, Proximal interphalangeal joint
PQ, Pronator quadratus
PROM, Passive Range of Motion
PT, Physical Therapy
PT, Pronator teres
PT, Prothrombin Time
PTB, Patellar tendon bearing
PTT, Partial Thromboplastin Time
PWB, Partial Weight Bearing
RA, Rheumatoid arthritis
RCL, Radial collateral ligament
RCR, Rotator cuff repair
RCT, Rotator cuff tear
ROM, Range of Motion
SAC, Short arm cast
SAS, Short arm splint
SC, Sternoclavicular joint
SCFE, Slipped capital femoral epiphysis
SER, Supination-external rotation (mechanism of ankle fracture)
SI, Sacroiliac joint

SLAP, Superior Labrum Anterior-Posterior
SLC, Short leg cast
SLS, Short leg splint
STS, Soft tissue swelling
TAM, Total Active Motion
TCDB, Turn, Cough, Deep Breathe
TDWB, Touch Down Weight Bearing
TEA, Total elbow arthroplasty
TFCC, Triangular fibrocartilage complex
THA, Total hip arthroplasty
THR, Total hip replacement
TKA, Total knee arthroplasty
TKR, Total knee replacement
TLSO, Thoraco-lumbo-sacral orthosis
TMA, Trans-metatarsal amputation
TMT, Tarso-metatarsal joint
TPM, Total Passive Motion
TSA, Total shoulder arthroplasty
TT, Tourniquet time
UCL, Ulnar collateral ligament
VSS, Vital signs stable
WBAT, Weight Bearing as Tolerated

References

1. Buckwalter JA, Glimcher MJ, et al. Bone biology I: structure, blood supply, cells, matrix and mineralization. Instruct Course Lect 1996;45:371–386.
2. Buckwalter JA, Glimcher MJ, et al. Bone biology II: formation, form, modeling, remodeling and regulation of cell function. Instruct Course Lect 1996;45:387–399.
3. Gamble JG. Development and maturation of the neuromusculoskeletal system. In: Morrissy RT, Weinstein SL, eds. Lovell and Winter's pediatric orthopaedics. Philadelphia: Lippincott-Raven, 1996.
4. Schenk RK. Biology of fracture repair. In: Browner BD, Jupiter JB, Levine AM, Trafton PG, eds. Skeletal trauma. Philadelphia: WB Saunders, 1992.
5. Hoppenfeld S. Physical examination of the spine and extremities. Norwalk, CT: Appleton-Century-Crofts, 1976.

Chapter 2

The Arthritides

Atraumatic painful afflictions of joints, categorized under the term *arthritides,* are common reasons for referrals to orthopaedic surgeons and can often be the presenting symptoms of systemic diseases. While rheumatologists provide the majority of nonoperative care for these disorders, it is important for the orthopaedic surgeon to have a basic understanding of these conditions since they are so commonly seen. Understanding these conditions also provides the orthopaedist with a framework upon which to decide which conditions would be more appropriately treated by a rheumatologist. This chapter will just go over the basics of the arthritic conditions.

The arthritides can basically be divided into noninflammatory, inflammatory, infectious, crystalline, and miscellaneous categories. An overview will be provided for the common conditions in each category. Infectious arthritis (septic arthritis) is discussed in Chapter 5, and the miscellaneous arthropathies will not be discussed, as they are not frequently encountered in orthopaedics.

DIAGNOSIS

A thorough history and physical examination with symptom specific laboratory and radiographic studies are necessary to determine the etiology of arthralgias. Even with advances in modern diagnostic techniques, the history and physical remain the most important tools for generating a working diagnosis for these disorders.

A detailed history often provides significant clues to the etiology of joint pain. Important pain-related factors include location (diffuse or localized), duration, intensity, radiation, and factors that mitigate or relieve pain. Past medical history, family history, and current medications are also important factors. The presence or absence of systemic symptoms such as nausea, weakness, fatigue, anorexia, weight loss, insomnia, depression, and fever should also be ascertained as they provide important information in formulating a working diagnosis.

The physical examination should include not only the painful joint, but also focus on the entire musculoskeletal system. Joints should be evaluated for warmth, swelling, deformity, range of motion, and crepitus. Fortunately, we have been provided with two upper and two lower extremities in most instances, allowing for comparison between bilateral structures. Any side-to-side differences should be recorded. Careful neurologic examination of the extremities including motor, sensory, and reflex testing should be performed to assess for any potential neurologic disorders or compression neuropathy. Muscles and bony prominences should be evaluated for point tenderness suggestive of a degenerative tendinopathy (lateral epicondylitis, Achilles tendonitis, patellar tendonitis) or fibromyalgia disorder. Systemic signs should also be recorded such as skin lesions, abnormal rashes, absent peripheral pulses, adenopathy, or abnormal pulmonary or cardiac exams.

Aspiration of a swollen joint, or arthrocentesis, is commonly performed by both orthopaedists and rheumatologists for diagnostic purposes. Specific techniques are discussed in Chapter 5. Sterile technique in any joint aspiration is of utmost importance in guaranteeing a pure (uncontaminated) specimen and in preventing a dreaded complication of inducing septic arthritis. Indications include uncertain diagnosis, hematoma evacuation for pain relief, injection of local anesthetic for analgesia or a procedure and corticosteroid injection for inflammatory arthropathies. The predominant indication for aspiration in orthopaedics is to rule out septic arthritis.

Synovial fluid, once obtained, should be grossly examined for color, presence of blood, opacity, and presence of particulate material[1]. Fluid viscosity and mucin clot measurements are not highly accurate, and although recommended in most older texts, are probably not necessary[1]. Sending fluid for a stat Gram stain and culture/sensitivity results is essential for evaluation of septic arthritis. Antibiotics should not be administered prior to obtaining synovial fluid if septic arthritis is suspected, as they can mask infection.

Cell count and differential are also important parameters in determining the etiology of an effusion. WBC counts of less than 10,000–20,000 are generally noninfectious, while WBC counts of 80,000–100,000 or higher should be presumed infectious until proved otherwise. Fluids with WBC counts in the 40,000–80,000 range can be confusing, and in these instances, the differential plays an important role. Noninflammatory effusions generally have <50% neutrophils, while infectious effusions are generally >90% neutrophils[2]. Confusion often occurs in crystalline-induced arthropathies, which can have intermediate WBC counts with high percentages of neutrophils. Crystal evaluation of synovial fluid is essential, but crystalline disease and infection can coexist; therefore, if the synovial analysis is suggestive of infection, it is best to err on the side of conservatism and treat for infection, as a missed infection can be disastrous. Another confusing circumstance is a low WBC count with a high percentage neutrophils in an immunocompromised patient. Once again, if infection is suspected, it should be treated accordingly.

Historically, glucose and protein measurements were made with low glucose and high protein being suggestive of infection but not necessarily proving it. For economic and practical purposes these tests can probably be eliminated, as other parameters can be used more accurately to diagnose infection[2,1].

LAB EVALUATION AND RADIOGRAPHS

Laboratory evaluation for a patient with a joint effusion should include CBC with differential and an ESR or CRP to measure systemic inflammation. These data will help determine if an infection or systemic inflammatory condition is present. Presence of anemia or thrombocytopenia can also be suggestive of a more systemic condition. In patients with a clinical presentation suggestive of an inflammatory arthropathy, other helpful tests include Rheumatoid factor (RF), antinuclear antibody (ANA) and uric acid. Interpretation of these tests and use of other more specific tests should remain under the realm of the rheumatologist, as that specialty is more experienced in that manner and would be directing the medical treatment of patients with these afflictions.

Radiographs of the affected painful joints should be obtained to evaluate for bony abnormalities. Different arthritides will have specific radiographic patterns that may aid in diagnosis[3,1] (Table 2.1).

Table 2.1
Radiographic Patterns in Arthritic Conditions

Disease	Sites	Radiographic Signs
RA	MCP, PIP, 1st CMC, wrist, foot, C-spine, knee, hip, elbow, shoulder	• Juxtaarticular erosions near insertion of capsule • Symmetric joint narrowing • Osteoporosis late • ST swelling large joints
Ankylosing Spondylitis	Vertebrae, hips and shoulders (50%); SI joints	• Progressive degen. changes SI joints • Vertebral squaring • Vertebral syndesmophytes (Bamboo spine) • Superficial erosions with reactive sclerosis and ankylosis
Psoriatic Arthritis	Hands—DIP, unilateral IP joint great toe SI joints (bilat symmetric involvement)	• Bone erosion beyond capsular attachment causing pencil-like tapering of bone • Bone apposition near involved joint • Resorption of terminal tufts • Segmental spine involvement (unlike AS) • Asymmetric bridging hyperostoses pencil-in-cup DIP deformity
Reiter's syndrome	Foot, knees, ankles, spine	• Difficult to distinguish from psoriatic • Periostitis • Metatarsal head erosions • Asymmetric nonbridging syndesmophytes
Gout	1st MTP, asymmetric large joints, spares spine	• Erosive bony changes (peri- or intraarticular) • Overhanging margin over eroded area • Uniform narrowing • No characteristic malalignments
Chondrocalcinosis	MPs, elbow, wrist, ankle, knee	• Calcified fibrocartilage • ST and synovial calcification

Table 2.1 (*continued*)

Disease	Sites	Radiographic Signs
OA	Knee, hip, 1st MTP, 1st CMC, spine, DIP	• Subchondral sclerosis and rarefactions • Can mimic synovial chondromatosis • Subchondral sclerosis • Subchondral cysts • Asymmetric jt. space narrowing • Marginal osteophytes • Malalignment with advanced disease

A brief discussion of the various arthritides will follow, with emphasis placed on osteoarthritis (OA) and rheumatoid arthritis (RA), as these are the entities most commonly treated by orthopaedic surgeons. Septic arthritis, an orthopaedic emergency in most instances, is discussed in detail in Chapter 5.

NONINFLAMMATORY ARTHROPATHIES[4,3,1]

Osteoarthritis (OA) is a noninflammatory degenerative joint condition associated with various degrees of cartilage degradation and associated bony deformity. It is the most common rheumatic disease. This process can result in altered joint mechanics with resultant alignment abnormalities (genu varum) and associated soft tissue contracture leading to limitations in motion. OA can be primary in nature or secondary to trauma or systemic disorders such as acromegaly, hemochromatosis, ochronosis, hyperparathyroidism, and epiphyseal dysplasia[1].

On a cellular level, the cartilage develops increased water content and decreased proteoglycan content (initially increased production then net degradation), which weakens the structure, making it more susceptible to injury[4]. Degradative enzymes (collagenases, metalloproteinases) released in response to injury can degrade the cartilage microstructure. Macroscopically, the cartilage develops fibrillation and fissures extending to subchondral bone. Sclerotic changes then occur in the subchondral bone from overload. Juxtaarticular cysts and marginal osteophytes eventually form, and joint space narrowing and sclerosis occur, giving the characteristic radiographic appearance of an osteoarthritic joint.

The prevalence of osteoarthritis increases with age and with the underlying conditions mentioned above. Those with underlying hip joint abnormalities (DDH, Perthes, SCFE) have a significantly increased prevalence of hip osteoarthrosis. In fact, Harris[5] feels that primary OA of the hip does not exist and that it only occurs in response to these underlying structural abnormalities.

The symptoms in OA are usually *unilateral, asymmetric, and not associated with significant effusions.* Initially pain is worsened by activity and relieved by rest, but eventually rest and night pain develop. Decreased range of motion and crepitus are also common in joints affected by OA. Commonly involved joints include the knee (genu varum), hip, first MTP, DIP (Heberden's nodes), PIP (Bouchard's nodes), and thumb carpometacarpal joint. OA also affects the spine at the facet joints and is associated with degenerative disc disease, degenerative scoliosis, and degenerative spondylolisthesis. This especially occurs in the lumbar spine most commonly at the L3–4 level.

Lab evaluation will reveal a normal ESR and CBC, and synovial fluid analysis may show a normal or slightly elevated WBC count (10,000–20,000) with normal differential. This pattern is found in most all of the noninflammatory arthropathies.

Treatment of OA differs with the stage of disease and the joints involved. The goals of treatment are pain relief, maintenance and restoration of function, and prevention of advanced changes. Canes are used for knee and hip OA to help unload the joint. Patients should be instructed to use their cane on the side opposite (contralateral) to their painful hip to help reduce the forces (joint reactive force) applied to the hip while ambulating. Pain can be alleviated with acetaminophen or NSAIDs. NSAIDs are effective in OA for their analgesic function, as the anti–inflammatory effect is not as crucial given OA is a noninflammatory arthropathy. Possible side effects of NSAID treatment (GI upset, peptic ulcer disease, renal insufficiency) should be reviewed with patients prior to initiating therapy.

Advanced cases of hip and knee OA can be successfully treated with joint replacement[6,7]. Osteotomy is an option in the hip and knee in young patients to help unload the degenerative cartilage. In the knee, high tibial osteotomy is an effective treatment for varus deformity with isolated medial compartment disease[8]. In the hip varus or valgus femoral osteotomy (depending on which effectively unloads the degenerative portion of the femoral head) or redirectional pelvic osteotomy can be an effective means of treatment in appropriate cases[9]. Advanced thumb CMC arthrosis can be effectively treated with a ligament reconstruction and tendon interposition (LRTI) procedure[10]. PIP and DIP changes rarely come to surgical treatment.

New frontiers for treatment and prevention of OA include identifying genetic and biochemical markers and attempting to modify any of these potential predisposing factors. These areas are currently under active investigation but are not yet applicable for any clinical situations. Chondrocyte transplantation has received significant press in recent years; however, this is intended for acute traumatic chondral defects as opposed to degenerative changes in articular cartilage.

Neuropathic arthropathy[11,1], or Charcot arthropathy, refers to a condition in which severe destruction of a peripheral joint occurs, presumed secondary to a disturbance in the sensory innervation of the joint. Spinal involvement is also common and can lead to gross instability. Underlying etiologies include **diabetes** (forefoot and midfoot), **tabes dorsalis** (70% lower extremity, 20% LS spine), **syringomyelia** (No. 1 cause, upper extremity neuropathic joint), myelomeningocoele and Hansen's disease (leprosy, mainly upper extremity).

Clinically, the affected joint undergoes rapid destruction and is generally *swollen, warm, and erythematous but painless or much less painful than expected*. It can easily be confused with infection and is differentiated by its normal synovial fluid analysis, normal ESR and WBC count, and minimal pain. Significant pain generally indicates pathologic fracture, or in the foot, a dysvascular condition. In the advanced destructive phase, instability develops. Radiographically, both sides of the joint are destroyed and bony fragments are visualized in the soft tissues.

Treatment is aimed at immobilizing the joint and minimizing weight bearing if the lower extremity is involved. In the upper extremity, the underlying cause is almost always syringomyelia; a cervical MRI should be ordered to evaluate for this condition. Surgery is generally not successful in neuropathic joints, and arthroplasty is contraindicated owing to the underlying instability and neuropathy predisposing to early failure[12].

Patients with **hemophilia**[4,1] (X-linked recessive factor VIII deficiency) are at risk for recurrent hemarthroses secondary to minor trauma. These lead to synovitis, cartilage destruction, and eventual joint deformity (**hemophilic arthropathy**). The joints most commonly involved, in order, are the knee, ankle, elbow, shoulder, and hip. During an acute attack, the joint will be warm and swollen. Patients should be treated with factor VIII replacement in the acute setting. Hemophiliacs have a high incidence of HIV secondary to exposure to blood products from multiple donors.

Treatment begins with synovectomy in the early stages to attempt to reduce the incidence of recurrent hemarthroses. In end stage joints, arthroplasty can be performed with fair results. Factor VIII levels must be maintained at 100%–120% for the first several days after surgery, 50%– 75% for the next 2 weeks, then 30%–50% for at least 6 weeks postoperatively. Perioperative management of the factor VIII levels should be directed by a hematologist.

The presence of a factor VIII inhibitor is an absolute contraindication to performing elective surgery in a hemophiliac, as such a patient will not respond to factor replacement and can bleed to death.

INFLAMMATORY ARTHROPATHIES[4,3,1]

The inflammatory arthropathies include a wide variety of rheumatologic conditions associated with joint swelling and destruction and usually associated with systemic symptoms. Synovial fluid generally will have a WBC count of 5000–75,000 with a normal differential and Gram stain showing no organisms. Crystal examination can help identify if the underlying condition is a crystalline arthropathy. The inflammatory arthropathies include rheumatoid arthritis (RA), systemic lupus erythematosus (SLE), juvenile rheumatoid arthritis (JRA), and the seronegative spondyloarthropathies. Rheumatoid arthritis and ankylosing spondylitis are the entities most frequently encountered by orthopaedic surgeons.

Rheumatoid arthritis is the most common inflammatory arthropathy and in its advanced stages can be physically, functionally, and emotionally incapacitiating. It occurs most commonly in females (2–3 : 1) around the 3rd to 5th decade of life and has been associated with genetic marker HLA-DR4 and positive rheumatoid factor (IgM antibodies against native IgG)[3,1]. In fact, high titers of rheumatoid factor are associated with more severe and active disease and more systemic involvement.

On a cellular level, the disease involves synovial proliferation, with eventual formation of the pannus consisting of fibroblasts, vessels, and various inflammatory cells (mononuclear early, then PMNs), which produce byproducts (collagenases, prostaglandins) capable of destroying collagen-containing tissues. The proliferating pannus causes the progressive destruction in RA with eventual degradation of articular cartilage, ligaments, tendons, and bone in advanced chronic cases[3,1].

Clinically, the disease presents with an insidious onset of morning stiffness, followed by pain in several joints. It generally presents with systemic involvement of multiple joints frequently beginning in the hands, wrists and feet, then later involving the spine (cervical), knees, elbows, hips, and shoulders. Systemic symptoms of fatigue, malaise, and diffuse soft tissue pain often precede the joint complaints. Initially, the patients develop stiffness in the morning and with inactivity, which will improve with activity and worsen with rest. This progressively worsens as the disease progresses.

Systemic involvement can occur with pericarditis, pulmonary fibrosis, splenomegaly/leukopenia (Felty's syndrome) and from complications related to a patient's rheumatoid medications. Eventually, if not arrested, the disease will lead to static joint deformities and soft tissue contractures with poor function.

Joint involvement in the upper extremity mainly affects the wrist and hand[13]. In the wrists, massive tenosynovitis can occur (usually dorsal > volar), which can cause pain and functional limitations, and can lead to extensor tendon rupture. The EPL and extensors to the small and ring fingers (Vaughn-Jackson syndrome) most commonly rupture. Generally, medical treatment is initiated first and if unsuccessful (usually >6 months without resolution) or if incapacitating pain or tendon rupture occur, a surgical synovectomy will be performed. Occasionally, destructive arthritis of the wrist may be severe enough to warrant arthrodesis or arthroplasty[13]. Distal radio-ulnar joint (DRUJ) involvement with instability or a degenerative distal ulna can necessitiate a distal ulna resection with stabilization using a variety of methods.

In the hand, the MCP joints are most commonly involved with swelling and later development of an ulnar deviation deformity. PIP involvement can also occur, but the DIPs will be spared, unlike in OA. Swan neck deformities (PIP hyperextension, DIP flexion) are common in advanced disease. Surgery is often necessary at the MCP level, with MCP arthroplasty being the most common procedure (usually silicon implants)[14]. This will serve to realign the fingers and reduce the tendency for subluxation or dislocation at the MCP joints. For the PIP joint, arthroplasty is not as successful as for the MCP[3]. For PIP involvement, fusion is usually performed in the radial digits and arthroplasty performed in the ulnar digits because of the importance of maintaining power grip.

In the elbow, flexion contractures and olecranon bursitis are common, with eventual joint destruction in advanced cases. Total elbow arthroplasty is a successful procedure in that circumstance.

Shoulder involvement generally occurs later in the disease course and can be successfully treated with arthroplasty. In cases with shoulder, elbow and hand involvement requiring surgery in all three areas, the proximal joints should be treated first.

RA can also affect the cervical spine. Involvement has been documented in 20%–90% of patients with moderate disease in various series[15]. The most common abnormality is **atlanto-axial instability (AAI)** secondary to pannus initiated destruction of the transverse and alar ligaments. *An atlanto-axial interval of > 3–4 mm is considered abnormal in an adult rheumatoid.* Other abnormalities include **cranial settling** (basilar settling, basilar invagination, superior migration of the dens) and **subaxial instability** (>3.5 mm listhesis)[15-17]. Controversy exists over routine screening with cervical radiographs; however, they should be performed in all rheumatoid patients undergoing major surgery to determine if the patient is at risk for neurologic compromise with positioning and intubation.

Cervical spine involvement can cause neurologic deficits. Ranawat et al[17] developed a neurologic classification with Class 1, no neural deficit; Class II, subjective weakness and dysesthesias with or without hyperreflexia; Class IIIA, objective weakness with ability to ambulate, and Class IIIB, objective weakness with quadriparesis and inability to ambulate. Patients with preexisting neurologic deficits are less likely to improve neurologically with surgery, but the deficit can potentially be stabilized with surgical treatment, if indicated.

Boden et al[11] found that the posterior atlanto-dens interval or space available for the cord (SAC) was more predictive of functional outcome than the anterior values. Patients with SAC less than or equal to 10 mm at C1–2 had no recovery if operated on, while those >10 mm did have some recovery. They recommended surgical stabilization with a SAC or posterior ADI less than or equal to 14 mm, as all patients with Class III deficits had SAC less than 14 mm.

Patients with neurologic symptoms and borderline values on plain radiographs including flexion/extension views should be considered for a dynamic MRI to see if cord impingement is occurring with flexion or extension. Obviously, the patient must be fully alert for this test, and it should be aborted if any neurologic symptoms develop during motion.

Cervical spine involvement is something that one must always be aware of while treating rheumatoid patients. An important point to remember is that if a functional patient progressively becomes nonambulatory, it should not immediately be attributed to progressive lower extremity disease, as cervical disease with myelopathy will frequently present with decreased ambulatory potential. In this setting, the cervical spine must be thoroughly imaged with plain films and, if necessary, MRI.

Lower extremity involvement frequently begins in the foot, which is one of the most common areas affected (90%) by rheumatoid disease[18]. The forefoot is most commonly involved, with hallux valgus and lesser MTP subluxation and dislocation, with eventual hammer or claw toe deformity. Orthoses can be used early in the course and advanced disease treated with first MTP fusion and metatarsal head resection with realignment of the lesser toes.

Posterior tibial tendon dysfunction is common in the mid/hindfoot, with potential for developing adult-acquired flatfoot deformity after collapse of the talonavicular joint. Early treatment involves synovectomy, orthoses, and possible tendon transfer, with talonavicular fusion being an option in advanced disease prior to collapse and triple arthrodesis being the option in more advanced cases. Ankle and subtalar involvement with valgus deformity is common and problematic and often necessitates ankle fusion or triple arthrodesis[18].

The knee is a common site of involvement in RA, which can lead to joint destruction and malalignment. Flexion contracture and valgus deformity are common. In cases of fixed valgus deformity, with correction back to normal alignment during arthroplasty procedures, peroneal nerve palsy can infrequently occur[19]. The hip is also frequently involved in RA. In cases of displaced femoral neck fractures, total hip arthroplasty is preferred over hemiarthroplasty because of rheumatoid involvement of the acetabular cartilage[20]. Arthroplasty represents successful surgical treatment in advanced cases of hip and knee arthritis[21,6,7,22].

RA also involves nonarticular structures, with tenosynovitis, tendon rupture, bursitis, and subcutaneous nodules being frequent manifestations.

Treatment of rheumatoid patients is aimed at maintaining function and preventing deformity. Initial management is with physical therapy and NSAIDs, with progression to methotrexate, anti-malarials, gold, penicillamine, corticosteroids, and newer experimental drugs. Methotrexate has represented a major improvement in medical therapy. Surgical treatment is performed secondary to failure of medical management, or from musculoskeletal complications of the disease, or from the medications used to treat the disease.

Systemic Lupus Erythematosis (SLE)[1] is an autoimmune inflammatory disease with multisystem organ involvement. Common features include classic malar butterfly rash, pericarditis, pleuritis, vasculitis, Raynaud's phenomenon, and glomerular nephritis, with renal failure requiring dialysis in many cases.

The most common presenting feature is symmetric arthralgias and synovitis. It can be confused with RA early in the disease course. The knee, MCP, and PIP joints are most frequently involved. The MCP joints are often ulnarly deviated and subluxated with a flexion deformity, with PIP hyperextension and DIP flexion (Jaccoud's arthropathy). Thumb IP hyperextension (Hitchhiker's thumb) and CMC subluxation are common. Joint destruction is less severe than in RA. AVN secondary to steroid treatment is the most common reason for orthopaedic intervention in this disease.

Juvenile Rheumatoid Arthritis (JRA)[23] is a systemic inflammatory arthropathy affecting children. Three major subsets of JRA exist with different degrees of involvement: systemic, polyarticular, and pauciarticular.

Systemic involvement (Still's disease) occurs in 20% of patients with fevers, rash, malaise, lymphadenopathy, hepatosplenomegaly, pericardial/pleural effusions, and muscle atrophy. Initially, myalgias and arthralgias occur during febrile episodes, then symmetric arthritis will occur within the first few months of symptoms. Males and females are equally involved, and patients are RF and ANA negative. Approximately 25% will have chronic severe arthritis, and the others will go into remission.

Polyarticular involvement occurs in 40%, more commonly females, with involvement of greater than four joints. Systemic symptoms occur but to a lesser extent than in Still's disease. The cervical spine must be evaluated, as it is frequently involved, especially at C2–3. Approximately 15%–20% of these patients will be RF positive and tend to have a worse prognosis, with 50% of them developing chronic destructive arthritis.

Pauciarticular disease occurs in 40% of patients and involves fewer than four joints. Two subtypes exist based on age of development. In the early childhood onset, females predominate, most commonly with involvement of the knees, wrists, elbows, and ankles. Thirty to fifty percent of patients have iridocyclitis, and frequent ophthalmologic slit lamp examination is necessary. In the late childhood onset, males predominate, with many being HLA-B27 positive. Clinically, hips and SI joints are frequently affected, and the pattern resembles a spondyloarthropathy. Iridocyclitis also occurs to a lesser extent than in the early childhood form but still requires ophthalmologic evaluation.

Overall, 75% of patients with JRA experience remission of disease. The main goals of treatment are maintenance of function and prevention of deformity. PT is important throughout the disease course. Aspirin is the most frequently used medication (discontinue during viral illnesses for fear of Reye's syndrome) followed by NSAIDs. Gold is used in severe cases, and steroids are avoided if at all possible.

Surgical treatment is occassionally necessary, and arthroplasty has been performed for severe arthritis, especially in the knees and hips. Results (longevity) do not approach those for arthroplasty in the older population[24]. Synovectomy is also occasionally performed. Generally, patients who come to surgical treatment are the polyarticular RF positive subset.

Spondyloarthropathies[3,1] represent a group of inflammatory arthropathies, seronegative (RF-negative) in nature, which are frequently associated with a positive HLA-B27 antigen. Inflammation most commonly involves the SI joints, but the spine and peripheral joints are also commonly involved. The inflammatory changes occur at the enthesis (ligament or tendon insertion onto bone), and these disorders are also termed enthesopathies. Nonenthesopathic changes also occur in the eyes, skin, aortic valve, and lung parenchyma. Conditions include ankylosing spondylitis (AS), Reiter's syndrome, psoriatic arthritis, and enteropathic arthritis. Frequently, there is clinical overlap between these disorders.

Ankylosing spondylitis (AS) predominantly affects males aged 20–40, beginning with **bilateral sacroiliitis** and progressing to disabling spinal deformity in many cases. Ninety percent of patients are HLA-B27 positive, and for individuals carrying this marker in the general population, there is a 10%–25% risk of developing AS. Systemic signs include **anterior uveitis,** prostatitis, conjunctivitis, and in severe cases pulmonary fibrosis and aortic insufficiency.

The hallmark of the disease is insidious onset of bilateral symmetric sacroiliitis with morning stiffness and improvement with exercise. This can progress to stiffness involving the entire spine and characteristic vertical syndesmophytes and "bamboo spine" appearance radiographically. Significant kyphosis can develop at the thoracolumbar and cervicothoracic junctions leading to the characteristic "chin on chest" deformity. Acute onset of severe back pain in advanced disease almost always indicates spinal fracture, which can be difficult to see radiographically, and is frequently associated with ascending epidural hematoma[25]. *Acute back pain in these patients must thus be taken seriously, and active attempts must be made (plain films, CT/MRI) to rule out fracture.* Other spinal deformities can be electively treated with corrective osteotomy to help straighten the kyphosis.

Other enthesopathic changes include plantar fasciitis, Achilles tendonitis, and costochondritis. Peripheral joint involvement occurs in 20%–30% of patients. Hips are most commonly involved with degenerative changes and protrusio acetabuli. Total hip arthroplasty is a challenge in these patients, who are at high risk for heterotopic ossification postoperatively and thus should be irradiated or treated with indomethacin for prophylaxis[26].

Initial treatment is with PT and NSAIDs. Patients with young age at onset and lower extremity involvement have the worst prognosis for this disease.

Reiter's syndrome classically presents in young males with a triad of conjunctivitis, urethritis, and arthritis. It is usually secondary to a GI infection with *Campylobacter, Salmonella, Yersinia* or *Shigella* and occurs 2–6 weeks after infection. The joints most commonly involved are the knees and ankles, but three typical musculoskeletal features are sausage digits, low back pain and Achilles tendonitis/plantar fasciitis.

Back involvement shows asymmetric sacroiliitis with asymmetric noncontiguous syndesmophytes. The back symptoms are not progressive, unlike those of AS. Metatarsal head erosion and periostitis frequently occur radiographically. HLA-B27 is positive in 80%–90% of patients.

Associated features include inflammatory eye lesions, balanitis, ulcers, and keratoderma. Treatment involves NSAIDs and PT. Most patients will have recurrent episodes of arthritis; some can have one self-limiting episode. Rarely will the course be continuous and unremitting.

Psoriatic arthritis affects 5%–10% of patients with psoriasis and generally involves peripheral joints in a pauciarticular asymmetric fashion. The DIP joints of the hand are most commonly affected, with radiographic erosions and classic "pencil-in-cup" deformity. Nail pitting and sausage digits are also hallmarks. Initially, if the arthritis is polyarticular, it can be difficult to distinguish from RA. Spine involvement also occurs, and cervical instability may result.

Treatment involves maintenance of motion and continuation of systemic treatment for psoriasis. Surgery, especially joint replacement, is associated with higher infection rates in these patients[27].

Enteropathic arthritis can occur in up to 15%–20% of patients with ulcerative colitis or Crohn's disease. The arthritis is mainly peripheral and affects the knees and ankles most commonly. It is nondeforming and generally shows a nonspecific pattern on synovial fluid analysis. A small percentage of patients may develop sacroiliitis without periphereal involvement. This subset of patients often has overlap with AS. Patients with enteropathic arthritis generally come to orthopaedic attention for problems related to corticosteroid therapy rather than from the disease itself.

CRYSTALLINE ARTHROPATHIES[3,1]

The crystalline arthropathies or crystalline deposition diseases represent a category of diseases in which arthritic changes occur secondary to a chronic inflammatory reaction triggered by abnormal crystalline deposits in tissue. They cause painful effusions that can be confused with infection, clinically and on synovial fluid analysis. Synovial analysis reveals cloudy, often yellow, thick fluid with 2000–100,000 WBCs and predominantly neutrophils. Gram stain and crystal analysis are often necessary to make a diagnosis, but infection and crystalline arthritis can coexist. Thus, if infection is highly suspected, it should be treated as though it were the primary problem. Gout and chondrocalcinosis are the major crystalline arthropathies.

Gout occurs secondary to abnormal nucleic acid metabolism, leading to increased serum uric acid with deposition of monosodium urate crystals in joints and soft tissues. These incite an inflammatory reaction with release of substances that can degrade cartilage. People with gout can be overproducers or underexcretors (90%) of uric acid.

Clinically, gout usually begins with an acute painful swelling of the great toe MTP joint (podagra). It can eventually involve any joint, but mainly affects the lower extremity. Significant degenerative changes and deformity can occur, occasionally necessitating arthroplasty procedures. Chronic gout can lead to crystal deposition in tissue (tophi), which commonly occurs at the ear pinna, eyelid, extensor elbow surface, and Achilles tendon.

Precipitating factors causing gouty attacks include trauma, ethanol abuse, drugs, surgical stresses, and acute medical illnesses. Generally, the attacks increase in frequency and intensity with time and can lead to chronic tophaceous gout, in which soft tissue involvement is present and bony changes can be advanced.

Diagnosis is based on history, examination, and synovial analysis. Synovial fluid will contain crystals that are *thin, tapered, and negatively birefringent.* These crystals are necessary to make the diagnosis of gout. Serum uric acid will also be elevated in the setting of an attack.

Treatment of acute episodes includes NSAIDs and colchicine. Colchicine can also be used for prophylaxis against recurrent attacks but is associated with GI toxicity. Corticosteroids are often necessary for acute attacks that do not respond to colchicine or NSAIDs. For patients who are uric acid underexcretors, uricosuric agents such as probenicid and sulfinpyrazone can be used; and, for overproducers, allopurinol is frequently utilized. The use of allopurinol can be limited by severe hypersensitivity reactions.

Chondrocalcinosis has many causes including ochronosis, hyperparathyroidism, hypothyroidism, hemochromatosis, and crystalline pyrophosphate deposition disease (CPPD). CPPD, also known as pseudogout, is probably the most common cause. It generally involves inflammation of one or more joints lasting several days, with abrupt onset and generally less pain than gout. The knee is most commonly affected.

Calcifications also occur in soft tissues and are frequently seen in cartilage, synovial fluid, and meniscus. Frequently, patients with these calcifications will be asymptomatic. Diagnosis is made by calcifications on radiographs and by synovial analysis revealing *short, rhomboid-shaped, positive birefringent crystals.*

Acute attacks are often precipitated by trauma, stress, and surgery. Treatment is symptomatic, as the attacks are usually self-limited, and surgery should be avoided in the acute setting, as it can precipitate further attacks.

In conclusion, this chapter reviews the basics about some of the more common arthropathies encountered in orthopaedics to help differentiate these entities in the acute setting and to know what to expect in a more advanced presentation. Chronic forms of arthritis should be managed in conjunction with a rheumatologist for optimal care.

References

1. Schumacher HR, ed. Primer on the rheumatic diseases. 9th ed. Atlanta: Arthritis Foundation, 1988.
2. Mikhail IS, Alarcon GS. Nongonococcal bacterial arthritis. Rheum Dis Clinics North Am 1993;19:311–331.
3. Kelley WN, Harris ED, Ruddy S, et al. Textbook of rheumatology. 5th ed. Philadelphia: WB Saunders, 1997.
4. Frymoyer JD, ed. Orthopaedic knowledge update 4. Rosemont: American Academy of Orthopaedic Surgeons, 1993.
5. Harris WH. Etiology of osteoarthritis of the hip. Clin Orthop 1986;213:20–33.
6. Rand JA, Ilstrup DM. Survivorship analysis of total knee arthroplasty. Cumulative rates of survival of 9200 total knee arthroplasties. J Bone Joint Surg 1991;73-A:397–408.
7. Sculte KR, Callahan JJ, et al. The outcome of Charnley total hip arthroplasty with cement after a minimum 20-year follow-up. J Bone Joint Surg 1993; 75-A:961–975.
8. Holden DL, James SL, et al. Proximal tibial osteotomy in patients who are fifty years old or less. A long-term follow-up study. J Bone Joint Surg 1988;70-A:977–982.

9. Millis MB, Murphy SB, Poss R. Osteotomies about the hip for the prevention and treatment of osteoarthritis. Instruct Course Lect 1996;45:209–226.

10. Burton RI, Pellegrini VD Jr. Surgical treatment of basal thumb arthritis of the hand. Part II: ligament reconstruction with tendon interposition arthroplasty. J Hand Surg 1986;11-A:324–332.

11. Alpert SW, Koval KJ, Zuckerman JD. Neuropathic arthropathy: review of current knowledge. J Am Acad Orthop Surg 1996;4:100–108.

12. Robb JE, Rymaszewski LA, et al. Total hip arthroplasty in a Charcot joint: brief report. J Bone Joint Surg 1988;70-B:489.

13. Terrono AL, Feldon PG, et al. Evaluation and treatment of the rheumatoid wrist. Instruct Course Lect 1996;45:15–26.

14. Stirrat CR. Metacarpophalangeal joints in rheumatoid arthritis of the hand. Hand Clin 1996;12:515–529.

15. Pellicci PM, Ranawat CS, et al. A prospective study of the progression of rheumatoid arthritis of the cervical spine. J Bone Joint Surg 1981;63-A:342–350.

16. Boden SD, Dodge LD, et al. Rheumatoid arthritis of the cervical spine. A long-term analysis with predictors of paralysis and recovery. J Bone Joint Surg 1993;75-A:1282–1297.

17. Ranawat CS, O'Leary P, et al. Cervical spine fusion in rheumatoid arthritis, J Bone Joint Surg 1979;61-A:1003–1010.

18. Abdo RV, Iorio LJ. Rheumatoid arthritis of the foot and ankle. J Am Acad Orthop Surg 1994;2:326–332.

19. Rose HA, Hood R, et al. Peroneal nerve palsy following total knee arthroplasty. A review of the Hospital for Special Surgery experience. J Bone Joint Surg 1982;64-A:347–351.

20. Koval KJ, Zuckerman JD. Hip fractures I: overview and evaluation and treatment of femoral neck fractures. J Am Acad Orthop Surg 1994;2:141–149.

21. Joshi AB, Porter ML, et al. Long-term results of Charnley low friction arthroplasty in young patients. J Bone Joint Surg 1993;75-B:616–623.

22. Severt R, Wood R, et al. Long-term follow-up of cemented total hip athroplasty in rheumatoid arthritis. Clin Orthop 1991;265:137–145.

23. Schaller JG. Chronic arthritis in children: juvenile rheumatoid arthritis. Clin Orthop 1984;182:79–89.

24. Chmell MJ, Scott RD, et al. Total hip arthroplasty with cement for juvenile rheumatoid arthritis. Results at a minimum of ten years in patients less than thirty years old. J Bone Joint Surg1997;79-A:44–52.

25. Graham B, Von Peteghem PK, et al. Fractures of the spine in ankylosing spondylitis. Diagnosis, treatment and complications. Spine 1989;14:803–807.

26. Lewallen DG. Heterotopic ossification following total hip arthroplasty. Instruct Course Lect 1995;44:287–292.

27. Stern SH, Insall JN, et al. Total knee arthroplasty in patients with psoriasis. Clin Orthop 1989;248:108–110.

Chapter 3

History and Physical Examination of the Orthopaedic Patient

THE ORTHOPAEDIC HISTORY[1]

A thorough history is an integral part of the diagnosis of musculo-skeletal injuries. The breadth and depth of the history should be dictated by the chief complaint. Musculoskeletal injuries can often be presenting symptoms of widespread disease processes.

Because the orthopaedic surgeon must frequently provide information about the injured patient to insurance carriers, employers, vocational rehabilitation counselors, and attorneys, specific details about the injury should be obtained and recorded, especially in work-related injuries. This information should include the following: date and exact mechanism of injury, time out of work, previous treatment and by whom, and referring physician or agency.

Acute Injury

The history of the acute injury should focus on the exact mechanism of the injury. Specific questions should be addressed toward body position when the injury occurred. An assessment of the force causing the injury should be made. For example, did the patient sustain the pelvic fracture in a fall in the bathroom or a motor vehicle accident? Is the onset of pain and limitation of range of motion immediate or gradual? When the injury occurred was there a sense of "giving way"? Did the patient hear or feel a "click" or a "pop"? If the patient has diminished or loss of sensibility or motor power, the onset of the neurologic change, i.e., immediate or gradual, must be obtained and documented.

Additional questions should focus on the patient's activities since the injury. Did the patient continue to participate in the game? Was the patient able to walk on an injured lower extremity after injury? Also, if the patient presents to the clinic some time after the injury, an effort should be undertaken to determine the patient's expectations and the reasons for delay in presentation.

Chronic Injury

Chronic injuries often require more extensive history taking. The pertinent history is often hidden in a maze of unrelated events. Many patients will unknowingly confuse dates and details. One effective way to sort out the details is to have two separate observers take the history, and then compare the details. The radiology film jacket will often help to put dates on previous trauma or visits to the clinic if old records are unavailable.

In nonacute injuries, the time frame should first be determined. When did the injury first occur? Have there been successive flares or episodes of reinjuries? What diagnostic and surgical procedures have been performed and what were the short- and long-term results? Has the presenting disability changed in character over time? As the history-taking progresses, often the open-ended question must be abandoned for more specific, detailed questions.

Constitutional symptoms should not be neglected. Questions should address signs and symptoms such as fever, chills, nausea, or vomiting.

Trauma

The orthopaedic history of the trauma patient focuses directly on the mechanism of injury. How much energy caused the injury? Are any other systems damaged? What injuries demand immediate surgical intervention and with what priority? What is the cardiopulmonary status of the patient? What are the risks of emergency anaesthesia? What is the tetanus status of the patient? Is the patient hemodynamically stable enough to permit a full evaluation in the emergency room? In all patients presenting to the emergency room who may require surgery, a full review of systems should be sought with emphasis on cardiopulmonary conditions that would increase anaesthetic risk.

Pain

Pain is a difficult symptom to describe or quantitate. The best description of the patient's pain should be detailed. The radiation of pain should be determined. Also ask the patient which movements and positions make him/her more comfortable and which make him worse. In chronic situations, it is important to understand when, during the day, the pain is greatest. It is also important to note how medicines affect the pain.

THE PHYSICAL EXAMINATION

The physical examination should begin in the examining room with the involved extremity well exposed for examination. An examination of the upper extremity requires that the entire forequarter be accessible. The patient should be draped to help maintain modesty. The lumbar spine cannot be examined without the patient in a hospital gown. Categorically, an unconscious trauma patient should be entirely undressed so that occult injury is not overlooked.

The optimum examining room places the examining table in the center of the room so that the patient can be approached from either side of the table with the patient either prone or supine.

The patient should be asked to demonstrate where the pain is most severe and the motions that aggravate or relieve the condition. Many patients will not localize their pain well, and in acute trauma, it is important to ask the patient to use the *one finger-one spot* rule to localize the point of maximum pain. The injured area should be examined for atrophy or asymmetry. Other observations should include abnormal posture, and the resting or "comfortable position."

After observation of the patient, the examiner should approach the patient and begin to palpate the area of interest. A useful technique is to progress from relatively pain-free areas to the most tender or sensitive regions. Any painful maneuvers should be avoided until the end of the examination (e.g., the straight leg raise in a suspected herniated nucleus pulposus). The examination should include a minimum of a joint above and below the injury.

In chronic diseases such as rheumatoid arthritis, an extensive evaluation of all joints may be necessary to follow the progression of the disease. Observations should include assessment of inflammation, extent of synovitis, warmth, and an accurate measurement of active and passive range of motion.

Range of Motion[1,2]

Examination of the range of motion (ROM) of the injured extremity often yields a wealth of diagnostic data, as well as qualitative measurement for future examinations. Normal values for range of motion of most joints are shown in Figures 3.1 to 3.7. A goniometer should be used to measure range of motion. An accurate range of motion assessment should include both active and passive ROM. When the the active range of motion is limited by pain, this should be noted. If the passive ROM is decreased, one should note if the endpoint is firm (i.e., a bony block to motion) or soft. Again, the examination should include a joint above and below the injury.

Motor Testing[1,2,3]

Examination of specific muscles or muscle groups will often give major diagnostic information to an injury or disease. Muscle strength is scored on a system of 0–5; 5 signifying normal strength, while 0 indicates no muscle activity, as shown in Table 3.1. Some examiners add a plus or minus to the grading system to denote more subtle differences in motor deficits. Normal motor strength is a somewhat enigmatic term—normal motor strength in an 88-year-old female is not normal motor strength in a professional athlete. An extremely helpful method of comparison is to measure the unaffected contralateral limb or muscle group to get a quantitative assessment of the normal. The motor examination will often give information about nerve root and peripheral nerve lesions. Although large muscle groups are innervated by contributions from several nerve roots, usually a single nerve root predominates. Tables 3.2 and 3.3 list the muscles and their innervation both by spinal root and peripheral nerves.

Reflexes[1,2,3]

No neurologic assessment is complete without deep tendon reflex testing. Reflex testing should be performed with the patient seated comfortably on the examining table with the feet off the ground. The primary reflexes are listed in Tables 3.4 and 3.5.

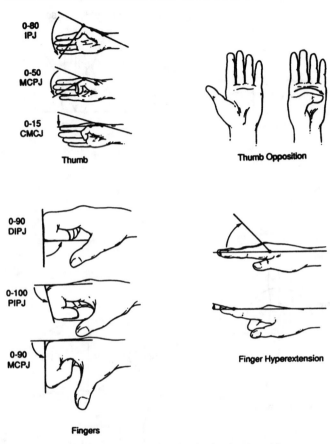

Figure 3.1.   Normal ranges of motion for the thumb and fingers.

The posterior tibialis reflex is included, although this reflex is difficult to demonstrate. The posterior tibialis reflex can be considered significant when it is present unilaterally.

In the patient with a suspected spinal cord injury, additional reflexes, especially the cremasteric and the bulbocavernosus reflexes should be tested. The absence of a bulbocavernosus reflex may indicate spinal shock for approximately 48 hours following trauma to the spine.

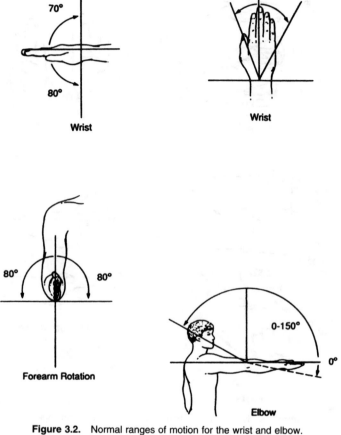

Figure 3.2. Normal ranges of motion for the wrist and elbow.

The bulbocavernosus reflex is tested by performing a rectal exam and, with the examining digit within the rectal vault, tugging on the glans penis, the clitoris, or an indwelling Foley catheter. An intact bulbocavernosus reflex exists when the anal sphincter contracts on the examining digit. The return of the bulbocavernosus reflex after a significant spinal injury signifies the end of spinal shock. If the patient has had absolutely no return of neurologic function below the injury level at the end of spinal shock, the prognosis for neurologic improvement is almost zero.

Sensory Testing[1,2,3]

Sensory testing should include a dermatomal examination for pin-prick and soft touch. Dermatomes are shown in Figures 3.8 and 3.9. The house officer should have a ready supply of safety

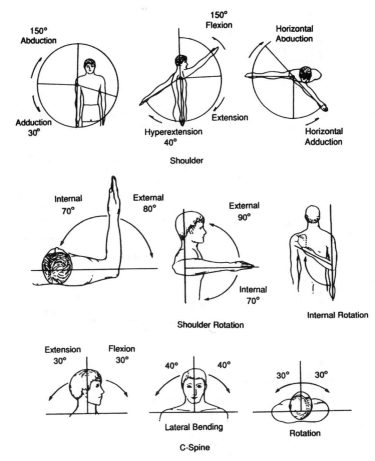

Figure 3.3. Normal ranges of motion for the shoulder and cervical spine.

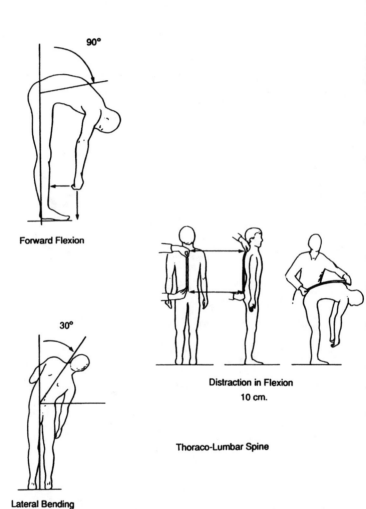

Forward Flexion

Distraction in Flexion
10 cm.

Thoraco-Lumbar Spine

Lateral Bending

Figure 3.4. Normal range of motion for the thoracolumbar spine.

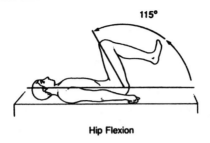

Hip Flexion

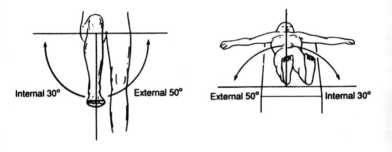

Hip Rotation in Flexion   **Hip Rotation in Extension**

Figure 3.5. Normal ranges of motion for the hip.

pins, which should be discarded after each use. In addition, the patient should be asked to perform sharp-dull discrimination in areas of question. Care should be taken to delineate an insensate area to determine whether it is dermatomal in pattern. This can be particularly difficult in patients with peripheral neuropathy secondary to diabetes, vascular insufficiency, heavy metal poisoning, or leprosy (Hansen's disease). A knowledge of the autogenous zones where there is no dermatomal overlap can be helpful in the examination.

Proprioception proceeds through different spinal tracts and should be tested separately. Proprioception is assessed by request-

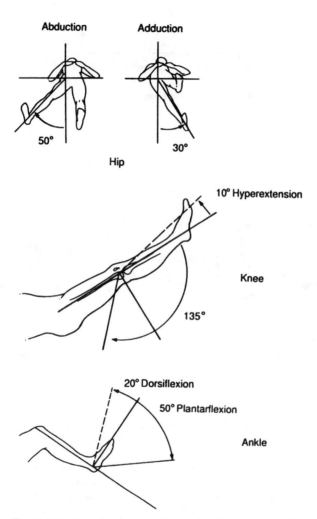

Figure 3.6. Normal ranges of motion for the hip, knee, and ankle.

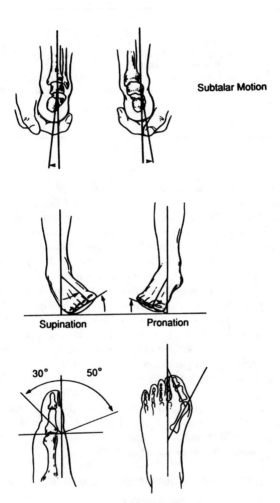

Subtalar Motion

Supination   Pronation

30°   50°

Figure 3.7. Normal ranges of motion for the foot and toes.

Table 3.1
Muscle Grading[2,3]

Grade	Description
5	Normal
4	Muscle contraction with full range of motion against gravity with some resistance
3	Muscle contraction with full range of motion against gravity
2	Muscle contraction with full range of motion with gravity eliminated
1	Flicker of muscle contraction
0	No activity

ing the patient to acknowledge the position of the extremity without vision. Grasp the toe or finger on either side rather than on the plantar and dorsal surface to eliminate pressure sensation.

In hand injuries, two-point discrimination allows for rapid and reproducible assessment of digital nerve function[5,6,7]. Two-point discrimination can be tested using blunted calipers or a paper clip bent into a "U." The patient's hand is rested palm up upon a table to maintain stability. The calipers are placed just lateral to the midline on the finger pad of the distal phalanx. The pressure used on the calipers is enough to just blanch the skin. The patient should then be asked to distinguish between "one" or "two" points. Unaffected or contralateral digits should be examined to gain patient confidence and to determine the normal discrimination for the patient. If the patient is able to discriminate between the two points of the caliper, the distance between the two points should be decreased and the process repeated. The distance is measured for each side of the digit, ulnar and radial. The normal distance for two-point discrimination in adults is 6 mm or less (Fig. 3.10).

SPECIFIC EXAMINATIONS AND SPECIAL MANEUVERS

Cervical Spine[1,2,3]

An examination of the upper extremity should always include an examination of the cervical spine. There are many reports of nerve compression at the cervical foramina that are discovered owing to persistent symptoms following a carpal tunnel release. The so-called *double crush syndrome refers to symptoms caused by nerve*

Table 3.2
Muscle Innervation—Upper Extremity[2-4]

Muscle	Peripheral Nerve	Nerve Root
Trapezius	Cranial nerve 11	Also $C_{2-4?}$
Rhomboids	Dorsal scapular	C_5
Levator scapulae	Nn. to levator scapulae	C_{3-4}
Pectoralis major	Medial and lateral pectoral	C_5-T_1
Deltoid	Axillary	C_{5-6}
Latissimus dorsi	Thoracodorsal	C_{6-8}
Supraspinatus	Suprascapular	C_{5-6}
Infraspinatus	Suprascapular	C_{5-6}
Teres major	Lower subscapular	C_{5-6}
Teres minor	Axillary	C_{5-6}
Subscapularis	Upper/lower subscapular	C_{5-6}
Serratus anterior	Long thoracic	C_{5-7}
Brachialis	Musculocutaneous	C_{5-6}
Biceps	Musculocutaneous	C_{5-6}
Triceps	Radial	C_{6-8}
Anconeus	Radial	C_{7-8}
Brachioradialis	Radial	C_{5-6}
ECRL, ECRB	Radial	C_{6-7}
Supinator	Radial [posterior interosseus]	C_{5-6}
AbPL	Radial [posterior interosseus]	C_{6-7}
ECU	Radial [posterior interosseus]	C_{6-8}
EDC	Radial [posterior interosseus]	C_{6-8}
EDQ	Radial [posterior interosseus]	C_{6-8}
EI	Radial [posterior interosseus]	C_{7-8}
EPB	Radial [posterior interosseus]	C_{6-7}
EPL	Radial [posterior interosseus]	C_{7-8}
FCR	Median	C_{6-7}
FCU	Ulnar	C_8-T_1
FDP [index, long]	Median [anterior interosseus]	C_7-T_1
FDP [ring, little]	Ulnar	C_7-T_1
FDS	Median	C_7-T_1
FPL	Median [anterior interosseus]	C_7-T_1
Pronator teres	Median	C_{6-7}
Pronator quadratus	Median [anterior interosseus]	C_7-T_1
Dorsal interossei	Ulnar	C_8-T_1
Palmar interossei	Ulnar	C_8-T_1
Lumbricals [index, long]	Median	C_7-T_1
Lumbricals [ring, little]	Ulnar	C_7-T_1
APB	Median	C_8-T_1
FPB	Median/ulnar	C_8-T_1
OpP	Median	C_8-T_1
AdP	Ulnar	C_8-T_1
Hypothenars	Ulnar	C_8-T_1

Table 3.3
Muscle Innervation—Lower Extremity[2-4]

Muscle	Peripheral Nerve	Nerve Root
Gluteus maximus	Inferior gluteal	L_4–S_1
Gluteus medius	Superior gluteal	L_4–S_1
Gluteus minimus	Superior gluteal	L_4–S_1
Hip external rotators	Nerves to . . .	L_4–S_2
Hip adductors	Obturator/tibial	L_{3-4}
Iliopsoas	Femoral	L_{2-3}
Quadriceps	Femoral	L_{2-4}
Sartorius	Femoral	L_{2-3}
Pectineus	Femoral	L_{2-3}
Semitendinosus	Sciatic [tibial]	L_5–S_1
Semimembranosus	Sciatic [tibial]	L_5–S_1
Biceps femoris	Sciatic [tibial/peroneal]	L_5–S_1
Tibialis anterior	Deep peroneal	L_{4-5}
Tibialis posterior	Tibial	L_5–S_1
EDL	Deep peroneal	L_{4-5}
EHL	Deep peroneal	L_5
Peroneus longus, brevis	Superficial peroneal	L_5–S_1
Gastrocnemius	Tibial	S_{1-2}
Soleus	Tibial	S_{1-2}
FDL	Tibial	L_5–S_1
FHL	Tibial	L_5–S_1
Foot intrinsics	Medial/lateral plantar [tibial]	L_5–S_2

Table 3.4
Deep Tendon Reflexes[2-4]

Muscle	Peripheral Nerve	Nerve Root
Biceps	Musculocutaneous	C_5
Brachioradialis	Radial	C_6
Triceps	Radial	C_7
Quadriceps (knee)	Femoral	L_4
Posterior tibialis	Deep peroneal (rarely elicited)	L_5
Gastroc/soleus	Tibial	S_1

Table 3.5
Superficial Reflexes[2-4]

Reflex	Peripheral Nerve	Nerve Root
Bulbocavernosus	Pudendal	S_{2-4}
Cremasteric	Genitofemoral	L_1
Babinski	Sciatic	S_1

compression at two different levels (e.g., the neck and the wrist). In any injury to the upper extremity, a minimum of a cursory exam of the cervical spine is warranted.

Palpation of the cervical spine should include posterior palpation of the spinous processes, as well as anterolateral palpation of the transverse processes. Excessive tenderness should be noted. Palpation of the anterior C-spine should include the lymphatic chain of the supraclavicular region. After the bony landmarks of the C-spine have been palpated, the examiner should examine the surrounding musculature of the neck. Specific attention should be paid to the upper trapezius and the sternocleidomastoid. These muscles are often exquisitely tender after hyperextension (whiplash) injuries.

The patient should be asked to flex his head to the chest, and the distance between the chin and chest should be noted. The patient should then be asked to fully extend his head, and the amount of extension should be noted. Do not confuse extension of the cervical spine with head rotation. At no time should the examiner force the C-spine into position. Rotation and lateral bending of the cervical spine should then be examined by asking the patient to touch his chin and subsequently his ear to his shoulder.

No examination of the cervical spine is complete without documentation of the deep tendon reflexes. The following is an outline for quick and accurate examination of the cervical spine.

C5 motor—deltoid (axillary n.), biceps (musculocutaneous n.) sensory—lat. arm (axillary n.)
DTR—biceps reflex

C6 motor—biceps (musculocutaneous n.), ECRB/ECRL (radial n.)

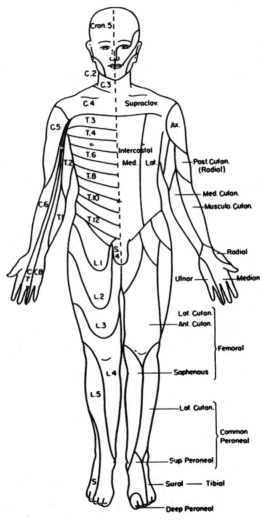

Figure 3.8. Sensory dermatomes (anterior).

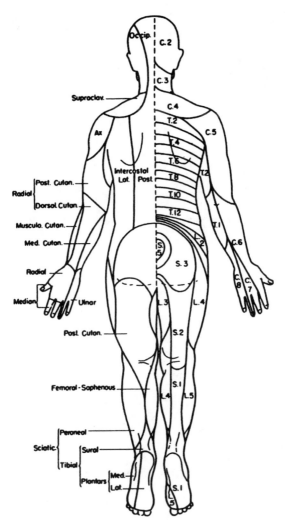

Figure 3.9. Sensory dermatomes (posterior).

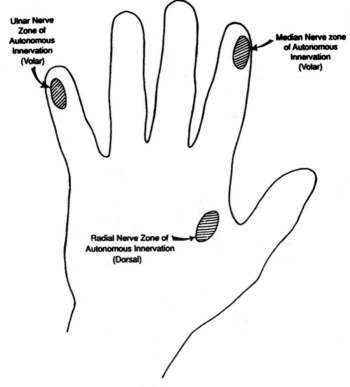

Figure 3.10. Zones of autonomous innervation for testing the nerves supplying the hand.

sensory—lat. forearm (musculocutaneous n.)
DTR—brachioradialis reflex

C7 motor—triceps (radial n.), FCR/FCU (median/ulnar nn.),
    MCP extension (radial n.)
sensory—long finger
DTR—triceps reflex

C8 motor—FDS (median n.), FDP (median/ulnar n.)
sensory—ring/little fingers (ulnar n.)
DTR—none

T1 motor—interossei mm. (ulnar n.)

sensory—medial arm around elbow (medial brachial cutaneous n.)

DTR—none

Upper Extremity

Shoulder[1,2]

The shoulder complex consists of the glenohumeral joint, acromioclavicular joint, the sternoclavicular joint, and the articulation of the scapula with the thorax. This joint has the largest range of motion of any joint in the body and is relatively superficial. The glenohumeral articulation is very small to allow for the large range of motion. The stability of the joint is provided by the soft tissues that surround the joint.

The shoulder is easily palpated, and significant landmarks include the acromioclavicular joint, the clavicle, the spine of the scapula, the bicipital groove of the humerus, and the acromion. The examination should begin with a visual inspection to determine abnormal contours or variance with the opposite shoulder.

Initial examination should include palpation of the bony skeleton and the shoulder girdle musculature. Specific attention should be paid to the deltoid, the pectorals, the long head of the biceps, and the rotator cuff musculature.

Observation and palpation of the acromioclavicular joint is a critical part of the examination to rule out acromioclavicular injury or arthritis. A positive cross-arm test is suggestive of arthritis or osteolysis. This test is performed by bringing the elbow on the affected side across the body near the contralateral shoulder. The test is positive if pain is elicited at the AC joint.

The rotator cuff is susceptible to damage, and several specific tests have been developed to examine this muscle group. The rotator cuff musculature forms a sleeve around the humeral head. These muscles serve as abductors and external rotators of the shoulder. Tears in the rotator cuff usually occur at the insertion of the supraspinatus tendon on the greater tuberosity. Tears often propagate along the tendon medially. Pain and/or tenderness around the greater tuberosity or anterior acromion is suggestive of a rotator cuff pathology (tear or tendinopathy), but patients with subacromial bursitis will often have pain in this region. The "drop-arm" test examines the rotator cuff. Have the patient abduct his arm to 90 degrees and then ask him to slowly lower his arm to his side. At approximately 30 degrees of abduction, the patient will no longer be able to gradually lower his arm and it will fall to the side. Unfortunately, the test is not always specific for a rotator cuff tear. One should compare the strength of the shoulder's external rotators to the contralateral side with the elbow at the patient's side. Ipsilateral external rotator weakness and pain, anterior acromion tenderness, and positive impingement signs are indicative of a cuff tear.

Shoulder impingement is a nonspecific sign of subacromial bursitis or rotator cuff pathology. This is often caused by hypertrophy of the acromion and impingement of the greater tuberosity and rotator cuff on the acromion. The Neer test is performed by internally rotating the patient's shoulder and forward flexing the shoulder. If this motion is painful at 90–100 degrees of forward flexion, it is a positive sign for impingement. The Hawkins' test is performed by forward flexing the shoulder to 90 degrees and internally rotating the shoulder to its endpoint. A painful endpoint is a positive test. Both of these tests are quite nonspecific, and a positive result is frequently followed by an impingement test. This test is performed by injecting the subacromial space with 10–15 cc of 1% lidocaine and repeating the Neer and Hawkins' tests. If, following the injection, they become negative, this suggests that the pathology is in the subacromial space or involves the rotator cuff.

Shoulder instability and labral tears are frequent causes of shoulder pain in adolescents and young adults. Unless the patient has a history of frank dislocations, these two entities are often difficult to distinguish in the clinic, especially in the athlete. Apprehension tests are usually performed with the patient supine in an effort to evaluate instability. Unfortunately, these tests are rarely conclusive because patients tend to "guard" on examination. Usually, the best clues come from the history. Many of these patients will not improve with PT and will ultimately be taken to the operating room. An examination under anaesthesia will often demonstrate shoulder instability, and arthroscopy can rule out labral tears and other intraarticular pathology.

Elbow[1,2]

Initially, one should inspect the skin to look for swelling and scars. The carrying angle of the elbow should then be observed.

The carrying angle is the amount of valgus with the elbow in full extension. This averages approximately 11 degrees with considerable variation about the mean. Males tend to have smaller carrying angles (5–10 degrees), and females have larger angles (10–15 degrees). Cubitus varus and cubitus valgus refer to excessive varus and valgus, respectively. Significant deviations from the normal carrying angle are usually the result of a physeal injury or fracture malunion during growth. Examination of the carrying angle with the elbow in less than full extension can lead to false measurements. The carrying angle is rarely a functional problem, but it can be a cosmetic one.

There are a number of significant landmarks that are easily palpated in the elbow. Laterally, the lateral epicondyle and the radial head are most easily palpated. Rotation of the radial head can be palpated during pronation and supination. The primary wrist extensors ("mobile wad") originate on the lateral condyle. Posteriorly, the major bony landmark is the olecranon, which is the site of insertion of the triceps. A bursa that is prone to excessive inflammation lies on top of the olecranon. Just medial to the olecranon is the ulnar groove in the humerus, which contains the ulnar nerve. The medial epicondyle marks the origin of the wrist flexors. The medial epicondyle of the humerus lies distally on the medial aspect of the elbow. Anteriorly, the biceps tendon is easily palpable. Just medial to the tendon are the brachial artery and median nerve.

Palpation of the triangle formed between the olecranon, the radial head, and the lateral epicondyle will often demonstrate an effusion if one is present. The center of this triangle is the easiest site for arthrocentesis when it is indicated.

The elbow is a complex hinge joint that normally has full extension, flexion to 145 degrees, and pronation and supination of about 80 degrees each. Limitations in motion, pain, or crepitus should be noted, as they may indicate pathology.

The medial collateral ligament originates from the medial epicondyle and is the major stabilizer of the elbow against valgus stress, while the radial head is the secondary stabilizer. The competence of the medial and lateral collateral ligaments is best tested by cupping and stabilizing the patient's affected elbow in the examiner's hand while flexing the elbow 20–30 degrees and applying varus and valgus stress to the ipsilateral forearm. Comparison should be made with the normal elbow.

Hand and Wrist[1,2,5,6]

Examination of the hand is extremely complex. The examination can only be as thorough as the examiner's knowledge of the anatomy and biomechanics. The first several paragraphs of this section will concentrate on the ER examination of the hand and upper extremity, and this will be followed by some specialized tests that will typically be performed in the office setting.

A good hand examination must include at least a brief cervical spine and brachial plexus examination, especially if there is any evidence of neurologic compromise. Nerve root compression or damage and brachial plexus lesions are frequently overlooked as sources of neurologic changes in the hand. The house officer should know the nerve root examination outlined in the cervical spine section and a diagram of the brachial plexus should always be near (Fig. 3.11) so one can pinpoint the location of a lesion.

Sensation in the hand is supplied by three nerves. The radial nerve supplies the radial-dorsal aspect, the median nerve supplies the volar aspect of the radial $3\frac{1}{2}$ digits (including the thumb),

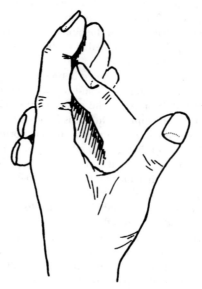

Figure 3.11. Testing the index finger FDP.

and the ulnar nerve supplies sensation to the ulnar half of the ring and the little fingers. There can be considerable overlap of the innervated areas. The sensory examination should include testing of the autonomous zones, as well as checking the radial and ulnar aspect of each digit for two-point distance discrimination (normal static value is <5–6 mm).

A quick and reliable motor examination is easy to perform. The following nerves innervate muscles moving the wrist and hand. Next to the listed nerves are muscles that are easy to check and can confirm or negate neurological function.

Radial n.—brachioradialis, ECRL/ECRB (wrist dorsiflexion)

Posterior Interosseous n. (branch of radial n.)—EPL (must hyperextend thumb IP), EDC (fully extend MCPs)

Median n.—FDS, opponens pollicis (thumb opposition)

Anterior Interosseous n. (branch of median n.)—FDP (index/long), FPL, pronator quadratus

Ulnar n.—adductor pollicis, interossei mm. (PIP extension or finger crossing)

It is sometimes difficult to perform an accurate examination for a variety of reasons. Occasionally, the patient is in pain, is hysterical, or he or she may be wearing a splint or cast that may cover autonomous zones or restrict motion. One must pay close attention to the subtleties of the hand examination in order to avoid obtaining incorrect data. For example, the patient must be able to hyperextend the thumb IP joint in order to demonstrate that the EPL is functioning. When testing the EDC, the patient should extend the MCPs while flexing the PIPs to eliminate any contribution by the intrinsic musculature. If checking thumb opposition, the patient should be able to oppose each digit. One should test the adductor pollicis m. by placing a piece of paper in the first webspace and asking the patient to squeeze it as you try to pull it out. If the patient has a weak adductor, the thumb IP joint will flex to attempt to compensate (positive Froment's sign). The lumbricals and the interossei are tested by having the patient flex the MCPs to 90 degrees while keeping the PIPs and DIPs fully extended. The interossei are also checked by abducting the fingers against resistance.

The Allen's test and the digital Allen's test are used to assess arterial blood flow in the hand. Simply confirming that there is both a radial and ulnar pulse does not rule out a compromise in the flow of one of the arteries. Pulsatile flow can occasionally be palpated in the radial or ulnar artery even when that particular artery is occluded proximally. This can occur because of flow through the palmar arch that serves as an anastomosis between the radial and ulnar arteries. To perform the Allen's test, one must occlude the radial and ulnar arteries on the volar aspect of the wrist and instruct the patient to make a tight fist, then open the hand 4–5 times in succession. Then, instruct the patient to completely open the hand (palm side up) and the palm should appear pale. The examiner should then release the pressure on one of the arteries and the palm should become pink within 1–2 seconds. One should then repeat the test for the other artery. If it takes longer than 1–2 seconds for either artery, there likely is diminished flow and one should time how long it takes for the palm to "pink up" and compare this with the time required when testing the same artery on the contralateral extremity. A modified version of this test can be used to check digital artery flow to an individual digit.

While testing the competence of the individual FDS tendons, it is important that all other digits besides the one being tested are fully extended in order to accurately test the structure and prevent a quadrigia effect. Since the FDP tendons tend to share muscle units and all the other tendons are kept on stretch except for the digit being tested, the FDP of that digit will not be able to contract and, therefore, only the FDS is being tested. On the other hand, the FDP tendon can be proved to be intact by merely flexing the DIP.

In order to evaluate any trauma to the dorsum of the hand or wrist, the house officer must know the locations of the six extensor compartments and the contents of each compartment. The first compartment contains the EPB and AbPL and forms the radial border of the anatomical snuffbox. The third compartment contains the EPL that passes just ulnar to Lister's tubercle on the dorsum of the wrist and continues distally to form the ulnar border of the anatomical snuffbox. The second compartment contains the ECRB and the ECRL and can be palpated just dorsal to the ulnar border of the snuffbox when a tight fist is made. The fourth compartment passes just ulnar to the EPL on the dorsum of the wrist and houses the EDC and the extensor indicis proprius. The fifth compartment contains the EDQ, and the sixth contains the ECU.

The distal ends of the fingers are very susceptible to infection because they are exposed to so much daily trauma in handling and manipulating a variety of objects, not to mention self-mutilating habits like nail-biting. A felon is an infection of the finger tuft that becomes increasingly painful with time because it is trapped between septa in the fingertip that attach the skin to the bone. A paronychia is an infection that starts on one edge of the nail and can spread around the entire nail base. Infections can also travel along the flexor tendon sheaths, resulting in a tenosynovitis that is demonstrated by the presence of Kanavel's signs. The four signs are: 1) fingers held in flexion, 2) uniform swelling of the finger, 3) intense pain with passive extension of the finger, and 4) extreme sensitivity to palpation along the course of the tendon sheath.

The bony architecture of the hand consists of the distal radius and ulna, the 8 carpal bones, 5 metacarpals, and 14 phalanges. Prominent bony landmarks that can be palpated include the radial styloid, the scaphoid (carpal navicular), trapezium, and first metacarpal along the radial border of the hand. On the radial palmar aspect of the wrist, the tuberosity of the scaphoid can be palpated. On the dorsal aspect of the radius is Lister's tubercle. Distal to Lister's tubercle, the depression of the capitate can be palpated. Along the ulnar side of the wrist and hand, the ulnar styloid and the triquetrum can be palpated. The pisiform bone is a sesamoid bone within the tendon of the flexor carpi ulnaris. All the bones must be palpated and the joints moved to rule out fracture or instability.

In order to perform a thorough ER evaluation, the house officer must carefully inspect the hand and any wounds. He or she must make sure that the hand and digits are neurovascularly intact and must rule out any fractures, dislocations, or infections. One should also evaluate the flexor and extensor tendons to make sure that they are working appropriately. The office hand examination will frequently involve many of the aforementioned tests, but there are several other specialized tests that will now be mentioned and are primarily used in the office setting.

Examination of the hand should include checking the active and passive range of motions for the wrist and digits. The range of motion for the MCP joint is 0–85 degrees, the PIP is 0–110 degrees, and the DIP is 0–65 degrees. A decrease in ROM can be because of a disruption of the articular surface, joint capsule tightness, or because of tight intrinsic or extrinsic musculature.

The Bunnell-Littler test evaluates the tightness of the intrinsic musculature as a possible source for decreased PIP range of motion. If the patient has limited PIP motion with the MCP joint in extension (intrinsics on stretch) and then has normal PIP motion when the intrinsics are relaxed by placing the MCP in flexion, the PIP tightness is likely owing to contraction of the intrinsic musculature (interossei, lumbricals).

Tightness of the extrinsic muscles of the hand can also be responsible for decreased range of motion in the digits. For example, increased digit extension when the wrist is volar flexed (extrinsic flexors are relaxed) compared with when it is extended may indicate that extrinsic muscle contracture is responsible for decreased MCP/PIP extension. The retinacular test is used to see if decreased DIP flexion is owing to a tight capsule or tight, oblique retinacular ligaments. If DIP flexion is substantially improved when the PIP is changed from an extended to a flexed position, the decreased ROM can likely be attributed to retinacular tightness.

Carpal tunnel syndrome is seen frequently in the office setting, and it is caused by compression of the median nerve by the transverse carpal ligament. Percussion of the ligament will cause parasthesias in the median nerve distribution in the affected patient (Tinel's sign or Percussion sign). A positive carpal compression sign is suggestive of CTS when pressure over the median nerve at the wrist causes parasthesias in a median nerve distribution. Phalen's sign is performed by flexing the wrists completely for 1 minute. If the patient develops symptoms consistent with carpal tunnel syndrome within that time, the test is positive for compression of the median nerve at the wrist. Many physicians also use a reverse Phalen's test, in which the same test is performed except that the wrist is dorsiflexed to put the carpal tunnel and its contents on stretch. Whenever one is evaluating a compression neuropathy in the hand, one must be sure to examine the cervical spine, brachial plexus, and entire extremity in order to rule out other sites of compression (a "double crush" syndrome) before making a surgical plan (Fig. 3.12).

Occasionally, patients will present complaining of decreased sensation, and the examination may be unclear or simply may not make sense. In these situations, the immersion test or the

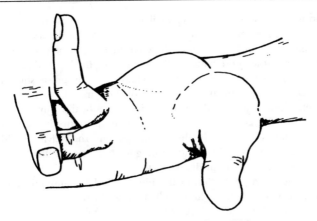

Figure 3.12. Testing the ring finger FDS.

betadine starch test can be useful. The immersion test is abnormal if skin that is immersed in water for 5 minutes does *not* wrinkle. The more reliable Betadine starch test is performed by first painting the hand with Betadine and allowing it to dry. One then mixes a corn starch/mineral oil slurry and applies it to the previously painted hand with a tongue depresser. If the hand is normally innervated, it will sweat and the hand will turn blue. If it is truly insensate, no blue color will be observed.

Lower Extremity

Pelvis and Hip[1,2]

The pelvis functions as a bony structure to transfer axial forces from the lower extremity to the spine. The pelvis is formed from the coalescence of three bones: the ilium, the ischium, and the pubis. The junction of these three bones forms the triradiate cartilage in the child. These bones eventually fuse and form part of the acetabulum. The femur is the longest bone in the body, and the proximal portion of the femur articulates with the acetabulum like a ball and socket to form the hip joint.

Anteriorly on the pelvis, significant landmarks include the anterior superior iliac spine, the iliac crest, the pubic tubercles, and the symphysis pubis. Posteriorly, the landmarks include the posterior superior iliac spine, the iliac crest, and the ischial tuberosity. The greater trochanter is the only palpable landmark of the proximal femur. Palpation of these landmarks can be extremely difficult in the obese patient. When palpating the hip and pelvis, the relationship of the greater trochanter to the pelvis should be checked to confirm the location of the femoral head in the acetabulum. Pain over the sacroiliac joints may be the only clinical evidence for sacroiliac (SI) joint ligamentous injury in light of a normal radiograph. In the trauma patient, the pelvis should be checked for stability by attempting to compress the iliac wings and noting any patient discomfort.

The range of motion of the hip should be examined in all planes. This should include abduction, adduction, flexion, and extension. Internal and external rotation of the femur should be checked with the hip flexed 90 degrees and fully extended. When testing the passive range of motion, the examiner should stabilize the pelvis so true hip motion is tested. In patients with osteoarthritis of the hip, the first limitation in range of motion is in internal rotation.

The patient's gait is important in the assessment of the hip, although gait disturbances can be caused by pathology anywhere in the lower extremity or in the lumbosacral spine. When examining the gait, observe one portion of the gait at a time. Specific notation should be made of any support the patient uses (i.e., crutch, cane, or walker). With the patient standing and the knees fully extended, leg lengths should be examined by palpating the iliac crests posteriorly. If the iliac crests are not of equal height with both knees straight and both feet together, a limb length discrepancy may be present. Scoliosis and contractures around the hip can also be causes of pelvic obliquity and should be ruled out. If a leg length discrepancy does exist, the most accurate method of measuring the discrepancy is by placing wooden blocks of standard sizes under the short leg.

Trendelenburg Test This test examines the strength of the gluteus medius. In the normal patient, the pelvis is level when the patient stands. When the patient is asked to stand on one leg, the gluteus medius on the supported side contracts and the pelvis will remain level or elevate on the unsupported side. If the pelvis cannot be maintained level on the unsupported side, the patient is said to have a "positive" Trendelenburg sign. Patients with gluteus medius weakness walk with a lurch because they attempt to shift their upper bodies laterally in order to compensate for weak hip abduction. This gait pattern is described as Trendelenburg gait. A Trendelenburg gait will be present in many painful conditions of the hip joint, as well as in cases of gluteus medius weakness.

Thomas Test This maneuver is used to determine if a fixed flexion contracture of the hip is present. The examiner locks the pelvis by bringing the contralateral leg into maximal flexion with the patient supine on the examining table. This eliminates any lumbar lordosis that can be used to compensate for a hip flexion contracture. The leg to be examined is then brought into maximal extension with the hip in slight adduction and internal rotation. If the leg does not fully extend to touch the examining table, then a fixed flexion contracture is present, and the angle of the flexion contracture can be estimated by measuring the lack of extension of the limb to touch the table.

Ober's Test[8,9] Since the widespread use of the polio vaccine, the incidence of iliotibial band contracture has decreased. The Ober test measures the amount of abduction contracture caused by the iliotibial band. The patient is placed on his side with the affected limb on the top. The pelvis is again locked by bringing the unaffected limb into maximal flexion. The affected limb is then brought into full extension and abduction. From the position of abduction, the leg is allowed to fall into adduction. If a contracture is present, the affected limb will not be able to move into adduction. In performing the test, the leg must be brought into full extension to place the iliotibial band over the greater trochanter. If the iliotibial band is permitted to move anterior to the greater trochanter, the test will yield a false-negative result.

Knee

The knee is one of the most commonly injured joints. Much of the diagnosis of soft-tissue pathology in the knee is made on the basis of the history and clinical examination (see Knee Injuries in Chapter 6). If the patient is examined immediately after an acute injury, tests for instability can be performed with minimal patient discomfort. In the presence of a tense knee effusion, performing an anterior drawer test can border on torture for the unanesthetized patient.

The knee consists of the articulations between the tibia and the distal femur. The femur has two articulations, which are the medial and lateral condyles. The tibia has a proximal flare or plateau, which is divided into medial and lateral compartments by the tibial eminence. The articulations between the tibia and femur contain both articular and meniscal cartilage.

Landmarks of the knee include the tibial tubercle and the patella anteriorly. The adductor tubercle is palpable on the medial femoral condyle. Posteriorly, the neurovascular bundle is found in the popliteal fossa between the insertions of the gastrocnemius. Gerdy's tubercle is palpable on the lateral tibia and the fibular head is obvious posterolaterally. Other anatomic structures include the insertion of the pes anserinus (sartorius, gracilis, and semitendinosus tendons) on the medial tibia; the insertion of the medial and lateral hamstrings on the tibia and fibula, respectively; and the iliotibial band, which is palpated laterally before its insertion at Gerdy's tubercle. The quadriceps tendon can be palpated as it inserts on the patella, and the patellar tendon completes the extensor mechanism as it links the patella and the tibial tubercle. The medial and lateral collateral ligaments are located on the respective sides of the knee. Pain over the origins of these ligaments with valgus and varus stress, respectively, can be associated with strain or rupture of these structures.

The presence or absence of an effusion is helpful in the diagnosis of a knee injury. The easiest way to demonstrate an effusion is to "milk" it from the suprapatellar pouch into the infrapatellar region, where it is appreciated as a fullness medial and lateral to the patellar tendon. The effusion is "milked" by pressing on the suprapatellar area, and sliding the hand distally. In a large effusion, the patella may be ballotable against the femoral condyles. This is performed by depressing the patella into the trochlear groove and then releasing it. The displaced effusion will cause the patella to rebound.

The majority of injuries to the knee are to soft tissue, although radiographs of the knee should be made to examine the bony architecture. For instance, in some anterior cruciate tears, the ligament is avulsed from its bony insertion with a small fragment of bone from the tibial eminence. The avulsion of the ligamentous insertion has prognostic significance in that a primary repair can be performed.

The major ligaments involved in knee injuries include the medial and lateral collateral ligaments, which are extraarticular, and the anterior and posterior cruciate ligaments, which are intraarticular. Many injuries to the major ligaments of the knee will be associated with injury to the meniscal cartilage, as these are secondary stabilizers of the knee.

The knee should initially be inspected to evaluate the skin, swelling, musculature (check for atrophy), and alignment. Swelling can be owing to an intraarticular effusion, a prepatellar bursitis, or a popliteal cyst (posterior). Alignment should be judged as normal, genu valgum (valgus), genu varum (varus), or genu recurvatum ("back knee").

Following inspection, the active and passive range of motion should be documented and the knee joint should be palpated. The localization of pain is often diagnostic. Tenderness along the joint line either medially or laterally suggests a meniscal injury or degenerative joint disease. Pain over Gerdy's tubercle is often associated with inflammation of the iliotibial band, known as *iliotibial band syndrome.* Lateral knee pain with the affected leg placed in the figure-4 position is often associated with lateral collateral ligament injury.

If range of motion is limited, its etiology should be determined. A locked knee can be caused by a meniscal tear or a cruciate ligament subluxated into the joint. Lack of full extension can be caused by an anterior meniscal lesion. Pain with flexion of the knee can be associated with posterior horn meniscal tears (these are commonly seen in football linemen and power lifting). Limitation of active extension can be caused by injury to the extensor mechanism, specifically a patella fracture, patellar tendon rupture, or quadriceps tendon rupture.

Lachman's Test[10,11] Lachman's test is the best test for assessing the anterior cruciate ligament. The test is performed with the patient in the supine position with the knee flexed about 30 degrees. The examiner supports the proximal tibia with one hand and grasps the distal femur with the other. With the patient as relaxed as possible, the examiner attempts to bring the tibia forward on the femur. Any motion of the joint will be seen and felt by the examiner. Again, the key to a successful assessment is relaxation of the musculature. Any findings should be compared with the contralateral limb.

Drawer Tests[10,11]   The drawer test examines the knee for instability of the cruciate ligaments. The anterior drawer tests the anterior cruciate, and the posterior drawer evaluates the posterior cruciate. To perform the anterior drawer test, have the patient lie in the supine position with the knee flexed 90 degrees and the foot flat on the examining table in the neutral position. Grasp the tibia with both hands, and place the thumbs on the anterior surface just above the joint line. The patient's foot is stabilized on the table by bracing it with the examiner's hip. With the patient relaxed, attempt to pull the tibia forward on the femur. If the tibia moves forward without a definite stopping point, the anterior cruciate may be damaged. The examiner should compare the anterior translation of the affected side with that of the uninjured knee. This test is not valid if the quadriceps and hamstrings are not relaxed. In the acutely injured patient, it may not be possible to perform this test secondary to patient discomfort. The posterior drawer test is performed in the same fashion, although pressure is applied to the anterior portion of the tibia in an attempt to translate the tibia posteriorly.

External and internal rotation of the foot in conjunction with the anterior drawer test can give information about the posteromedial and posterolateral capsular stability, respectively. The posteromedial knee capsule tightens with the foot in external rotation, and the anterior drawer should be less even in the presence of a torn anterior cruciate. If the amount of forward motion is the same as with the foot in neutral postion, posteromedial capsule damage can be suspected. With the foot in internal rotation, the posterolateral structures tighten, and the amount of forward motion with the anterior drawer test should be diminished despite an anterior cruciate injury. Again, if forward motion is the same as when the foot is in the neutral position, there may be injury to the posterolateral capsule.

Varus and Valgus Stress[10]   The medial collateral ligament (MCL) can be tested by applying forced valgus stress on the limb. With the patient supine, the leg to be examined is supported under the proximal tibia by the examiner's contralateral hand. With the knee flexed 20 degrees, a valgus force is applied gradually to the knee joint with the other hand. If the MCL is injured, the patient will have pain in the anatomic region that will increase with stress. Using the same method, a varus force is applied to the knee to test the lateral collateral ligament. Asymmetric laxity is often indicative of a partial or complete collateral ligament tear.

Pivot Shift[10,11] The femoral condyle is shaped in the form of a cam. Motion at the knee joint is a combination of rotation and gliding of the femoral condyle over the tibia. In the presence of an anterior cruciate deficiency, there is a delay of posterior gliding of the tibia on the femur. The pivot shift test is performed by placing the patient supine and straightening the affected lower extremity. One then applies a valgus stress on the knee while axially loading the extremity and flexing it. The absence of an ACL causes the tibia to remain excessively anterior in extension. The tibia is actually subluxated anteriorly until a certain amount of flexion is reached and the tibia "pops" back into position (relocates). This test is difficult to perform by the inexperienced examiner, especially if the patient is guarding. Again, findings should be compared with the contralateral extremity.

McMurray Test[2] This test examines the knee for a tear in the posterior horn of the medial meniscus. The test is performed with the patient supine, and the knee flexed. The foot is internally and externally rotated to loosen the knee joint. The knee is then brought into extension with the foot held in external rotation and a steady valgus force applied. If a click or pop is appreciated during extension, the test is suggestive for a posterior medial meniscus tear.

Foot and Ankle[1,2]

The foot and ankle include a complex series of bones, joints, and soft tissues that require a great deal of skill and experience to examine. Examination begins by inspecting and comparing the two feet to determine any asymmetry between them. One should look for callosities, as these may indicate sites of excessive wear.

After inspecting the feet, the foot and ankle are palpated to determine any areas of tenderness. The palpation should proceed along well-known anatomic landmarks and should include the heelcord, the lateral and medial malleoli, the talar head, the deltoid ligament, the anterior talofibular ligament, the sustentaculum tali (along the medial aspect of the calcaneus), and the plantar aspect of the metatarsal heads.

Since the foot and ankle consist of multiple joints, it is important to assess the motion of only the major, more mobile joints. It is important to document the dorsi- and plantar flexion of the talocrural (ankle) joint, the inversion and eversion of the subtalar joint (performed by stabilizing the talus in the ankle mortise with one hand while testing motion of the subtalar joint with the other hand), the motion of the midfoot (the talonavicular and calcaneocuboid joints, which are tested by stabilizing the heel with one hand and testing eversion and inversion, and adduction and abduction of the forefoot with the other hand), and the motion of the metatarsophalangeal and interphalangeal joints.

Motion can be recorded both passively and actively. More commonly, it is measured passively by the examiner. However, active motion is also tested during the muscle testing portion of the foot and ankle examination. The following muscles are usually tested: ankle plantar flexion (gastroc/soleus complex), ankle dorsiflexion (peroneals and anterior tibial), foot eversion (peroneals), foot inversion (anterior and posterior tibial), toe extension (extensor digitorum longus and extensor hallucis longus), and toe flexion (flexor digitorum longus and brevis). In addition to providing information about each individual muscle, this portion of the examination may help identify any problems relating to lumbar nerve roots, as the muscle groups are innervated by specific nerve roots (Tables 3.2 and 3.3).

In cases of acute or chronic ankle sprains, specific tests of the foot and ankle include the anterior and posterior drawer tests to test the anterior talofibular ligament (ATFL) and the calcaneofibular ligament (CFL), respectively. Stress radiographs are sometimes indicated in order to diagnose chronic ankle instability. These tests and radiographs are described in the section describing ankle sprains in Chapter 6.

THE PEDIATRIC EXAMINATION[8,9,12,13]

Examination of children is not simply the examination of a smaller-sized version of an adult. Children are different both physiologically and psychologically and the differences must be kept in mind by the examiner. Although it is always a good idea to examine the "normal" extremity when one is presented with a unilateral complaint, this practice is of paramount importance in children in order to establish some trust between the child and the examiner. Failure to gain trust initially and immediate examination of the injured, painful area will make the child distrustful. This will lead to frustration for the examiner and the parents. After examining the normal extremity, the examination of the injured limb should begin in an area that is not injured and only at the end of the examination should the injured area be palpated and examined.

Neonates have certain musculoskeletal differences that change gradually as the child grows. Many of the initial differences are related to positioning of the fetus in the uterus. In order to understand what is normal and abnormal in children, it is absolutely necessary to understand the varying growth patterns of the extremities in children.

Prior to examining a child, one must first obtain a clear history. In addition to finding out why the parents have brought the child for evaluation and when that condition started, one must obtain a clear pregnancy history (length, type of delivery), birth history (weight, Apgars, days in hospital), family history, PMH, PSH, current medications, and allergies. It is also important to obtain a good history about developmental landmarks. This helps assess neurologic development. The parents should be questioned about when the child first began to sit up, to crawl, to attempt to stand, and to walk. Normal milestones are approximately as follows:[8,9,13]

Head control—about 3 months
Sitting up—about 6 months
Independent sitting, crawling—about 8 months
Pulling to stand—about 10 months
Walking independently—about 12 months
Handedness—18 months
Knows full name—2 years

The neonatal spine has a long, kyphotic C-curve with no areas of lordosis initially present. This is because of the "curled up" position that the child had in the womb. As children grow and begin to sit and raise their heads, the spine will develop the normal lumbar and cervical lordosis. The cervical lordosis develops as the child begins to raise his head at about 2–3 months. The lumbar curve develops when the child is sitting up and beginning to stand, usually by 10–12 months.

The neonatal spine must also be examined to rule out bony anomalies, skin defects, skin discoloration, or hair tufts. All of these are suggestive of spinal dysraphism, such as myelomeningo-coele or diastamatomyelia. Neonatal neck range of motion should be evaluated to rule out motion loss that may be indicative of a torticollis or a congenital anomaly such as Klippel-Feil syndrome.

In adolescents, the forward bending position can give one a better view of a rib hump or lumbar fullness that may result from a curvature of the spine. The size of the rib hump or lumbar fullness can be quantified with a scoliometer giving the physician an idea of how much rotation is associated with the spine curvature. In evaluating a patient with scoliosis, it is important to note shoulder asymmetry, as it may affect surgical management. It is also important to note the height of the iliac crests, since a leg length discrepancy can cause an apparent curvature of the spine.

In utero, the fetal upper extremities are usually positioned with the arms across the chest and the elbows flexed. Thus, most neonates have flexion contractures at the elbows and slight internal rotation contractures of the shoulders. These correct as the child begins to use his hands and should be fully corrected by 6 months to 1 year of age. Evaluation of the shoulder should initially ensure that the scapula is not elevated or winged. Additionally, one needs to confirm that range of motion is appropriate. Glenohumeral to scapulothoracic motion should have a ratio of about 3:2. Primary examination of the hands mainly involves neurovascular status and notation of deletions or supernumerary digits.

In the newborn, the most important musculoskeletal assessment is the hip joint. The incidence of instability of the hip in the newborn has been reported as 1 in 60 by Barlow. Early detection of hip instability will often allow for simple closed management of the problem with minimal late sequelae.

The child should be examined when he/she is cooperative. Little information will be gained from the examination of a crying infant. All examinations of the hip should be made with the child entirely disrobed, including removal of the diaper. With the child in the supine position and the legs extended, the skin should be examined for asymmetric skin folds, as well as any other gross abnormality.

Barlow's Test[8,9,12]

With the child in the supine position and the hips flexed 90 degrees, the distal femur is controlled by the thumb, and the fingers are placed over the greater trochanter. The examiner's other hand stabilizes the pelvis while he adducts the femur and gently applies a posteriorly directed, axial load on the femur. Instability is noted by a click as the femoral head subluxates over the rim of the acetabulum. Sometimes a clunk is felt as the hip completely dislocates with this maneuver. One should distinguish between hips that are "subluxatable" and those that are "dislocatable."

Ortolani's test[8,9,12]

For this test, the child is again in the supine position with one of the examiner's hands stabilizing the pelvis and the other gripping the femur with the thumb on the medial distal femur and the fingers over the greater trochanter. The hip is then slowly abducted. If the hip is dislocated, the examiner will feel a clunk as the hip relocates into the acetabulum. A helpful mnemonic for recalling the position of the femoral head is that in Ortolani's test the femoral head starts "out" and is reduced "in." OUT-IN, O-I, O-rtolan-I. These hips are dislocated but are "relocatable." The Barlow and Ortalani tests are effectively used in the newborn infant.

Galeazzi's Sign

The child is again placed supine on the examining table. The knees should be brought together with the hips flexed 90 degrees. A dislocation should be suspected if there is an apparent discrepancy in femoral length with the affected side being shorter (pediatric hip dislocations are typically lateral and superior). The femoral length discrepency is known as a positive Galeazzi sign. This test is more sensitive in older children.

The presence of the greater trochanter above the line (Nelaton's line) between the anterior superior iliac spine and the ischial tuberosity signifies a dislocation of the hip. Asymmetric hip abduction is a sign of dislocation that develops at around 3 months owing to an adduction contracture on the same side as the dislocation.

Examination for hip flexion contracture is performed in one of two ways in children. In the Thomas test, the patient is supine and both hips are flexed maximally. One then brings the hip to be tested into extension while the other hip is maintained in full flexion. The amount of hip flexion still present on the side being tested when the pelvis starts to tilt forward is the amount of the hip flexion contracture. The other method is the Staheli test. The patient is placed in the prone position with the lower extremities flexed over the edge of the table. The side to be tested is slowly extended, while one hand stabilizes the pelvis. The degree of contracture is the angle remaining when the pelvis starts to tilt.

With the child supine, the hips should be flexed and internally and externally rotated. The child should then be placed prone and have internal and external rotation checked. The complete rotation arc should be around 90–100 degrees. In adults, the hips internally rotate less than they externally rotate. Neonates usually have a slight external rotation contracture. However, this is compensated by the fact that the femoral neck is anteverted more in children than it is in adults. Femoral anteversion measures the relationship of the femoral neck to the knee axis. As the child begins to stand, the external rotation contracture stretches out and the excessive anteversion causes the child to stand with the legs slightly internally rotated and the toes thus pointing inwardly ("toeing-in").

Toeing-in is a common reason for parents to bring their child to clinic. Femoral anteversion is the most common cause of toeing-in, followed by tibial torsion and metatarsus adductus. This diagnosis is made by noting a disproportionate amount of bilateral hip internal rotation compared with external rotation. The Ryder test also assesses femoral anteversion. The patient is placed prone with the hips extended and the knees flexed 90 degrees. The examiner then internally rotates the hip to the position at which the greater trochanter is most prominent on the lateral aspect of the hip. The patient's femoral anteversion is equal to the angle that the tibia is making with a line perpendicular to the examining table when the greater trochanter is most prominent.

The knee examination in children is usually performed when anxious parents bring the child to clinic concerned about knock-knees (genu valgum) or bowlegs (genu varum). Virtually all children will have genu varum when they first begin to stand. This usually corrects at about age 2, and most children then develop genu valgum until they are about 4–5. Again, this usually corrects to a normal physiologic appearance. One should place the child supine and measure the distance between the right and left medial femoral condyles with the knees extended and the ankles brought together to follow genu varum clinically. Likewise, to clinically evaluate genu valgum, the child is placed supine with the knees extended and touching each other and the distance betwen the medial malleoli is measured (the intermalleolar distance). The femorotibial angle should be measured using a goniometer while evaluating both of these conditions.

Two causes of severe bowing at the knees are rickets and Blount's disease[11,13]. If rickets is suspected, appropriate blood and urine tests can be performed to diagnose it. Blount's disease is a growth disorder of the proximal tibial physis that results in severe genu varum. It usually also presents with a varus thrust during gait and requires radiographic confirmation for accurate diagnosis. On examination, the varus should be limited to the proximal one-third of the tibia or the diagnosis should be questioned. Excessive tibial torsion can also give the appearance of Blount's disease, so one must be careful.

Internal tibial torsion is a common cause of toeing-in. Tibial torsion measures the relationship of the knee axis to the ankle axis and can be determined by flexing the knee about 10 degrees, aligning the patella to be directed anteriorly. One then compares the angle formed between the line connecting the peaks of the lateral and medial malleoli and the line that the knee hinges on. Normally, the ankle is externally rotated about 20–25 degrees relative to the knee and the femur. Less than this would indicate some degree of internal tibial torsion and the foot would point in or toe-in.

Children's feet can have many abnormalities. The most common severe abnormality is a clubfoot, or talipes equinovarus. This is manifested by the hindfoot being plantarflexed (equinus) and the forefoot adducted (varus). The equinovarus is of varying severity and rigidity. There are often posterior and medial creases. The interval between the medial malleolus and the navicular is diminished and fixed. The sinus tarsi is obliterated and not palpable. The heel pad seems to be "empty" because the hindfoot is in severe equinus.

The third cause of in-toeing is metatarsus adductus. This occurs when the forefoot turns slightly inward. This can be evaluated by examining the plantar aspect of the foot. A line drawn plantarly between the hindfoot and midfoot, if extended distally, should pass between the second and third toes. If this line passes lateral to that web space, metatarsus adductus of varying severity is present. An indication of severe metatarsus adductus is the presence of a medial skin crease.

The Coleman block test used in the evaluation of the cavus foot to determine whether the deformity is stiff or flexible. In this test, the patient places the lateral half of his foot on a block and thus allows his first metatarsal to flex as much as possible without touching the floor. One then should evaluate the hindfoot to see if any of the varus deformity previously seen has disappeared. In a stiff foot, the varus hindfoot will remain. In a flexible foot, the varus hindfoot should become valgus as soon as the first metatarsal lost the support of the ground.

Leg length discrepancies are often encountered in pediatric orthopaedics. The classic method of measurement compares the distances from the anterior superior iliac spine to the medial malleolus with the patient in the supine position and the hips and knees extended. The other method of measuring leg length discrepancy involves getting the patient in a standing position with both hips and knees completely extended and putting one's fingertips on the patient's posterior iliac crest. One should palpate and visualize the iliac crest and put blocks under the deficient side until the crests become level. One should then measure the height of the blocks utilized in order to quantify the leg length discrepancy.

Observational gait analysis is a crucial aspect of the pediatric orthopaedic examination. One should observe the child's velocity by visualizing his cadence and his stride length. After this, one should visualize the ankle, knee, hip, and trunk positions during heel strike, stance phase, toe-off, and swing phase. Observation of the gait can help evaluate the child's balance, muscular strength, contractures, and out-of-phase function. Gait analysis by video, electromyography, and force plate studies is becoming increasingly popular prior to surgical intervention in many conditions, especially cerebral palsy.

An important part of the orthopaedic examination includes the assessment of joint range of motion. This enables the orthopaedist to identify joint and muscle contractures. Motion loss can be owing to either bony anomaly, as is found with a slipped capital femoral epiphysis, a muscular defect such as tight hamstrings in a child with CP, or a capsular contraction as is often found in the posterior knee capsule of the child with spina bifida. In muscles spanning two joints, one of the joints must be immobilized while the other's motion is being assessed. For example, when one is testing the popliteal angle in order to assess hamstring contracture, one places the femur on the ipsilateral side directly perpindicular to the patient and the examination table, while the patient is in the supine position. After this is done, the knee is extended to the point at which contracture stops further extension. When checking for heelcord contractures, one must test the dorsiflexion of the ankle with the knee both in a flexed and extended position, and record both of these measurements since the gastroc/soleus complex spans the knee and ankle.

Spasticity is frequently seen in conditions such as cerebral palsy, and this can make assessment of range of motion quite difficult. The increase in tone of a muscle can vary from one examination to the next, causing inconsistencies in measurement. It is important for the clinician to decide whether or not the contracture is static or dynamic, because treatment may differ. An example of a static contracture is when a patient is lying supine and one cannot get the ankle to dorsiflex beyond neutral with the knee flexed. A dynamic contracture of the same muscle would be noted if the patient were able to dorsiflex the ankle 20 degrees with the knee flexed, but then proceeded to walk on his toes.

Finally, the pediatric examination should include a detailed neurologic evaluation. While it is important to test the strength of the various muscle groups, this is not always possible to do in children because they cannot follow instructions well. In these cases, information can be gained by watching the child play or hold objects, to see which muscle groups appear to be active. In addition, the foot can be stimulated by stroking the plantar surface and seeing which muscles react to pull the foot away from this noxious stimulus.

The neurologic examination includes testing of the deep tendon reflexes, as in the adult. Babinski testing and testing for clonus should be performed. The presence of hyperreflexia, clonus, a stretch reflex (often termed claspknife rigidity) and/

or upgoing toes on the Babinski test are the four hallmarks of spasticity and will support a diagnosis of spastic cerebral palsy.

In addition, certain infantile reflexes should be tested if there is any suspicion of a developmental delay. If any two of these reflexes are abnormal after 12 months of age, the prognosis for unassisted ambulation is poor[5]. The infantile reflexes are as follows: Moro reflex, head-turning reflex, asymmetric tonic neck reflex, symmetric tonic neck reflex, foot-placement reaction, extensor thrust, and the parachute reaction [5,11,13].

The Moro reflex is tested by jarring the table, or dropping the infant's head into extension. The Moro reflex is sudden extension or spreading of the upper extremities. This reflex appears by 6 months but should disappear by 12 to 16 months.

The head-turning reflex is tested with the child in the side-lying position. The head is tilted downward and rotated toward the floor. A positive head-turning reflex is present if the lower extremity on the same side flexes at the hip and knee. The asymmetric tonic neck reflex is tested in the supine position. The head is rotated toward one side, and the reflex is present if the extremities extend on the face-turned side and flex on the occiput side. The symmetric tonic neck reflex is tested with the child prone. The reflex is present if extension of the head causes extension of the forelimbs and flexion of the hindlimbs. The three neck reflexes should all disappear in the normal infant at about 6 months.

The foot-placement reaction is tested by holding the child with the feet dangling such that they just touch the edge of the examining table. Normal infants will lift the feet and place them on the table. An abnormal reaction is to simply allow the feet to continue to hang loosely.

Extensor thrust is present if, when the child is held in a weight-bearing position, the legs extend at the ankle, knees, and hips and adduct and cross.

The parachute reaction is tested by holding the child under his arms and tilting him downward and forward. Normally the child will extend the upper extremities as if to break the fall. The parachute reaction normally appears at about 9 months of age. It is abnormal if it is not present after that age.

References

1. Urbaniak J. Manual of orthopaedic surgery. Chicago: American Academy of Orthopaedic Surgeons, 1979.

2. Hoppenfeld S. Physical examination of the spine and extremities. New York: Appleton-Century-Crofts, 1976.
3. Hoppenfeld S. Orthopaedic neurology. New York: Appleton-Century-Crofts, 1979.
4. Hollinshead WH. Anatomy for surgeons: Vol. 3. The back and limbs. 2nd ed. New York: Harper & Row, 1969.
5. American Society for Surgery of the Hand. The hand: examination and diagnosis. Edinburgh: Churchill-Livingstone, 1983.
6. American Society for Surgery of the Hand. Syllabus—regional review course in hand surgery, Durham, NC, 1984.
7. Moberg E. Methods of examining sensibility of the hand. In: Flynn JE, ed. Hand surgery. Baltimore: Williams & Wilkins, 1966.
8. Lovell WW, Winter RB. Pediatric orthopaedics. Philadelphia: JB Lippincott, 1986.
9. Tachdjian MO, ed. Pediatric orthopaedics. Philadelphia: WB Saunders, 1972.
10. Feagin JA Jr, ed. The crucial ligaments. New York: Churchill-Livingstone, 1988.
11. Torg JS, Conrad W, Kalen J. Clinical diagnosis of anterior cruciate ligament instability in the athlete. Am J Sports Med 1976;4:84.
12. Barlow TG. Early diagnosis and treatment of congenital dislocation of the hip. J Bone Joint Surg 1962;44B:292.
13. Bleck EE. Locomotor prognosis in cerebral palsy. Develop Med Child Neurol 1975;17:18.

Chapter 4
___

Radiologic Evaluation of the Orthopaedic Patient

Radiographic imaging is a useful and, in many cases, necessary tool in the diagnosis of orthopaedic injuries. Adequate imaging is needed not only for diagnosis, but also for evaluation of open and closed reduction maneuvers. The physician should select the appropriate views so that a diagnosis is not missed.

Special mention is warranted in the examination of the unresponsive trauma patient. Additional screening films are necessary so that occult injuries are not overlooked. These views should always include a minimum of a lateral cervical spine film, which includes the cervicothoracic junction, and an anteroposterior view of the pelvis. Additionally, A-P and lateral views of the thoracic, lumbar, and sacral spines are often indicated in unresponsive patients.

PLAIN RADIOGRAPHS

Radiographs evaluate the bones in a single plane. In order to adequately evaluate the bony skeleton, the part to be examined should be viewed in a minimum of two planes that are 90 degrees apart. The following paragraphs list the routine views for the evaluation of orthopaedic trauma. These lists are merely introductory guidelines, and additional views including "cone-down" and oblique views can yield additional information about fractures.

C-spine: A-P, lateral, open-mouth odontoid, bilateral obliques. The study is not considered adequate unless the cervicothoracic junction is visualized, including the superior portion of the body of T1. A "swimmer's view" is sometimes helpful in visualizing the cevicothoracic junction.

Trauma C-spine: A-P, lateral, bilateral trauma obliques, odontoid view. These views are obtained with the patient immobilized in the supine position. After interpretation of these films, formal obliques and lateral views are performed with the patient in the upright position (if the patient can cooperate). If there appears to be a fracture of the C-spine, additional imaging can be performed using a computed tomogram (CT) scan (1.5–3.0 mm axial cuts with reconstructions).

If the trauma patient is alert and denies neck pain and has a normal range of motion without tenderness, no neck films are needed. If the patient is alert and complains of neck pain or has an examination that reveals tenderness or decreased range of motion, the neck should be immobilized and a trauma series should be performed. If plain radiographs are normal, the patient's neck still requires immobilization until adequate lateral flexion-extension views of the cervical spine are performed to rule out ligamentous injury. *The patient must flex and extend his own neck without assistance from the physician or technician.* If the patient is not able to flex and extend his or her neck enough, the Philadelphia collar must remain in position until pain or spasm decreases enough to allow the patient to be studied adequately (usually 7–10 days). If flexion-extension views reveal instability, an MRI is indicated for further evaluation. If the trauma patient is not alert but neck films are normal (comatose, intoxicated, on drugs), the Philadelphia collar must remain in position until he or she is considered alert enough to cooperate with a physical examination.

Shoulder: For an elective shoulder series, the standard is a true A-P view, an outlet (Bigliani) view, an axillary lateral view, and occasionally, an A-C joint view. The trauma series includes a true A-P (shot perpendicular to the scapular blade rather than the coronal plane of the body and also termed a *glenoid fossa view*), a Y-lateral view, and an axillary lateral view. To determine the presence or absence of a Hill-Sachs lesion in the evaluation of shoulder instability, two views often ordered are a Stryker notch and a West Point view.

Clavicle: A-P of the clavicle. Fractures of the distal clavicle can be seen on routine views of the shoulder. If additional views are indicated, the tube can be aimed cephalad and caudad 45 degrees to obtain 2 orthogonal views of the clavicle.

Acromioclavicular Joint: AP of the A-C joint (A-P view aimed 15° cephalad), axillary lateral view. The AP view easily demonstrates superior or inferior displacement of the clavicle relative to the acromion. The axillary lateral is required for assessing anterior or posterior displacement. Stress radiographs are used by some to distinguish between type II and type III separations. These views are an A-P view of the shoulders with both shoulders included on the same film. The view is then repeated with 10 pounds of weight secured to the patient's wrists. The patient should not hold the weights, as this tenses the shoulder musculature. When imaging this joint, the roentgen beam needs to be angled such that it aims 15 degrees cephalad.

Humerus: A-P, lateral views.

Elbow: A-P and lateral views of the elbow are usually sufficient; however, an oblique view may give additional information about the radial head. When the elbow cannot be fully extended, the A-P view should center on the elbow joint, not the humeral shaft. Elbow films should also include a sufficient amount of the humerus and forearm, so that assessment of alignment can be made.

Wrist: A-P, lateral, and oblique views of the wrist are adequate in most cases. When a distal radius fracture is suspected, the film must contain a sufficient length of the radius to assess the alignment of the fracture in both the lateral and A-P planes. When carpal pathology is seen on routine views or suspected based on clinical examination, six additional views can be helpful. These views are A-P views in maximal radial and ulnar deviation, lateral views in maximal volar and dorsal flexion, and a clenched-fist P-A and lateral.

Hand and Digits: A-P, lateral and oblique views constitute the initial examination. When there is damage to a separate digit, a lateral of the specific digit is necessary for the measurement of alignment.

Thoracic Spine: A-P and lateral views.

Lumbosacral Spine: The full series includes seven views: A-P, lateral, bilateral 30-degree obliques, a coccyx view, a cone-down view of the lumbosacral junction, and an A-P pelvis. When possible, the films should be obtained in the standing position.

Trauma Lumbosacral Series: This includes the above series, with specific attention to the thoracolumbar junction. When instability is suspected, lateral flexion and extension views should be obtained.

Scoliosis Series: These films include a P-A and lateral of the spine. Left and right lateral bending views shot in a P-A direction are used preoperatively to assess curve flexibility. These views should include all curves on a single film (i.e., thoracolumbosacral). Whenever possible, these films should be obtained with the patient in the weight-bearing position. P-A views, as opposed to A-P views, decrease the amount of radiation to the radiosensitive breast and thyroid tissue in the adolescent.

Pelvis: In pelvic trauma, a complete pelvic series includes an A-P view, Judet views, and inlet/outlet views. Judet views are oblique projections with the pelvis rotated 45 degrees in each direction. The iliac oblique (medial anterior oblique) brings the posterior column and anterior acetabular wall into profile, and the obturator oblique (lateral anterior oblique) allows visualization of the anterior column and the posterior acetabular wall. Inlet/outlet are A-P projections with the tube directed 60 degrees caudad and 45 degrees cephalad. In acetabular fractures, a CT of the pelvis is necessary for an assessment of joint congruity.

Hip: A-P pelvis, A-P hip, and cross table lateral. The lateral view demonstrates the femoral head and the acetabular articulation. A standing true lateral view of the hip demonstrates the relationship of the femur to the pelvis (pelvic flexion). This view is helpful in the preoperative planning of hip arthroplasty. Another view often performed in a standard series is a frog-leg lateral. This is very useful in pediatric conditions, especially evaluation of Legg-Calvé-Perthes disease and slipped capital femoral epiphyses. However, in the adult or in the trauma patient, it yields minimal information, as it provides a lateral of the proximal femur rather than of the pelvis and acetabulum. One exception is that a frog-leg lateral radiograph should be used to evaluate avascular necrosis of the femoral head in the adult.

Knee: Standing A-P and lateral views. Supplemental views include intercondylar notch and patellar sunrise views. Several different methods of imaging the patella tangentially (the sunrise view) have been described. Many of them carry eponyms, but there is minimal difference among the various views.

Ankle: A-P, lateral, and mortise (oblique) views.

Foot: A-P, lateral, and oblique. A number of special views of the foot highlight various aspects of the skeleton. The three views just mentioned should be used to localize the injury, and target specific views. The Harris heel view allows examination of the calcaneus and subtalar joint in suspected calcaneal fractures.

TOMOGRAPHY

Tomography remains a useful tool in the imaging of the articular surfaces, such as the tibial plateau and the elbow. In addition, it can be used to image the cervicothoracic junction in the patient where it cannot be seen on plain film. Computed tomography has displaced much of the routine use of tomography, although its usefulness should not be overlooked. Tomography is often used when hardware causes too much metal artifact on CT scan. An accurate knowledge of the topographical anatomy is necessary for interpretation.

COMPUTED TOMOGRAPHY

Computed tomography offers improved skeletal imaging especially in the spine, pelvis, and in the evaluation of articular anatomy. In the spine, visualization of degenerative disease, as well as imaging of trauma has been improved. CT scan with myelography is invasive but gives accurate information regarding bony and neural anatomy. CT scans are performed on spine trauma to further assess fracture patterns, subluxations and dislocations, listhesis, and spinal cord compromise or root impingement.

Three-dimensional reconstructions are often used in studying pelvic and acetabular fractures. CT accurately assesses the congruity of the acetabulum, and bone fragments in the joint can be accurately identified. Three-dimensional reconstruction also facilitates improved preoperative planning for reduction and fixation of all intraarticular fractures.

MAGNETIC RESONANCE IMAGING

Magnetic resonance imaging (MRI) has revolutionized soft-tissue imaging of the musculoskeletal system. This modality does not use radiation and thus can be safely used on pregnant women and young children. Its current orthopaedic uses are extremely varied and include evaluation of soft-tissue tumors, imaging of the spinal cord and its roots, and assessment of the cartilage and ligaments of the knee, shoulder, and wrist, to name a few. It is also used to rule out nondisplaced femoral neck fractures in the elderly and to assess osteonecrosis of the femoral head, talus, and scaphoid. Magnetic resonance arthrogram is currently being evaluated to see if it can offer improved intraarticular imaging (e.g., labral tears in the shoulder).

ULTRASOUND

Ultrasound is an operator-dependent diagnostic modality that is noninvasive and does not expose the patient to any radiation. It is used primarily in orthopaedics for diagnosing rotator cuff tears in the shoulder and for ruling out deep vein thrombosis in the thigh. It is often used to rule out a hip effusion in an infant or toddler. In Europe and in a few centers in the United States, it is used as a screening tool to evaluate a congenital hip dislocation.

RADIONUCLIDE IMAGING

Radionuclide imaging, in the form of bone scans or skeletal scintigraphy, is used often in orthopaedics. The technique involves injection of a radioactive tracer into the blood, followed by imaging the entire body or parts of the body at set intervals to measure the uptake of the tracer. Several different techniques exist, but the most commonly used tracer is a technetium compound (99Tcm), usually either a pertechnate or phosphate salt. Another commonly used tracer is gallium (67Ga). Gallium is more costly and requires more radiation exposure but can be more sensitive in the diagnosis of osteomyelitis.

Bone scans are quite helpful in the diagnosis of osteomyelitis and stress fractures. Osteomyelitis may not demonstrate any plain film changes for up to 2 weeks, but a bone scan will often show increased uptake in the first 2–3 days. Stress fractures that are undetectable on the plain radiograph can often be diagnosed by bone scan within 1–2 days.

Bone scans are sometimes performed by injection of the tracer, with a static phase whole-body scan being performed approximately 3 hours later. Usually, a three-phase bone scan is performed simply because it tends to yield more data. The three-phase bone scan consists of a localized static blood pool image immediately after injection, a dynamic flow curve performed immediately after injection (the radionuclide angiogram or the "poor man's arteriogram"), and a whole-body static bone scan performed 3 hours after injection. Osteomyelitis will demonstrate increased uptake in both the late and immediate images, while cellulitis will usually show increased uptake only on the immediate images.

Bone scans are also helpful in the diagnosis and staging of bone and soft-tissue tumors. In this instance, the scan can show satellite or metastatic lesions, as well as demonstrate evidence of bone invasion by a soft-tissue lesion.

Indium labeled white blood cell scans are helpful in the diagnosis of infection. Indium scans are performed over a 24–48-hour period. They are often used to confirm a diagnosis of osteomyelitis following a positive bone scan.

INVASIVE IMAGING

MRI is noninvasive and has replaced many of the invasive imaging modalities that were used in the past. Despite MRI, there are still some uses for arthrography, myelography, discography, and angiography, especially when patients have small metallic implants (e.g., aneurysmal clip) that may contraindicate an MRI procedure.

Arthrography

Arthrography involves the injection of a radiopaque iodinated contrast material into a joint followed by plain radiographs of the joint. It is useful in multiple joint complaints, but its use has been largely supplanted by MRI. Arthrography is sometimes used to help diagnose a rotator cuff tear, though an MRI gives more information (muscle appearance, amount of tendon retraction). It is very useful in evaluating children's elbow and hip problems because of the lack of epiphyseal ossification makes plain radiographs less helpful.

Myelography

Myelography involves injection of a radiopaque iodinated contrast material into the epidural space via a lumbar puncture. It is used with CT to evaluate the spinal canal and neural foramina for stenosis and other sources of neural impingement that may explain neurogenic pain. The procedure formerly carried a very high complication rate of postmyelogram headaches and nausea, but newer, water-soluble, nonionic, low osmolality agents have lessened the incidence of these problems.

Discography

Discography consists of injecting a radiopaque iodinated contrast material directly into the nucleus pulposus, usually via a lateral approach using fluoroscopy. The procedure is performed for possible disc pathology, mostly degenerative disc disease. Although the appearance of the disc on radiograph is important, equally important is the amount of dye accepted by the disk, as degenerated disks will accept more. A normal lumbar disk accepts only 1.0 to 1.5 milliliters. Most important is the patient's response to the injection. When the injection exactly re-creates the patient's typical back pain, this is presumptive evidence that the disc being injected is the source of the patient's pain.

Angiography

Angiography, primarily arteriography, has multiple uses in orthopaedics. It is used in trauma to evaluate the integrity of major arteries near the sites of fracture or puncture wounds. It is used in the work-up of bone or soft-tissue tumors to determine the proximity of the major vessels and the resectability of lesions. The advent of CT and MRI has slightly decreased this indication. However, arteriography is now often used in orthopaedic oncology for evaluating the possibility of intraarterial injection of chemotherapeutic agents directly into a lesion. It is also used to assess and perform embolization of large feeding vessels for tumors prior to resection to decrease blood loss. In addition, arteriography can be used to evaluate multiple vascular syndromes of the upper and lower extremities, including Raynaud's phenomenon, ulnar artery thrombosis, true and false aneurysms, and atherosclerotic disease. Arteriograms are also useful in the preoperative planning for elective microsurgical free tissue transfers.

A pulmonary arteriogram remains the gold standard for the evaluation of pulmonary embolism. Likewise, a lower extremity venogram is the gold standard for the diagnosis of deep vein thrombosis.

Selected Readings

1. Ballinger PW. Merrill's atlas of radiographic positions and radiologic procedures. 6th ed. 3 vols. St. Louis: CV Mosby, 1986.
2. Gehweiler JA, Osborne RL, Becker RF. The radiology of vertebral trauma. Philadelphia: WB Saunders, 1980.

3. Putman CE, Ravin CE. Textbook of diagnostic imaging. 3 vols. Philadelphia: WB Saunders, 1988.
4. Resnick D. Bone and joint imaging. Philadelphia: WB Saunders, 1989.
5. Rogers LF. Radiology of skeletal trauma. 2 vols. New York: Churchill-Livingstone, 1982.
6. Sandler MP et al. Correlative imaging: nuclear medicine—magnetic resonance—computed tomography—ultrasound. Baltimore: Williams & Wilkins, 1989.

Chapter 5

Orthopaedic Emergencies

OPEN FRACTURES, JOINTS, AND DISLOCATIONS[1]

An open fracture is one in which a break in the skin communicates with a fracture or fracture hematoma. Similarly, an open dislocation or open joint will have communication between the articular surfaces and the outside environment. The term compound fracture has been synonymous with open fracture; however, use of this term is essentially outdated.

Open fractures constitute a surgical emergency in that the injured surface is exposed to the outside environment and is thus prone to bacterial contamination. These injuries are often high energy in nature and can lead to soft-tissue and periosteal stripping and devascularization. The presence of devascularized tissue also makes this environment more prone to infection and creates difficulty in fracture healing secondary to loss of blood supply and loss of sources of osteoprogenitor cells. Open joints are prone to articular cartilage damage, which can be irreversible, and experience the same contamination as open fractures, which can lead to septic arthritis, as discussed later in this chapter.

The main determinants of outcome in open injuries *are the amount of bacterial contamination and the amount of soft-tissue devitalization.* These wounds must be meticulously handled in the emergency setting to minimize further contamination. Gustilo and Anderson[2] have provided a useful classification for open fractures based on the factors of contamination, bony comminution, and soft-tissue injury:

Grade I—Wound <1 cm; minimal soft-tissue injury; minimal bony comminution

Grade II—Wound 1–10 cm; moderate soft-tissue injury; moderate bony comminution

Grade III—Wound >10 cm; high energy injury with contamination and extensive soft-tissue loss; usually highly comminuted fracture

Grade III-A—Grade III injury without extensive soft-tissue loss or periosteal stripping; Soft-tissue coverage of bone is possible

Grade III-B—Grade III injury with extensive soft-tissue loss and periosteal stripping; poor bone coverage, which usually requires soft-tissue reconstructive surgery

Grade III-C—Grade III injury with vascular injury requiring repair; usually requires additonal soft-tissue reconstructive surgery

Grade III wounds are also characterized by high levels of contamination. Open fractures caused by 1) shotgun wounds, 2) high-velocity gunshot wounds, 3) segmental fractures with displacement or diaphyseal bone loss, 4) high energy crush injuries, and 5) barnyard injuries are always considered Grade III fractures regardless of the size of the wound, because of the energy and contamination involved in these circumstances. The true extent of soft-tissue damage cannot be evaluated in the emergency room setting and must be determined at surgery. A seemingly small and benign wound on initial superficial examination can actually be associated with significant soft-tissue stripping and devitalization once assessed in the operating room setting.

Assessment of the patient with an open injury begins with a thorough history and physical examination if the patient is capable of providing one. The history is important to determine the mechanism of injury, amount of time it has been open, type of potential contaminants (barnyard, fresh water, salt water), medical co-morbidities, allergies, and history of tetanus administration.

In highly contaminated wounds, 250–500 units of tetanus immune globulin should be administered with tetanus toxoid if the patient has had less than three lifetime immunizations, or if their last immunization was greater than 5 years ago[3]. If the patient has had greater than three lifetime tetanus immunizations with the last one less than 5 years ago, then only toxoid needs to be administered. In minor wounds, the toxoid vaccine should be administered if the last dose was greater than 10 years ago.

Emergency room personnel are usually well-schooled in the indications for tetanus administration; however, this topic must be addressed by the treating physician in all open injuries.

On examination the ABCs (Airway, Breathing, Circulation) must first be assessed and stabilized generally under the direction of a general or trauma surgeon. Once the primary evaluation is complete, the orthopaedic evaluation may proceed. An entire musculoskeletal trauma examination must be performed, as patients with open fractures often have other associated injuries. Any laceration or wound over a joint or extremity segment with an associated fracture must be considered an open joint or fracture until proved otherwise. A thorough neurovascular examination is essential for the injured extremity, and the nature of the wound must be accurately assessed and documented within the limits of the emergency room setting.

The true extent of the open injury cannot be completely assessed in the emergency room in most instances. In the case of a laceration over a joint, one can inject saline and methylene blue into the joint to see if extravasation occurs through the wound, but this is not always completely accurate. Lacerations can also be probed to see if they communicate with an underlying fracture, but, once again, this is not always accurate; and, it is safest to treat these injuries as open fractures or open joints. Wounds with gross contamination can be superficially irrigated in the emergency room if not immediately taken to the operating room. All wounds should be dressed with a moist saline or Betadine-soaked gauze. The use of Betadine is controversial, as it may be associated with decreased osteoblast function. Patients should not be sent for additional studies without having their wounds dressed, as this can possibly expose them to hospital-acquired pathogens.

Patients with obvious fractures or dislocations (open or closed) and neurovascular compromise should have a formal attempt at reduction prior to splinting and obtaining radiographs. Injuries with gross displacement should also be gently manipulated and splinted in near-normal alignment with plaster or prefabricated splints prior to obtaining radiographs. A neurovascular examination should be performed after any manipulation to see if changes have occurred. Fractures without gross displacement or neurovascular compromise can be splinted in situ and then undergo radiographic evaluation, as blind reduction in these circumstances can actually worsen the fracture configuration, especially if it has an intraarticular component.

Radiographic evaluation should include chest, A-P pelvis, and lateral cervical spine for any trauma victim. Radiographic examination of the fractured extremity should then be performed. Although splints can obscure the fine details of a fracture, they are necessary to prevent gross fracture motion and displacement and also provide some comfort by immobilizing the fracture.

Antibiotics should be administered upon initial diagnosis of an open skeletal injury. In Grade I and Grade II wounds without gross contamination, a first-generation cephalosporin is sufficient, while for Grade III injuries or any injury with gross contamination, an aminoglycoside should be added. The aminoglycoside dose should be adjusted based on the patient's renal status initially and then based on peak and trough levels for continued treatment. An aminoglycoside should also be administered preoperatively in cases delayed for surgery. For any barnyard type injury, Penicillin G should be administered intravenously every 4 to 6 hours to cover for clostridial infection.

Patients with open fractures and joints should be taken to the operating room as soon as possible for surgical debridement and fracture stabilization. If the surgery is to be delayed, then further irrigation should be performed in the emergency room with a pulsatile lavage irrigation system, if possible. The wound should then be redressed and the extremity again splinted. The practice of obtaining preoperative wound cultures is controversial.

Any case of delayed surgery warrants frequent examinations to assess for changes in neurovascular function, for impending compartment syndrome, or for rapidly aggressive soft-tissue infection. Preoperative planning for debridement and fixation should also be occurring at this time.

Assessment and initial treatment of open skeletal injuries thus requires rapid and thorough evaluation of the overall patient status and injured extremity with meticulous wound inspection and dressing and proper splinting of the extremity. Even with optimal initial treatment, these injuries can be extremely difficult to definitively treat and can be associated with significant complications.

COMPLETE OR PARTIAL AMPUTATION

Complete or partial amputation of an extremity or digit is a common injury, especially in industrialized areas. Prior to the use of modern microsurgical techniques, most of these injuries were treated with revision amputation; however, many amputated parts can now be replanted with good functional results utilizing these microsurgical techniques. An essential component of this process is proper transportation of the amputated part, as an improperly handled part can drastically alter its viability.

A completely amputated digit or portion of an extremity can be packaged for transport by using one of the following methods: 1) wrapping the part in a gauze sponge soaked in normal saline or lactated Ringer's and placing the bundle on ice, or 2) immersing the part in saline or Ringer's solution in a plastic bag and placing the bag on ice[4]. These instructions must be clearly communicated to the referring physician or emergency medical technician to ensure proper preservation during the transportation process.

The immersion method is preferable in that the part is less likely to become frozen and less likely to be strangled in the wrapping. This method is also easier to explain, and digital maceration has not been a problem with immersion.

If properly handled, a digit can survive up to 24–30 hours of cool ischemia time, and a more proximal specimen can survive up to 12 hours of cool ischemia. If not cooled, the parts undergo warm ischemia time and a proximal amputation may potentially survive only 6 hours and a digit 12 hours[4]. Proper cooling is thus essential for transportation, as the procedures themselves may take several hours before revascularization is achieved. The digits survive longer than more proximal amputations because they do not have muscle.

Those considered the best candidates for replantation include patients with amputated thumbs, multiple digits, partial hand (through palm), wrist, elbow or above elbow, individual digit distal to flexor digitorum superficialis insertion and any part in a child. Those considered poor candidates include amputations with crushed or mangled parts with multiple amputation levels, arteriosclerotic vessels, mentally unstable patients, and those with cool or warm ischemia times longer than those mentioned in the above paragraphs[4]. If there is any doubt as to whether a patient is a candidate for replantation, then it is probably best to transfer the patient to an institution proficient in replantation, so a surgeon experienced in performing these procedures can examine the patient and make an educated decision whether to proceed with replantation or revision amputation.

In partial amputations, revascularization, rather than replantation, is the term applied to extremity or digital reconstruction. By definition, vascular repair is necessary to prevent necrosis of the partially amputated part. In these cases even small bridges of tissue should be left intact as they may contain structures or venous channels that may aid in the reconstruction process. Generally, revascularization procedures are less demanding than replantations, with a better chance of eventual viability.

In cases of partial amputation, the soft tissues must again be handled with great care. A neurovascular examination should be performed to assess for any viable function. The exposed soft tissues should then be covered with a moist gauze dressing soaked in saline or dilute Betadine solution. This will help prevent dessication of tissues, and the Betadine may potentially provide an antibacterial effect. The dressing should be loose to prevent strangulation of the part, and the part should be cooled with an ice bag to prevent warm ischemia. If the injury is proximal to the digital level and a long bone fracture involved with malalignment, then the extremity should be carefully splinted until surgery is performed.

In any proximal revascularization or replantation, myonecrosis and infection are potentially fatal complications and an arterial shunt will frequently be necessary to minimize ischemic time and lessen the likelihood of these complications. Fasciotomy of the distal compartments should be considered if arterial repair or grafting is performed.

In complete or partial amputations associated with major hemorrhage, survival of the patient takes far greater precedence than that of the limb, and measures must be taken to stop the hemorrhage regardless of its effect on the potential for limb reconstruction. Direct pressure should be attempted to control bleeding, and if unsuccessful, then the patient should go urgently to the operating room. If this is not possible, then attempts should be made to isolate and clamp or ligate the vessel. This is not ideally performed in the emergency room as exposure is poor and there is a high likelihood of clamping other vital structures (nerves) or causing irreparable intimal damage to the vessel. The bottom line remains that survival of the patient takes far greater precedence than survival of the limb.

With respect to severe lower extremity injuries, the decision between reconstruction and amputation can be extremely difficult, as reconstruction can involve multiple procedures over an extended period of time, often with poor results, while amputation can provide rapid return of functional status with the use of modern prostheses and rehabilitation regimens. Injuries in question are Grade III-B and III-C open fractures that require vascular or significant soft-tissue reconstruction. Patient factors such as age, co-morbidities, and preoperative status of the leg are all important considerations.

Multiple systems have been devised to grade the extent of injury in a mangled extremity and predict candidates for reconstruction versus amputation; however, none has been extremely accurate or reproducible[5]. The question of amputation or limb salvage in a mangled lower extremity is perhaps one of the most difficult ones an orthopaedic surgeon must face. Even those with significant experience at Level One trauma centers have difficulty with this decision and cannot provide clear-cut guidelines to solve this dilemma.

Factors that have been shown to provide poor functional and limb survival results with salvage include severe soft-tissue injury that cannot promptly be covered; vascular injury at or below the trifurcation of vessels; vascular injury with extensive soft-tissue crush injury (muscle will die even if revascularized); warm ischemia greater than 6 hours; and posterior tibial nerve disruption (loss of plantar sensation). Patients with co-morbidities such as diabetes, tobacco abuse, peripheral vascular disease, COPD, and severe cardiac disease are also poor candidates, in that limb salvage in extreme circumstances can be a threat to their lives[1,5]. These patients should be advised of their greater potential for failure.

Ultimately, this emotionally charged decision for lower extremity reconstruction versus amputation must be made by the physician, patient, and patient's family after consideration of the options and their likelihood for successful outcome. In a training program, this data should be conveyed by the attending physician, as that individual will be the one directly responsible for the outcome of whatever pathway is chosen by the patient or the patient's family.

COMPARTMENT SYNDROME[6]

A compartment syndrome refers to a clinical condition in an extremity in which the circulation and function of tissues in a closed space are compromised by increased pressure within that space[1]. A compartment consists of muscle and neurovascular structures surrounded by dense fibrous tissue (fascia). Elevation of pressure within this closed, inflexible space compromises blood flow and nerve function, and if the pressure is not relieved, then permanent, irreversible damage may occur. Sequelae of untreated compartment syndromes are functionally devastating and a major source of malpractice liability. All acute care personnel must be familiar with this syndrome and diligent in recognizing it to prevent disastrous consequences.

The basic etiologies are decreased compartment size owing to tight dressings or closure of fascial defects and increased compartment content secondary to bleeding, muscle hypertrophy, increased capillary permeability (trauma), and increased capillary pressure. Specific etiologies include complications of open and closed fractures (especially tibial shaft, pediatric supracondylar humerus), arterial injury, reperfusion injury after revascularization, snake bites, burns, acute and chronic exertional states, gunshot wounds and intraosseus fluid administration in infants. Muscle injury is the most common cause leading to edema and thus increased compartment content. Tight dressings and splints are a possible, though rare, iatrogenic cause.

Once the compartment pressure becomes elevated beyond a threshold level, ischemia to the muscle and nerve occurs. This critical pressure may be as low as 20 mm Hg below diastolic pressure, which is a level documented to produce ischemia in injured muscle[7]. In the setting of total ischemia, skeletal muscle can survive for 4 hours without irreversible changes, but at 8 hours suffers complete irreversible changes[6]. The changes at 6 hours are variable. Peripheral nerves can survive 4 hours of ischemic time with just neurapraxic changes, but after 8 hours axonotmesis and irreversible changes can occur. Neural tissue has greater capacity to survive ischemic damage than muscle and can potentially survive up to 12 hours without complete irreversible damage. Early diagnosis and treatment are essential to avoid permanent, irreversible damage.

Diagnosis is made by history and physical examination in the conscious patient and can be confirmed with intracompartmental pressure measurements. In the unconscious patient and in those who have a postoperative nerve block, the clinical examination will not be accurate and pressure measurements may be the only means of diagnosis. The five "P's" of pain, paresthesia, pallor, paralysis, and pulselessness are classically considered the hallmark of compartment syndrome; however, if all five of these signs are already present, especially pulselessness, then the process has probably reached the point where changes are irreversible.

Pain, often severe and unremitting in nature, is the most sensitive and earliest indication of an impending or ongoing compartment syndrome. This pain is more severe than that expected for the underlying injury and generally will not respond to the usual analgesics. *Pain with passive stretching of the muscles in the compartment in question is the key finding in diagnosing a compartment syndrome.* Generally, this will also be one of the earliest signs, and intervention at this point may prevent serious sequelae. In addition, the involved compartment should be palpated and will be firm and swollen in a compartment syndrome.

Paresthesias also begin to occur relatively early in the course of this syndrome. Initially, the changes are sensory in the distribution of the cutaneous nerves running through that compartment. These are still generally reversible. Once motor changes or paralysis occur, then the syndrome is usually well established and irreversible changes may have already occurred. Intervention at this point may not provide full functional recovery but can prevent further functional loss.

Pallor is a nonspecific sign and should not be used to diagnose compartment syndrome. The extremity will often appear cyanotic early in the course of injury, and pallor may not occur until after major arterial occlusion has occurred. *Pulselessness must not be used as a means of diagnosing compartment syndrome.* It is generally the last sign to occur, and ischemia could have already caused irreversible changes. Irreversible tissue changes can even happen in the setting of palpable pulses. Perhaps the only situation in which pulselessness will be an early sign prior to irreversible changes is when arterial injury has occurred with associated bleeding into the compartment. Exploration with attempted vascular reconstruction and fasciotomy are indicated in these circumstances.

In equivocal cases and in patients who cannot provide an accurate physical examination, intracompartmental tissue monitoring is indicated. Techniques include the Whitesides infusion method, Slit catheter, Wick catheter, and Stryker STIC device. The latter device is most commonly used at this time. Regardless of technique, the device must be zeroed prior to each reading. Each compartment in the affected extremity should be measured. In addition, pressures immediately adjacent to a fracture will be higher that those throughout the remainder of the compartment, and several sites should be measured if the diagnosis remains in question[8]. Several measurements may also be necessary in cases where initial pressures are low or equivocal and the symptoms acutely worsen or continue on their course.

Treatment of any acute compartment syndrome involves fasciotomy of the affected compartment(s). The sites most commonly involved in compartment syndrome include the lower leg, forearm, foot, and hand. The thigh and upper arm generally have larger compartments with more flexibility for swelling and rarely have compartment syndromes. The leg has four compartments (anterior, lateral, deep and superficial posterior) and forearm three (dorsal, volar, mobile wad) (Fig. 5.1). The foot has medial, central, lateral, and interossei compartments of relevance, as well as other small compartments with less clinical relevance (Fig. 5.2). Foot compartment syndromes are commonly associated with crush injuries, Lisfranc fracture-dislocations, and calcaneal fractures[9]. The hand has thenar, hypothenar, dorsal, and volar interossei, and an adductor pollicis compartment. Hand compartment syndromes most commonly occur secondary to burns, infection, trauma, and arterial injury[10].

The cutoff pressure for considering fasciotomy is controversial and a standard pressure (classically 30–40 mm Hg) should not be utilized, as in hypotensive patients the critical pressure may indeed be lower, and in hypertensive patients this pressure may not affect flow at all. Whitesides et al[6] will perform fasciotomy if intracompartmental pressures rise to a level of 20 mm Hg below the patient's diastolic pressure. This level has been associated with ischemia to injured muscle in experimental models.

Common techniques for all fasciotomies include skin incisions long enough to allow adequate exposure for fascial incision over the entire extent of the compartment. Cutaneous nerves should be avoided when making the fascial incisions. Skin and fascia must not be closed at the time of fasciotomy, because if closed, they may provide enough constriction to reinstitute a compartment syndrome. Skin closure can eventually be per-

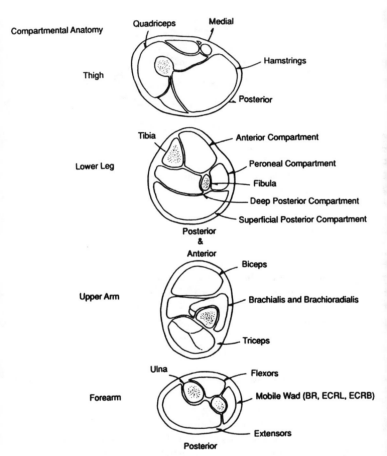

Figure 5.1. Anatomy of the compartments of the thigh, lower leg, upper arm, and forearm.

Compartments of the foot

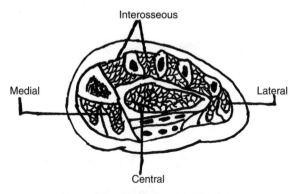

Figure 5.2. Compartments of the foot.

formed in delayed primary fashion (48–72 hours) if the soft tissues will allow for it, or the defect can be treated with split thickness skin grafting. Specific fasciotomy techniques for each compartment can be found in standard orthopaedic texts.

Some patients will have continued signs of compartment syndrome postfasciotomy. In these cases, one must question the completeness of the initial fasciotomy and consider exploration and fasciotomy extension. *Patients with signs or symptoms of compartment syndrome secondary to tight casts or dressings should have these materials split all the way to the skin level to allow for swelling and expansion in the given compartment.* In most cases this will be sufficient to relieve symptoms, but if this does not help and if pressures are elevated, then fasciotomy is indicated.

Sequelae of a missed compartment syndrome are disastrous and include myonecrosis with possible myoglobinuria and renal failure, infection, ischemic contractures, chronic pain, limb paralysis and dry gangrene in severe unrecognized cases. This problem should not be missed, and these complications should never occur. Fasciotomy, once the syndrome is established and paralysis has occurred, is not indicated, as infection can easily occur in a bed of dead exposed muscle.

AGGRESSIVE SOFT-TISSUE INFECTION[3]

Necrotizing fasciitis and clostridial myonecrosis (gas gangrene) represent two clinical scenarios in which soft-tissue infection, which initially may appear benign, can rapidly and aggressively spread throughout an extremity (and beyond) and potentially be fatal[3]. These situations must be promptly treated once recognized to prevent loss of limb and life.

Necrotizing fasciitis (NF), first described in the United States by a Confederate soldier in the Civil War, is a relatively uncommon infection but one that has gained considerable recognition recently because of media reports of epidemics of "flesh-eating *strep*." In the extremity it is usually acquired through open wounds, abrasions (often unrecognized), and injection sites in intravenous drug abusers. It can also rarely occur in the postoperative setting (usually postabdominal surgery). Patients at increased risk for developing NF are diabetics, intravenous drug abusers, alcoholics, those with peripheral vascular disease, and the malnourished.

The bacteria most frequently responsible for these infections are Group A streptococcus. Another bacterial subtype involves mixed anaerobic and facultative bacteria including enterobacteriaceae and non-Group A streptococci. *Vibrio* species are also a potential cause from a marine environment.

Clinically, the patient will initially present with high fever, local edema and erythema, and pain out of proportion to the local findings. The affected area will initially be red, shiny, edematous, without sharp margins, and exquisitely tender. This subsequently progresses to cutaneous bullae and necrosis over 2–5 days, at which point the skin is anesthetic owing to necrosis of superficial nerves. The defining characteristic of NF is fascial necrosis with widespread undermining of the skin, usually beyond the region that appears involved superficially. At this point, muscle or bone can become involved and the patient may become tachypneic, tachycardic, and hypotensive. In cases caused by mixed organisms, subcutaneous crepitation may exist. Unfortunately, most patients present with the disease at a relatively advanced stage. If seen at an early stage, the extremity can be imaged with CT or MRI to rule out abcesses or edematous changes along fascial planes. If present, then treatment must be initiated without delay.

Treatment involves aggressive debridement and fluid and electrolyte resuscitation. All necrotic skin and fascia must be debrided and exploration repeated at frequent intervals (24–48 hours or sooner, if symptoms dictate). Antibiotics should be started immediately, beginning with triple therapy or ampicillin/ sulbactam and then tailoring therapy to the culture/sensitivity results. Even with aggressive debridement, 25% of patients in one series with upper extremity NF went on to amputation. In that series, an average of three debridements was necessary to control the infection[11]. Mortality rates in the United States were 28% for NF from 1989–1991. Mortality is increased for late diagnosis. Hyperbaric oxygen may decrease mortality when used in conjunction with surgical debridement, but it is not an alternative to aggressive surgical debridement as a sole means of treatment.

Clostridial myonecrosis (gas gangrene) differs from NF in that the infection crosses fascial planes and is characterized by gas production and necrosis in muscle. In addition, it is more rapidly progressive than NF and can be fatal even within 12 hours of infection[3]. It is caused by clostridial species, most commonly *Clostridium perfringens* in an orthopaedic setting. These organisms produce exotoxins that are highly virulent and cause the myonecrosis, which can lead to necrotizing gangrene within hours. These organisms require a low oxygen tension environment to multiply, which is why they thrive in contaminated traumatic wounds.

Clinically, these patients present with severe pain and systemic toxicity in most instances. The pain can be sudden in onset, similar to acute vascular occlusion, and the wound appearance can rapidly change. Subcutaneous crepitation is a hallmark of this disease. Patients often develop mental status changes early and paradoxically have improvements in mental status prior to succumbing to the infection. The skin may initially appear bronze-brown and then mottled, edematous and covered with multiple bullae with profuse drainage.

Treatment must be initiated immediately to save the patient's life. Aggressive debridement, which in many cases involves amputation, must be done to stop the rapid spread of exotoxins and infection. Gas is usually encountered upon entering a muscular compartment, and the muscle will usually be dead. Penicillin must be started immediately and clindamycin or Flagyl utilized in penicillin-allergic patients.

Hyperbaric oxygen is a useful adjunct in gas gangrene, as it kills clostridia and arrests toxin production. It can be used preoperatively to better define the necrotic area and stabilize the patient, but only if it is readily available. Delays to transfer a patient to a facility with hyperbaric oxygen prior to surgery are not advised given the rapid progression to mortality if not treated rapidly. Hyperbaric oxygen is also a useful postoperative adjunct. Mortality with rapid debridement in extremity myonecrosis is less than 20%.

An important fact to remember with any open laceration or soft-tissue infection caused by an open wound is tetanus prophylaxis. This is reviewed in the section on open fractures in this chapter.

SEPTIC ARTHRITIS[12,13]

Infection of a joint space, also referred to as septic arthritis, represents an orthopaedic emergency in that delay in diagnosis or treatment can lead to an adverse outcome with significant disability to the affected joint. Those at increased risk for septic arthritis include the elderly and immunocompromised (HIV, RA, SLE), patients with preexisting joint disease, intravenous drug abusers, and patients with a history of direct open or closed trauma to the affected joint. Most cases of septic arthritis come from hematogenous seeding from a distant site. Other mechanisms involve direct inoculation from trauma, surgery or arthrocentesis, and spread of contiguous soft-tissue infection into the synovial cavity. The knee is the most common joint infected in adults, followed by the hip, shoulder, elbow, and ankle. Intravenous drug abusers will develop infections at unusual sites generally not amenable to surgical drainage, such as the sternoclavicular, manubriosternal and sacroiliac joints. Children can get direct spread of metaphyseal osteomyelitis into the joint especially in the hip, ankle, shoulder and elbow, where the metaphysis is intracapsular[14].

Once bacteria enter the synovial cavity, they release toxins that contribute to cartilage degradation. In addition, PMNs (polymorphonuclear leukocytes) proliferate and release proteolytic enzymes and inflammatory by-products such as interleukin-1 and tumor necrosis factor-alpha that degrade cartilage. These events occur within the first 24–48 hours postinfection. Intraarticular effusion ensues with a direct pressure effect on the cartilage. Microscopic degradation occurs, and cartilage softening and fissuring can be seen by day seven postinfection. The pressure leads to capsular distension, which can also diminish joint blood supply, especially in the hip, and which predisposes the joint to further insult. The goal of treatment is elimination of toxins and organisms with joint sterilization. Best results occur if intervention happens early in the time course of the infection.

The organisms responsible for joint infection vary based on patient characteristics. Infants and neonates generally develop *Staphylococcus aureus* and methicillin-resistant *Staphylococcus aureus* (MRSA) infections, while children 6 months to 2 years old most commonly develop *Hemophilus influenzae* and *Staphylococcus aureus*. Older children predominantly develop *Staphylococcus aureus*. In adults, *Neisseria gonorrheae* and *Staphylococcus aureus* are most common. Gonococcal arthritis is most common in sexually active young adults and can be polyarticular in presentation but is classically considered monoarticular. These patients generally have other signs of gonococcal infection such as rash or genitourinary discharge[15]. MRSA joint infections are increasing, especially in hospitalized patients. *Staphylococcus epidermidis* is common in periprosthetic joint infections. Gram-negative infections may provide a clue to an immunocompromised state or intravenous drug abuse. Antibiotic therapy will be based on the infectious organism and its sensitivity.

Patients generally present with fever, chills, malaise, and significant joint pain and tenderness. The pain is usually monoarticular in nongonococcal infection. Swelling and erythema will often be noticeable on the more superficial joints, but the most consistent sign on examination is *limitation of active and passive range of motion with severe pain on attempted motion*. The examination generally provides enough information to suspect septic arthritis but elderly debilitated individuals and neonates often do not provide such a classic presentation.

Children often present a diagnostic dilemma, as their presenting symptom may only be a limp or refusal to ambulate. Septic arthritis must be suspected until proved otherwise, as a missed infection, especially in the hip, can be disastrous. Approximately 50% of cases of septic arthritis in children are preceded by an upper respiratory infection[14].

The key to definitively diagnosing an infected joint is arthrocentesis (joint aspiration). Synovial fluid should be sent for stat Gram stain, culture and sensitivity, and cell count with differential. Crystals should be analyzed in suspected cases of crystalline arthritis. Gram stains reveal positive results in 50%–75% of patients with nongonococcal arthritis and in 25% of patients with gonococcal arthritis, while synovial fluid cultures are >85% positive in nongonococcal and 25% positive in gonococcal arthritis. Blood cultures should also be ordered, as well as serum CBC with differential and ESR or CRP. A broad-spectrum antibiotic can be administered once cultures are obtained. Earlier administration of antibiotics could potentially alter the culture yield. If gonorrhea is suspected, then synovial fluid should be sent for culture on a chocolate agar medium. Urethral cultures and cultures of any skin lesions should also be sent in these instances[15].

Arthrocentesis is an extremely important procedure for an orthopaedist to master. It is a necessity in the diagnosis of a septic joint, but it is also useful for hematoma aspiration and corticosteroid injection. *Central to any arthrocentesis procedure is maintaining diligent sterile technique.* The site should be sterilely prepped and draped and sterile gloves and needles used for aspiration. Unsterile technique increases the risk of contaminating the joint with bacteria, which is a dreaded and avoidable complication. Subcutaneous infiltration of a local anesthetic may help diminish the pain associated with the needle stick, as an 18-gauge or larger bore needle must be used to aspirate large joints since the fluid can be loculated and highly viscous. Neurovascular structures are to be avoided, and the procedure should be performed in a controlled manner to avoid damage to the underlying articular surfaces.

Arthrocentesis requires a thorough understanding of bony landmarks surrounding joints[16]. Techniques for aspiration and injection of various joints and spaces are discussed as follows:

Shoulder: The glenohumeral joint can be aspirated from either an anterior or posterior approach. Anterior approaches risk injury to the brachial plexus or cephalic vein if the needle is placed too far inferior or medial. The posterior approach can injure the axillary nerve and posterior humeral circumflex artery if the entry point is too inferior, but this is a rare complication.

From an anterior approach, an 18-gauge spinal needle is inserted at a point approximately 1 cm lateral to the coracoid process and the joint space located by translating the humeral head anteriorly and posteriorly while palpating for the space. The needle is directed toward the joint space and should enter the joint with minimal resistance. If any resistance is met, the needle should be redirected.

The posterior approach is familiar to those who perform shoulder arthroscopy. The posterolateral tip of the acromion is palpated and an entry point marked 1–2 cm inferior and 1–2 cm medial to this landmark. The joint line is found as above and the tip of the coracoid process palpated with the examiner's opposite hand. The needle is then directed into the joint by aiming toward the coracoid. Once again, minimal resistance is met with entering the joint.

Subacromial bursa: The posterolateral tip of the acromion is again palpated and an entry point made 1 cm inferior to this. The needle should aim for the undersurface of the acromion. The injection should flow easily into the subacromial space.

An alternative method is to palpate the lateral border of the acromion and start the injection site approximately 2 cm below this point, again aiming for the undersurface of the acromion. Injection should not be met with resistance. If the needle is aimed too superiorly, the subcutaneous space may be injected and a visible wheal will demonstrate this error.

Acromioclavicular joint: This is a difficult joint to accurately enter for injection. The joint can usually be palpated just anterior to the triangular junction between the clavicle, acromion, and scapular spine. A 20- to 22-gauge needle can be used to enter the joint from a superior inclination. The needle can be "walked along" the distal clavicle until the joint is entered. Rarely will synovial fluid be encountered. AC injection is usually utilized to help differentiate the source of shoulder pain.

Elbow (Fig. 5.3): The joint should be flexed 90 degrees and the lateral humeral epicondyle, radial head, and olecranon should be palpated on the radial side of the joint. The radial head can be identified by feeling it rotate during forearm pronation and supination. The needle should enter perpendicular to the skin in the center of the triangle, aiming between the radial head and the lateral humeral epicondyle.

Wrist (Fig. 5.4): One must understand the anatomy of the extensor compartments of the forearm at the wrist level when aspirating or injecting this joint, as the procedure is done on the

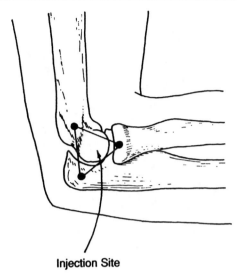

Injection Site

Figure 5.3. The site for aspiration of the elbow joint. The triangle's land-marks correspond to the lateral epicondyle, the radial head, and the ole-cranon.

dorsal surface. The easiest site of entry is between the third and fourth compartments corresponding to the EPL and EDC/EIP, respectively. The needle can be placed perpendicular to the skin and just ulnar and distal to Lister's tubercle. The wrist should be placed in flexion and distracted to open the dorsal side of the joint.

Alternative sites are between compartments four and five (EDQ), but there is no bony landmark to palpate, so it can be difficult to differentiate between the compartments based on superficial palpation alone. Thus, this site is not recommended for inexperienced examiners. Another potential site is radial or ulnar to the ECU tendon just distal to the ulnar styloid, corresponding to the 6-U interval of wrist arthroscopy.

Fingers: It is rare to inject the MCP and IP joints of the fingers. The joint can be palpated dorsally with the finger in slight flexion and then a 24–26-gauge needle can enter dorsomedially or dorsolaterally immediately below the extensor mechanism. Manual traction can be applied longitudinally on

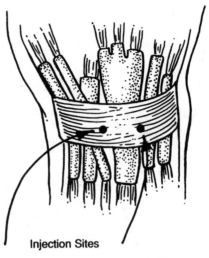

Injection Sites

Figure 5.4. The 3–4 (left) and 4–5 (right) portals for aspiration of the wrist joint.

the finger to open the joint space. One must be certain not to stray in a volar direction, as this can injure the neurovascular structures. The toe joints can be injected in similar fashion.

Hip (Fig. 5.5): The hip is a difficult joint to aspirate or inject and should be done in the presence of someone experienced in this technique, as the needle is in close proximity to major neurovascular structures. It is often recommended to perform this under fluoroscopic guidance with injection of radiopaque contrast to make sure the needle is in the joint. An anterior (more common) or lateral approach can be used.

In the anterior approach with the patient in the supine position, the anterior superior iliac spine (ASIS) and pubic tubercle are palpated to mark the course of the inguinal ligament. The femoral artery is then palpated along this line and a point is marked 2–3 cm lateral to the pulse. This point is also usually 2–3 cm inferior to the ASIS. The needle is then placed perpendicular to the skin and directed posterior or posteromedial until bone is encountered. If any difficulty is encountered, fluoroscopy should be used.

In the lateral approach, the tip of the greater trochanter is palpated with the patient in the supine position. The needle enters perpendicular to the skin just anterior and superior to the trochanteric tip and is directed parallel to the examination table in a medial direction slightly cephalad. One will often slide along the femoral neck until the joint is entered.

Knee: Multiple approaches can be made for knee aspiration. With the knee in full extension and the patient in the supine position, the joint can be entered either medial or lateral to the patella, with medial usually being easier. The patella can then be palpated and the needle placed medial to it and in a slightly posterior direction. It often has to be redirected to enter pockets of fluid.

With the knee slightly flexed (20–45 degrees), the inferomedial and inferolateral borders of the patella are marked and there are often soft spots present at these points. The needle is then directed toward the intercondylar notch after entering at either site, and fluid is aspirated. This approach often yields more fluid than the other. It can also be done in a supine position with a pillow placed under the knee to allow for flexion.

Ankle: The ankle can be entered from a medial or lateral approach just anterior to the medial or lateral malleolus, respec-

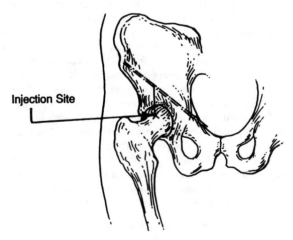

Injection Site

Figure 5.5. Injection site for aspirating the hip joint.

tively. The foot can be plantar or dorsiflexed to identify the joint line and then placed in neutral position for needle entry. The needles should be passed in a posterior direction and aimed slightly toward the center of the ankle.

An essential component of any joint aspiration is **sterile technique**. If any difficulty is encountered upon attempting to enter a joint, fluoroscopy can be a helpful tool.

Treatment of a septic joint involves antibiotics and drainage. Antibiotics should be broad-spectrum until an organism is cultured. Generally in community-acquired infections in adults, penicillinase-resistant antistaphylococcal antibiotics should be administered, while in nosocomial cases, which frequently involve MRSA, vancomycin should be administered. In intravenous drug abusers, Gram-negative infections are common and a second- or third-generation cephalosporin and aminoglycoside should be administered. If gonococcus is suspected, ceftriaxone or penicillin G should be administered. Once sensitivities are available, antibiotic choice should be tailored to them. Length of recommended intravenous treatment is generally 4 to 6 weeks in adults (shorter in gonococcus) and shorter in children, followed by oral medications in both groups.

Controversy exists as to the best method of drainage of infected joints. Repeat aspiration, arthroscopy and arthrotomy are the methods commonly used. Aspiration until the effusion is gone and cultures are sterile is a possible treatment in low virulence infections in superficial joints amenable to repeated aspirations. It is especially useful in gonococcal knee infections, as these are not usually aggressive and the knee can be easily aspirated. Surgical drainage is indicated for *Staphylococcus aureus,* Gram-negative infections, hip infections, anatomically altered joints, no response to antibiotics, and suspected loculation of synovial fluid[17]. Arthroscopy has demonstrated good results in the treatment of these infections but is not adequate enough to eradicate prosthetic joint infections[18,19]. Arthroscopy also avoids the morbidity associated with open procedures, but further study needs to be performed to determine which method is most effective.

Rapid recognition and treatment of these infections can help avoid the dreaded complications of erosive arthritis and loss of motion associated with untreated septic arthritis.

KNEE DISLOCATIONS[20,21]

Knee dislocations are not common injuries, but when encountered require diligent attention and evaluation, as vascular compromise is frequent with high risk of eventual amputation. Dislocations can be high or low energy injuries, with the high energy varieties frequently associated with multiple injuries and the low energy ones frequently isolated sequelae of sports trauma.

The direction of a dislocation can be anterior, posterior, medial, lateral, or rotary. The most common directions are anterior and posterior, and the most common rotary direction is posterolateral. When a dislocation is encountered, closed reduction should be performed after assessment of vascular status. Posterolateral dislocations are associated with the medial femoral condyle buttonholing through the capsule, making them irreducible by closed means. These can be recognized by a transverse skin infolding over the anteromedial knee. A dislocated knee can often reduce spontaneously prior to evaluation and thus thorough knee evaluation is necessary for any patient with multiple trauma or with potential mechanism for knee injury. A knee is considered dislocated if three or more ligaments (ACL, MCL, PCL, LCL) have laxity of 6 mm or greater in comparison with the ligaments of the opposite knee.

A thorough neurovascular examination is essential for any patient with a suspected knee dislocation. Major popliteal artery injury occurs in 30%–40% of knee dislocations and peroneal nerve injury occurs in up to 25% of injuries (especially lateral dislocations). Anterior dislocations are associated with traction injuries to the popliteal artery causing intimal tears, and posterior dislocations are associated with contusion to the vessel with potential disruption. Even if pulses are palpable, arterial injury can still be present. Measurement of Doppler pressures (ankle-brachial index) on both extremities is required to determine if any vascular insufficiency is present on the dislocated side. Vascular injury is a surgical emergency, as collateral flow cannot support the lower extremity.

If pulses are absent or diminished on the dislocated side, urgent vascular surgery consultation is required. An intraoperative arteriogram, although of lower quality, is preferred over one in the radiology suite, and, if it is abnormal or equivocal, surgical exploration is urgently undertaken. Any delay in surgical revascularization threatens extremity survival, as ischemia of 8 hours of duration or longer is associated with subsequent amputation rates of greater than 85%[22]. A pulseless extremity should be explored without an arteriogram to avoid any further delays. Amputation is a preventable complication in most circumstances if vascular insufficiency is promptly recognized. Even if patients have normal pulses on presentation, some surgeons recommend an arteriogram on a nonemergent basis, as occult damage with delayed arterial insufficiency may occur.

Other immediate surgical indications are open dislocations and compartment syndromes. Neurologic injury, although common, is not considered an emergent surgical indication, as it is not limb threatening. Timing of ligamentous reconstruction remains controversial and beyond the scope of this text.

Knee dislocations thus represent an orthopaedic emergency, as the associated vascular complications can be limb threatening.

UNSTABLE PELVIC FRACTURES[23,24]

Hemodynamic instability in a trauma patient that cannot be corrected with volume resuscitation is indicative of internal injuries, with pelvic fractures representing a potential site of massive bleeding causing hemodynamic changes. The multitrauma patient must undergo assessment for pelvic fractures in the initial evaluation period after assessing the ABCs (Airway, Breathing, Circulation), as an unstable pelvic fracture can lead to life-threatening blood loss.

On physical examination, pressure can be applied to the anterior iliac crests to see if motion occurs in the iliac wings, suggesting pelvic disruption. If the extremities are not fractured, then any shortening or abnormal rotation indicates pelvic displacement. Longitudinal traction should also be applied to the lower extremities (if uninjured) with subsequent iliac motion indicating vertical displacement. Bony palpation should be performed to search for crepitance or abnormal motion indicative of fracture or dislocation. The skin should also be checked for open wounds or severe contusions. Open pelvic injury can be disastrous with mortality rates up to 50%.

If open injury is suspected, the assessment should include general surgery-directed sigmoidoscopy to rule out rectal/colonic laceration and visual vaginal and digital examination in a female to rule out laceration. In the presence of a bowel laceration, diverting colostomy should be performed (preferably in the left upper quadrant to avoid potential pelvic incisions) to prevent soiling of the open pelvic wound. Urologic evaluation is also necessary to rule out urethral or bladder injury. A thorough extremity neurovascular examination is essential, as lumbosacral plexus injuries are common, especially with unstable fractures.

Radiographic assessment is also essential to define the injury. An A-P pelvis radiograph is part of the standard trauma series (chest, pelvis, lateral cervical spine) and will demonstrate most pelvic trauma. Other useful plain radiographs include the inlet view, to assess for pelvic ring disruption, and the outlet view to assess for sacral fractures and vertical shear injuries. Radiographic signs of instability include pubic symphysis disruption >2.5 cm, opening of the SI joints (open book injury), 1 cm or more of vertical or posterior displacement of the iliac wings in relation to the sacrum, and avulsion fractures of the sacrum, ischial spine or the L-5 transverse process[24]. CT scan with or without 3-D reconstruction is an important addition for planning definitive reconstruction once the patient is provisionally stabilized.

Provisional stabilization is indicated for unstable fracture patterns with associated hemodynamic instability. Pelvic stabilization closes the potential space for bleeding, allowing for a tamponade effect on injured vessels. Open book injuries with symphyseal and SI joint disruption can be effectively stabilized with an anterior pelvic frame. A frame is placed by applying two to three Schanz screws into each iliac crest (starting 2 cm posterior to the ASIS), and then manually closing the widened pelvis and applying an anterior external fixator to the screws. Pelvic clamps perform the same function. Application of a frame must be coordinated with the trauma surgeons to allow them access to perform laparotomy, if indicated. In certain instances (spinal injury, laparotomy prior to frame placement), anterior plating of the pubis can provide provisional fixation in an open book injury without posterior displacement. Posterior ligamentous injuries without pelvic widening are generally not life threatening and are safer to stabilize after the initial resuscitation procedure.

In fractures involving vertical or posterior SI displacement (vertical shear injuries), external fixators will not provide adequate stabilization. A traction pin should be placed in the distal femur or proximal tibia to help reduce the vertical displacement with longitudinal traction through the pin, and then once reduced, a frame can temporarily stabilize the injury or open reduction and internal fixation can be performed for definitive stabilization. Vertical injuries are highly unstable and even if a patient is initially hemodynamically stable, they can suddenly develop massive hemorrhage if the fracture is not reduced and displaces further (disrupts pelvic hematoma).

In patients who continue to be unstable after application of an external fixator or in those who have instability with fracture patterns not amenable to external fixation, arteriogram with embolization of any bleeding vessels may be a life-saving procedure.

The goal after initial resuscitation and stabilization is application of stable definitive fixation to allow for rapid mobilization of the patient. For percutaneous techniques, this can be done relatively early postinjury; however, for open techniques, this should be delayed at least 48 hours to prevent disruption of the pelvic hematoma with associated massive bleeding. Delay should not be excessive, as these patients are at high risk for ARDS, pulmonary emboli, and multisystem organ failure.

THE UNSTABLE SPINE[25–27]

An unstable spine injury, while generally not life threatening, represents a true orthopaedic emergency, as the patient's immediate and ultimate neurologic status can be affected by the initial management of the injury. Most spine injuries occur secondary to motor vehicle accidents, falls, gunshot wounds, and sports-related accidents. Most high-velocity injuries will have other associated injuries, and assessment of the entire patient is necessary. In addition, injury at one spinal level is associated with additional noncontiguous spinal injuries in 10%–15% of cases[25,26]. These noncontiguous injuries are often overlooked, with subsequent delays in diagnosis and treatment.

Initial assessment of the patient with spinal injury most frequently occurs at the injury scene, and it is rare for the orthopaedic surgeon to be performing the initial immobilization. Most prehospital emergency medical personnel are now well trained in initial immobilization techniques and understand the importance of neck and trunk stabilization in anyone with suspected spinal injury.

Immediate assessment, however, begins with the ABCs. The airway must be established, and if intubation is necessary, the nasotracheal route is preferred to avoid neck extension during the intubation process. The neck must be stabilized during all resuscitation maneuvers. Patients should be maintained on oxygen on transport to the hospital to help prevent hypoxemia and resultant tissue and neuronal injury.

Once the ABCs are assessed, spinal immobilization becomes essential[28]. With any moving of the patient, the neck must be stabilized in a neutral position by the hands of the person directing the movements and once feasible a hard cervical collar should be placed for additional support. Preferably, the collar should have an opening anteriorly in case emergent tracheostomy is necessary. The patient should then be placed on a rigid backboard from head to toes in length and belted to the board around the thorax, head and extremities, to immobilize the thoracic and lumbar spine. The scoop backboard is the most effective for patient transport. Care must be taken to prevent excess movement. Log rolling has now been associated with significant fracture site motion and is not recommended. Assessment should be performed rapidly by a physician in a controlled environment to minimize the time spent on the backboard, as it has been associated with decubitus formation, especially in insensate patients.

For children with suspected cervical spine injuries, the standard backboard can be hazardous[29]. Children up to age 6 have disproportionately large heads and while lying on a flat board are at risk of developing flexion, kyphosis, and anterior translation in unstable cervical injuries. They should thus be placed in a position to raise the thorax 2–4 cm, thus lowering the occiput. This can be done by placing a pad beneath their shoulders. This can effectively reduce displaced fractures and make them more difficult to diagnose. Further stabilization is done with cervical and head side supports.

Patients with spinal cord injury will frequently be hemodynamically unstable, especially in cervical and upper thoracic injuries above T-6. One must differentiate the instability of neurogenic shock from that of hemorrhagic shock, as the treatment differs. In neurogenic shock the hypotension is associated with bradycardia and a regular pulse, while in hemorrhagic shock it is associated with tachycardia and an irregular pulse. Hemorrhagic shock is initially managed with fluid resuscitation, which is not helpful in patients with neurogenic shock, as their volume status is not deficient and excess fluid can cause congestive heart failure. Neurogenic shock is managed by maintaining peripheral vascular tone frequently with dopamine and sometimes using atropine for its vagolytic effect. Maintaining normal blood pressure will minimize ischemic damage to the spinal cord.

Once stabilized, a thorough neurologic examination must be performed for any multitrauma patient or any patient with suspected spinal injuries. The examination must include motor, sensory, and reflex testing. In the intubated, unconscious patient, reflex testing may be the only possibility on examination. The spine should then be palpated (while keeping the neck stable) to check for bony step-off and in the awake patient for tenderness. In addition, any contusions or lacerations should be noted. The bulbocavernosus reflex should be tested in all patients with spinal injuries. If absent, it indicates that the patient is in spinal shock and the definitive neurologic status is still in question. Spinal shock resolves within 48 hours in nearly all cases.

When performing the neurologic examination, the most caudad level of normal sensory and motor function must be documented. The patient's neurologic level will be the most caudad level with muscle function sufficient to provide anti-gravity function. The level above this must be normal. Patients with an *incomplete neurologic injury have preservation of some motor or sensory function below the level of the injury, while those with complete injuries have no motor or sensory function below the level of the injury.* Once again, spinal shock must be assessed to determine if the information is accurate and definitive. If a patient has a complete injury for greater than 48 hours, then no return of function is expected.

One must also assess for injuries during the secondary trauma survey. Patients with upper thoracic spinal injuries frequently have lung injuries or can have aortic transection. Any mediastinal widening on chest radiograph should be considered an aortic injury until proved otherwise and assessed further with an aortogram. Low thoracic and thoracolumbar flexion-distraction injuries are associated with intraabdominal trauma, and a diagnostic peritoneal lavage or abdominal CT should be performed in these injuries. Noncontiguous spinal injuries are common, thus the entire spine should be imaged with plain radiographs if a high velocity mechanism is present, especially in an unconscious patient.

A lateral cervical radiograph is part of the initial trauma series of films and will help identify any fractures, unstable segments, and soft-tissue swelling about the spine. For patients with cervical spinal cord injury levels or those with neck pain, a full cervical series (A-P, odontoid, obliques) is indicated. The cervicothoracic junction must be visualized and, if not well seen on standard lateral radiographs, a swimmer's view should be ordered. Thoracic and lumbar films should be ordered as indicated by examination or if there is a high speed mechanism of injury. CT scans are helpful adjuncts for defining canal compromise and further delineating the fracture pattern. MRI scans are used to define canal compromise in patients with neurologic deficits, to assess for suspected disc retropulsion and to define cord contusion and epidural hematoma. Occasionally, patients will present with neurologic deficits without plain film evidence of injury. This is termed spinal cord injury without obvious radiographic abnormality (SCIWORA), and it most commonly occurs in children. This represents another indication for MRI.

Patients with spinal cord injury may benefit from administration of methylprednisolone if given within 8 hours of injury[30]. A 30 mg/kg bolus is given followed by a continuous infusion of 5.4 mg/kg/hr for 23 hours. Its mechanism of action is reduction of edema, stabilization of neuronal membranes from free radicals and potent antiinflammatory effect. Potential risks include a statistically insignificant increase in gastrointestinal bleeding and wound healing problems. Use of this regimen has demonstrated improvement in motor and sensory function if given within 8 hours of injury.

Management of unstable spinal injuries initially revolves around effective stabilization. In the thoracolumbar spine, this involves lying flat on a rigid surface initially, with mobilization in a rigid orthosis for stable fractures and immobilization on a rotary-type bed versus emergency operative stabilization in unstable fractures. The rotary bed will help prevent atelectasis in the perioperative period. The timing of surgery is controversial, but most sources agree that emergent surgery is indicated in cases of progressive neurologic deficit and in cases of incomplete neurologic deficit secondary to neural compression, translational injury, and kyphotic deformity.

In the cervical spine, initial immobilization is provided by a rigid cervical orthosis. For subluxations and facet dislocations, which will require traction for reduction, a halo ring or Gardner-Wells tongs should be placed as described in the next section. The halo ring should also be placed for any injury that may be definitively treated in a halo vest/jacket. Prior to placing a patient in traction, one must consider the mechanism of injury. For unilateral or bilateral facet dislocations, there can be an associated disc herniation, which can lead to disastrous consequences if the facet dislocation is reduced and the patient becomes quadriplegic[31]. An MRI is indicated prior to reduction and if a herniated disc is present, the level should be decompressed anteriorly prior to reduction. If there is no disc herniation, then weights can be added in 5- to 10-pound increments, with lateral radiographs and physical examinations performed after each weight is added. Once reduced, the patient should remain in traction at that weight until a halo vest/jacket is applied or until surgery.

Emergency surgery in cervical spine injuries is indicated with progressive neurologic deterioration in the setting of canal compromise. Other operative indications include a stable neurologic deficit with irreducible canal compromise, incomplete lesion with initial improvement and early plateau and grossly unstable osseous or ligamentous injuries.

HALO PLACEMENT[28,32]

Although halo placement is not an emergency in most instances, it is discussed here in relation to its use in unstable cervical spine injuries.

Application of a halo fixator is among the most common procedures performed by an orthopaedic house officer. It was first introduced by Perry and Nickel in 1959[33] and remains the most effective type of cervical orthosis for providing rigid immobilization. Indications for usage are many and include treatment of many cervical fractures, immobilization for arthrodesis and a means for traction and immobilization in unstable cervical injuries prior to operative fixation. Contraindications to usage include unstable skull fractures and infection of proposed pin sites. Complications of treatment (pin tract infection, pin loosening) are common, thus meticulous attention to detail is necessary.

Halo application should not be performed alone and ideally is done with two other people; however, this is not always possible, and one assistant is usually sufficient. Most institutions in which halos are routinely applied will have sterile halo application trays. The ring application must be performed under sterile conditions to minimize the risk of pin tract infections.

The ring is placed with the patient in the supine position and head resting on a head ring support with the neck stabilized. For complete ring halos (circumferential), the head should rest beyond the edge of the bed on a ring support and for incomplete rings (crown-type halo) the head can remain supported on the bed. The hard cervical collar should remain intact until both the halo ring and vest are applied.

The halo ring should be sized so that it will rest 1 cm off the skin surface in all areas. Once proposed pin sites are chosen, the hair is shaved all around that region and the skin thoroughly prepped with a Betadine solution. Optimal placement of anterior pins is 1 cm superior to the orbital rim along the lateral two-thirds of the orbit. They should be placed below the level of greatest skull diameter to prevent cephalad pin migration, especially in patients with long, sloped foreheads. Pin placement medial to the safe zone can injure the supraorbital and supra-trochlear nerves and frontal sinus. Pin placement lateral to the safe zone can injure the temporalis muscle (thin cortical bone with easy skull penetration) or zygomaticotemporal nerve. The posterior pins should be placed roughly diagonal to the anterior pins and the ring should rest 1 cm above the ear pinnae.

Once the skin is prepped, the pin sites should be infiltrated subcutaneously down to the skull periosteum with 1% lidocaine with epinephrine. The pins are then placed through the ring (no incision necessary) perpendicular to the skin and the patient is asked to gently close their eyes and relax their forehead during anterior pin placement. The pins are sequentially tightened alternating in diagonal fashion at 2 in-lb increments until each has reached 8 in-lb. Most modern systems will have plastic applicators that break off once this torque is reached, and it can be confirmed with a torque wrench. The locknuts are then placed and gently tightened. Pins should be tightened to 8 in-lbs 24–48 hours after application. Some people advocate more frequent tightening up to once a day for 3 days postapplication.

In children, halo rings should be applied to a lower torque of 2–5 in-lb given the thin nature of their skulls. Multiple pins are recommended in children less than 3 years of age. Some people would recommend multiple pins up to the ages of 6 to 7. Custom devices may be required if the standard ones are too large, and a Minerva cast can be used as an alternative form of immobilization if an appropriate halo cannot be placed.

Once the ring is applied, the patient will be placed in traction for reduction or placed into a vest. The vest is sized by measuring chest circumference at the level of the xiphoid process. The posterior portion of the vest is applied first with the trunk elevated off the bed and neck strictly supported. The posts are stabilized to the ring and then the anterior portion is applied and anterior posts stabilized to the ring. A lateral radiograph is then obtained to check alignment and any necessary adjustments made. Excess extension should be avoided to prevent dysphagia. Radiographs and neurologic examinations should be performed after each adjustment.

After application, the pins should be cleansed with a diluted Betadine or hydrogen peroxide solution daily. Pin site infection occurs in up to 20% of cases and can be treated with local pin care and oral antibiotics if painful or minimally draining, but a pin should be removed if cellulitis or an abscess develops. This should be treated with intravenous antibiotics until it clears. If a pin is removed, a new pin should be placed at an alternate site free of swelling and erythema.

Other complications include pin loosening (30%–60%), which can be treated with placement of a new pin; loss of reduction; pressure sores from the vest; and dural puncture (rare). This device thus provides the most rigid cervical immobilization of any orthosis but care must be taken in application as complications, although minor, are common.

References

1. Chapman MW, Olson SA. Open fractures. In: Rockwood CA Jr, Green DP, eds. Fractures in adults. Philadelphia: Lippincott-Raven, 1996.
2. Gustilo RB, Anderson JT. Prevention of infection in the treatment of one thousand and twenty five open fractures of long bones: retrospective and prospective analyses. J Bone Joint Surg 1976;58-A:453–458.
3. Chapnick EK, Abter EI. Necrotizing soft tissue infections. Inf Dis Clin North Am 1996;10(4):835–855.
4. Urbaniak JR. Replantation. In: Green DP, ed. Operative hand surgery. New York: Churchill Livingstone, 1993.
5. Tornetta P III, Olson SA. Amputation versus limb salvage. Instruct Course Lect 1997;46:511–518.
6. Whitesides TE, Heckmann MM. Acute compartment syndrome. Update on diagnosis and treatment. J Am Acad Orthop Surg 1996;4:209–218.
7. Heckmann MM, Whitesides TE, et al. Histologic determination of the ischemic threshold of muscle in the canine compartment syndrome model. J Orthop Trauma 1993;7:199–210.

8. Heckmann MM, Whitesides TE, et al. Compartment pressure in association with closed tibial fractures. The relationship between tissue pressure, compartment and the distance from the site of the fracture. J Bone Joint Surg 1994;76-A:1285–1292.

9. Myerson M. Soft-tissue trauma—acute and chronic management. In: Mann RA, Coughlin MJ, eds. Surgery of the foot and ankle. 6th ed. St. Louis: CV Mosby, 1993.

10. Rowland SA. Fasciotomy. The treatment of compartment syndrome. In: Green DP, ed. Operative hand surgery. New York: Churchill Livingstone, 1993.

11. Gonzalez MH, Kay T, et al. Necrotizing fasciitis of the upper extremity. J Hand Surg 1996;21-A:689–692.

12. Esterhai JL, Gelb I. Adult septic arthritis. Orthop Clin North Am 1991;22:503–514.

13. Mikhail IS, Alarcon GS. Nongonococcal bacterial arthritis. Rheum Dis Clinics North Am 1993;19:311–331.

14. Sonnen GM, Henry NK. Pediatric bone and joint infections. Diagnosis and antimicrobial management. Pediatr Clin North Am 1996;43: 933–947.

15. Scopelitis E, Martinez-Osuna P. Gonococcal arthritis. Rheum Dis Clinics North Am 1993;19:363–374.

16. Kelley WN, Harris ED, Ruddy S, et al. Textbook of rheumatology. 5th ed. Philadelphia: WB Saunders, 1997.

17. Lane JG, Falahee MH, et al. Pyarthrosis of the knee. Treatment considerations. Clin Orthop 1990;252:198–204.

18. Parisien JS, Shaffer B. Arthroscopic management of pyarthrosis. Clin Orthop 1992;275:243–247.

19. Thiery JA. Arthroscopic drainage of septic arthritides of the knee. A multicenter study. Arthroscopy 1989;5:65–69.

20. Good L, Johnson RJ. The dislocated knee. J Am Acad Orthop Surg 1995;3:284–292.

21. Schenck RC. The dislocated knee. Instruct Course Lect 1994;43: 127–136.

22. Green NE, Allen BL. Vascular injuries associated with dislocation of the knee. J Bone Joint Surg 1977;59-A:236–239.

23. Bone LB, Stegemann P, Babikian G. Management of the multiply injured patient with fractures. Instruct Course Lect 1995;44:477–485.

24. Tile M. Acute pelvic fractures II. Principles and management. J Am Acad Orthop Surg 1996;4:152–161.

25. Levine AM, McAfee PC, Anderson PA. Evaluation and emergency treatment of patients with thoracolumbar trauma. Instruct Course Lect 1995;44:33–45.

26. Slucky AV, Eismont FJ. Treatment of acute injury of the cervical spine. Instruct Course Lect 1995;44:67–80.

27. Spivak JM, Vaccaro AR, Cotler JM. Thoracolumbar spine trauma II. Principles of management. J Am Acad Orthop Surg 1995;3:353–360.

28. Vaccaro AF, An HS, et al. The management of acute spinal trauma. Prehospital and in-hospital emergency care. Instruct Course Lect 1997;46:113–125.

29. Herzenberg JE, Hensiger RN, et al. Emergency transport and positioning of young children who have an injury of the cervical spine. The standard backboard may be hazardous. J Bone Joint Surg 1989;71-A:15–22.

30. Bracken MB, Shepard MJ, et al. A randomized controlled trial of methylprednisolone or naloxone in the treatment of acute spinal injury: Results of the Second National Acute Spinal Cord Injury Study. N Engl J Med 1990;322:1405–1411.

31. Eismont FJ, Arena MJ, Green BA. Extrusion of an intervertebral disc associated with traumatic subluxation or dislocation of cervical facets:case report. J Bone Joint Surg 1991;73-A:1555–1560.

32. Botte MJ, Byrne TP, et al: Halo skeletal fixation: techniques of application and prevention of complications. J Am Acad Orthop Surg 1996;4:44–53.

33. Perry JL, Nickel VI. Total cervical spine fusion for neck paralysis. J Bone Joint Surg 1959;41-A:37–60.

Chapter 6

Fractures, Dislocations, and Other Musculoskeletal Injuries

THE LANGUAGE OF FRACTURES

As with all branches of medicine, fractures are discussed in a language peculiar to the specialty involved. It is imperative that the physician or medical student learn this language in order to accurately describe a fracture to the senior resident or attending physician. Without such an accurate description, effective communication about treatment modalities is not possible.

Fractures are classified according to: 1) the bone involved; 2) the location of the fracture; 3) the pattern of the fracture fragments; and 4) the amount of anatomic disruption. Following are the four main locations in which a fracture can occur:

Fracture Location

Diaphysis: The diaphysis is the main shaft of long, tubular bones (Fig. 6.1).

Metaphysis: The metaphysis is the flared end of a long bone, and is located between the diaphysis and the physis (Fig. 6.1).

Physis: The physis is present only in a growing bone. It is the cartilaginous growth plate that occurs near the end of a long bone. At skeletal maturity, the physis ossifies and fuses with the epiphysis and the metaphysis (Fig. 6.1).

Epiphysis: The epiphysis is the end of a long bone between the physeal cartilage and the articular cartilage (Fig. 6.1).

Fracture Patterns

Closed Fracture: A closed fracture is one in which the skin is intact overlying the fracture and its hematoma.

117

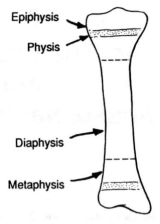

Figure 6.1. The four main parts of a long bone.

Open Fracture: An open fracture is one in which there is a break in the integument that communicates with the fracture site or fracture hematoma. The size of the break in the integument is immaterial in classification as an open fracture, although it carries prognostic significance. See Table 5.1 and the section on Open Fractures in Chapter 5 (Orthopaedic Emergencies) for a discussion of the prognostic significance.

Comminuted Fracture: A comminuted fracture is one in which the bone is divided into more than two fragments by the fracture lines. There are subclassifications of comminuted long bone fractures, but it is important to remember that a fracture with 100 fragments and one with two large fragments and a smaller one are both considered comminuted. However, there is a difference in prognostic significance (Fig. 6.2).

Extraarticular Fracture: An extraarticular fracture is one in which the fracture line does not enter a joint cavity (Fig. 6.3).

Intraarticular Fracture: An intraarticular fracture is one in which the fracture line enters a joint cavity (Fig. 6.3).

Transverse Fracture: A transverse fracture is one in which the fracture line is perpendicular to the long axis of the involved bone (Fig. 6.4).

Oblique Fracture: An oblique fracture is one in which the fracture line subtends an oblique angle with the long axis of the involved bone (Fig. 6.4).

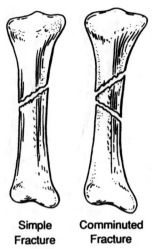

**Simple
Fracture**

**Comminuted
Fracture**

Figure 6.2.   Simple and comminuted fractures.

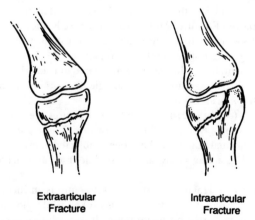

**Extraarticular
Fracture**

**Intraarticular
Fracture**

Figure 6.3.   Extra- and intraarticular fracture patterns.

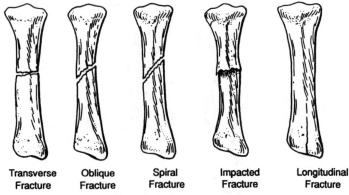

| Transverse | Oblique | Spiral | Impacted | Longitudinal |
| Fracture | Fracture | Fracture | Fracture | Fracture |

Figure 6.4. The five main directions of fracture patterns.

Spiral Fracture: A spiral fracture is an extreme case of an oblique fracture in which the plane of the fracture through the bone rotates about the long axis of the bone (Fig. 6.4).

Longitudinal Fracture: A longitudinal fracture is parallel to, or nearly parallel to, the long axis of the involved bone (Fig. 6.4).

Impacted Fracture: An impacted fracture is one caused by a compressive force that causes the end of a bone to be driven into the contiguous metaphyseal region of the bone without displacement. It may, however, be angulated or rotated (Fig. 6.4).

Pathologic Fracture: A pathologic fracture is a fracture through abnormal bone.

Stress (or Fatigue) Fracture: Stress fractures are considered by some to be a type of pathologic fracture. These are fractures through normal bones that have been subjected to cyclic loading at loads that, acting singly, are not sufficient to cause acute fractures.

Greenstick Fracture: A greenstick fracture is an incomplete fracture in which only one cortex is broken while the opposite cortex and periosteum remain intact. It is much more common in children (Fig. 6.5).

Torus Fracture: A torus fracture is also more common in children. It is an impaction injury in which the cortex of a long bone buckles with no loss of cortical continuity (Fig. 6.5).

Plastic Deformation: Plastic deformation is an injury occurring exclusively in children's bones. It occurs when a child's bones simply bend with no break in either cortex. This occurs because children's bones are more porous and, consequently, less brittle (Fig. 6.5).

Physeal Injury: This is an injury through the physeal plate in a developing child. These injuries have their own system of description and are discussed in more detail below.

Dislocation: Dislocation is technically defined as total loss of congruity between the articular surfaces of a joint. Anything less than total loss of congruity should be strictly termed a subluxation. However, extreme subluxations are often termed dislocations, but this is not technically correct.

In addition to describing the location of the fracture and the pattern of the fracture lines and fragments, it is necessary to be able to describe the degree of anatomic disruption. Loss of normal anatomy can occur because of displacement, angulation, rotation, and separation.

Anatomic Disruption

Displacement: This is a measure of the translational distance between the corresponding cortices of the fracture fragments.

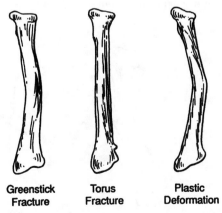

Greenstick   Torus   Plastic
Fracture   Fracture   Deformation

Figure 6.5. Special fracture patterns seen in children.

An example can be seen in Figure 6.6 (left). The tibia has two fracture fragments. The distal fragment has moved with no angular change in the longitudinal axis of the fragment. It has been translated laterally.

Angulation: Angulation measures the angle between the longitudinal axes of the main fracture fragments (Fig. 6.6 [middle]). Here the two tibial fragments are angulated and lines are drawn through each fragment corresponding to their longitudinal axis. These lines intersect with an angle of 20 degrees, which is the measure of the angulation of the fracture. It is important to be able to describe the direction of angulation, and this can cause difficulty. The reason is that different texts describe angulation in different methods.

In Figure 6.6, the tibial fragments are angulated such that the distal end of the distal fragment points laterally. Although it would be proper to say that the fracture is angulated into valgus (distal fragment directed laterally), there is no similar analogy to describe anterior-posterior angulation. Some authors describe this fracture as angulated laterally, meaning that the distal fragment is directed laterally, while others would call this medial angulation, meaning that the apex of the fracture is directed medially. For consistency, we recommend describing the direction of the apex of an angulated fracture (e.g., apex medial, apex dorsal).

It is best to simply describe the fracture pattern and not attempt what may be an ambiguous short-cut in terminology. In

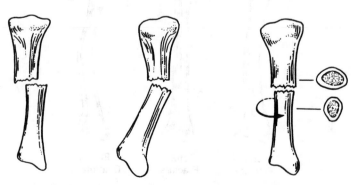

Figure 6.6. Fracture displacement, angulation, and rotation.

Figure 6.6, if you say, "It is angulated with the apex directed laterally," there is less chance for misinterpretation.

Rotation: Rotation is a twisting about the longitudinal axis of one of the fracture fragments. It is the most difficult type of fracture disruption to see on radiographs, and it is also the deformity that remodels the least as the fracture heals. Rotation can be evaluated better clinically than it can be radiographically. One clue to rotatory deformity can be seen in Figure 6.6 (right). Here the fracture is not angulated or displaced, but the apparent diameter of the bone changes on opposite sides of the fracture line.

Separation: Separation describes the situation in which there is a gap between the fracture fragments.

It is now possible to fully describe an adult fracture. When calling a senior resident or attending physician to describe an injury, a complete description might be as follows, "The fracture is a closed, simple, transverse, extraarticular fracture of the distal radial metaphysis. The distal fragment is displaced dorsally 1 centimeter, and the fracture is angulated 20 degrees with the apex directed volarly." The common eponym of this fracture is a Colles' fracture, but the above description conveys much more information.

Physeal Injuries

Children's fractures can be more difficult to describe accurately because of the presence of the growth plate. There are several classification systems for fractures involving the physis. By far the most widely used is the Salter-Harris system, which is as follows:

Salter-Harris Type I: In this injury, the fracture line goes directly through the physis. There may be a slight gap between the fragments, but since the physis is not radiopaque, the gap can usually only be appreciated by a comparison film of the opposite extremity. The diagnosis is often a clinical one, and immobilization and no weight bearing until the child is symptomatically better are usually sufficient (Fig. 6.7).

Salter-Harris Type II: In this injury, the fracture line is mostly through the physis, but it exits one cortex such that a small fragment of metaphysis is included with the fracture fragment containing the physis and epiphysis (Fig. 6.7).

Salter-Harris Type III: In this injury, the fracture line is mostly through the physis, but it exits one cortex such that a small

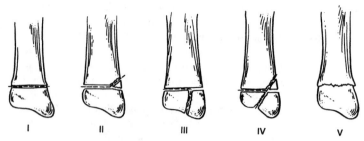

Figure 6.7. Salter-Harris classification.

fragment of epiphysis is included with the fracture fragment containing the metaphysis and diaphysis (Fig. 6.7).

Salter-Harris Type IV: In this injury, a fracture line crosses the physis such that both fracture fragments contain portions of the metaphysis, physis, and epiphysis (Fig. 6.7).

Salter-Harris Type V: In this injury, there is no definite fracture line, and like the Salter-Harris Type I, this injury cannot be easily diagnosed radiographically. The injury involves a crush injury to the physis in which the metaphysis and epiphysis are acutely impacted upon one another. Unfortunately, the diagnosis is often a retrospective one, and this injury carries a very high risk of growth plate arrest (Fig. 6.7).

The Salter-Harris classification is an excellent system in that it conveys prognostic information about each injury. As one goes from a Type I to a Type V, the risk of growth arrest or deformity of the growth plate greatly increases. There have been descriptions of a few, very rare, injuries to the growth plate, which some authors term Types VI or VII. In addition, the above classification has been broken down further by Ogden. However, the above five categories are sufficient for most pediatric physeal injuries.

RADIOLOGY OF FRACTURES

While it might seem a simple matter to diagnose a fracture from a radiograph, certain points can be made. If a fracture is diagnosed, it is imperative to evaluate the joints proximal and distal to the fracture with radiographs. Many concurrent fractures and dislocations have been missed because this rule was not followed.

While often a good examination of those joints will determine the need for a radiograph, many times the patient will be in too much pain to allow a good examination, and it is safer to simply radiograph the adjacent joints.

There are standard views that radiologic technicians use for each joint, usually beginning with A-P (anteroposterior) and lateral views. Often the physician will desire additional views. The standard views and certain special views are discussed in Chapter 4. In addition, certain special views will also be mentioned below in discussing the individual fracture types.

Basic Fracture Biomechanics[1]

Fractures occur because of four main types of forces acting on bones—tension, compression, bending, and torsion[1]. It is important to understand the difference in the forces, because they cause characteristic fracture patterns, especially in long bones. Often, it is possible to deduce the force causing the fracture by analyzing the fracture pattern. This information can then be used to aid in reducing a fracture by reversing the force that caused it.

Tension: Tension is a force applied to a bone or a portion of the bone such that the portion under tension is increasing in length.

Compression: Compression is a force applied to a bone or a portion of the bone such that the portion under compression is decreasing in length.

Bending: Bending forces can be termed either pure two-point bending or three-point bending forces. In pure bending, forces are applied to opposite ends of a bone in the same direction. In three-point bending, two forces are applied as in pure bending and a third force is applied between the other two but in the opposite direction (Fig. 6.8).

Torsion: Torsion is a force applied that causes a bone to rotate about its long axis.

One must remember that the above forces rarely occur in isolation. Specifically, when a bone is subjected to three-point bending forces, the cortex from which two forces are applied will be in tension and the opposite cortex will be under compression (Fig. 6.9).

The characteristic patterns produced by the four main forces are as follows[1]:

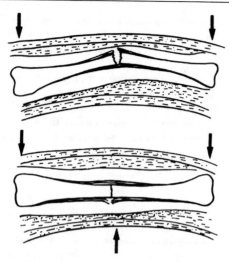

Figure 6.8. Examples of a poorly applied cast (top) and a properly applied cast (bottom). Cast at bottom shows the use of three-point bending applied against a soft-tissue hinge.

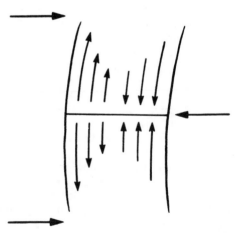

Figure 6.9. The three-point bending principle. The side on which two forces are applied is under tension, while the opposite cortex is under compression.

Tension: The fracture pattern is straight transverse. Usually, tension occurs only about a portion of the bone. Pure tension applied to a bone is extremely rare.

Compression: Compression causes an oblique fracture pattern. If there are no other forces involved, the oblique fracture will subtend an angle of 45 degrees with the long axis of the bone.

Bending: As mentioned, bending causes one cortex to be under tension and one cortex to be under compression. Consequently, the fracture pattern will be a combination of the two patterns. The fracture pattern will be mostly transverse (along the tension side) but will propagate obliquely on the compression surface.

Torsion: The fracture pattern will be a spiral or long oblique type.

Closed Reduction—Basic Techniques[2]

After one has evaluated the fracture pattern carefully and decided if it can be treated by closed reduction and immobilization, it is necessary to know how to perform a reduction. Every fracture is different, and the exact technique of reduction depends on the individual fracture. However, there are well-established principles that guide practitioners in reducing fractures and dislocations.

First, by studying the fracture pattern and applying the biomechanical principles mentioned above, one should be able to deduce the mechanism of injury that caused the fracture. Second, it must be realized that stability of a fracture, after reduction, depends on the fracture pattern to a degree, but also depends a great deal on the soft-tissue envelope surrounding the fracture. Simply stated, closed reduction of fractures involves reversing the original injury mechanism and holding the fracture by using the cast or bandage to apply proper pressure to the soft-tissue envelope.

Reduction of the fracture actually is a bit more difficult than simply reversing the mechanism of injury. In Figure 6.10 (top), an example of a fracture is shown, and the fracture site shows that the ends of a fracture are never purely linear but rather have multiple areas of interdigitations. Attempting to merely reverse the fracture will cause these bone shards to impinge on one another and prevent reduction.

Impaction of the fragments on one another during reduction is prevented by first longitudinally distracting the fracture frag-

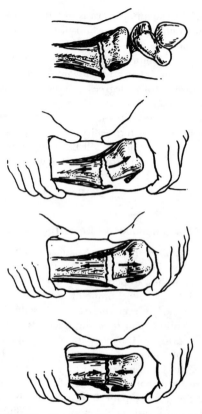

Figure 6.10. The basic steps in fracture reduction.

ments, then gently exaggerating the mechanism of injury to disengage the ends of the fracture. Reduction is then performed by reversing the mechanism. The best example of such a reduction is shown in the closed manipulation of a Colles' fracture shown in Fig. 6.10. Here the physician's hands are placed on opposite ends of the fracture site, with the thumbs gently palpating the fracture ends opposite the apex of the fracture. Both hands pull longitudinally in opposite directions to distract the fracture (Fig. 6.10), then the fracture angulation is slightly increased, and finally, the fracture is reduced by reversing the mechanism, pushing volarly with both thumbs at the ends of the fracture fragments.

Several points must be followed concerning this basic method of reduction: 1) the three steps (distraction, exaggerate mechanism, reverse mechanism) should be done in one smooth, continuous motion; 2) it usually requires more force than one might imagine; and 3) pain will cause muscle spasm, and reduction will not be possible without adequate anesthesia in the form of a hematoma block, digital block, axillary block, intravenous xylocaine (Bier block), or some other appropriate form of analgesia.

Further elaboration concerning the soft tissues is necessary. Commonly, attention is directed only to the bones since they are so easily seen on radiographs. One must always remember that the reduction is maintained using the soft-tissue hinge. This soft-tissue hinge is illustrated in Figure 6.11. Most long bone fractures will have a hinge of soft tissue (periosteum) on one cortex of the fracture. Usually, the hinge overlies the cortex opposite the apex of an angulated fracture.

When a soft-tissue hinge exists on one cortex of a fracture, it is almost impossible to overreduce the fracture. The hinge will remain intact and prevent this. However, the fracture can redisplace if the soft tissues are not used properly to maintain the reduction. Maintenence of the reduction is performed by applying a cast or splint such that the principle of three-point

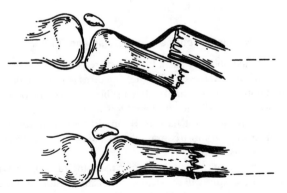

Figure 6.11. Fractured tibia with an intact soft-tissue hinge on the anterior surface (top). This is used to maintain fracture reduction (bottom).

bending is used. Figure 6.8 shows examples of properly (bottom) and improperly (top) applied casts.

The first cast shown (Fig. 6.8 [top]) fits the limb well but does not apply pressure properly against the soft-tissue hinge. Therefore, nothing is holding the fracture stable, as the soft tissue is loose and the fracture can displace. In the second example (Fig. 6.8 [bottom]), the cast is bent against the cylinder of the leg and illustrates the principle of three-point bending. The ends of the cast provide a force against the same cortex that contains the soft-tissue hinge. The middle of the cast pushes against the fracture site at its apex such that the soft-tissue hinge is maintained under tension. This will prevent the fracture from redisplacing. Charnley has stated, "Curved plaster makes straight bones"[2].

Should one apply plaster before or after reducing the fracture? It depends on the amount of help available, the fracture pattern, and the practitioner's experience. Charnley recommends applying a few layers of plaster, reducing the fracture in the wet cast, and then finishing the cast[2]. This requires excellent and quick casting ability, and the ability to reduce the fracture quickly. To do this, there should be minimal swelling so that the fracture ends can be felt through the early layers of plaster. In lieu of applying plaster first, it is helpful to have an assistant maintain the reduction while the practitioner applies the cast or splint. While learning to reduce fractures, it is probably better to reduce the fracture and then apply the cast or splint; in fact, we routinely prefer this sequence.

Special Fractures—Pathologic and Stress

As mentioned above, a pathologic fracture is a fracture through abnormal bone. A stress (or fatigue) fracture is a fracture through normal bone, but one that has been subjected to cyclic overloading at loads normally not sufficient to cause a fracture. A pathologic fracture does not have to occur through a tumor in the bone. In fact, the most common cause of pathologic fractures is osteoporosis.

It is important to always recognize pathologic fractures. While certain radiographs will show an unmistakable lesion in the area of the fracture, it is critical that a high index of suspicion be maintained for those fractures occurring with minimal trauma in seemingly healthy patients. This should always arouse suspicion of a pathologic fracture.

In cases of bone tumors, treatment of the fracture depends on establishing the correct diagnosis. Occasionally, the radiographic appearance is pathognomonic and biopsy is not necessary. Radiographic diagnosis of bone tumors is aided by evaluating four aspects of the lesion: 1) the margins of the lesion; 2) the periosteal reaction to the lesion; 3) the matrix pattern of the lesion; and 4) the location of the lesion[3].

The margins of a bone tumor are classified as either a geographic pattern, a moth-eaten pattern, or a permeative pattern. Examples of each are shown in Figure 6.12. A geographic pattern, especially one with thick, sclerotic borders, suggests a slow-growing benign process, which allows the bone time to wall off the lesion. Both moth-eaten and permeative patterns suggest a more aggressive lesion and can be suggestive of a malignancy[3].

The periosteum can react to a bone lesion in several manners, which are shown in Figure 6.13. Generally, more benign lesions

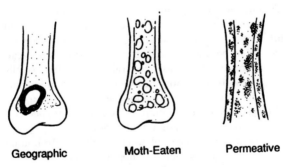

Geographic   **Moth-Eaten**   **Permeative**

Figure 6.12.   Patterns of bone destruction by tumors.

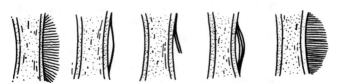

Figure 6.13.   Types of periosteal elevation.

cause less reaction, which is usually manifested as a thickening or very slight elevation. More aggressive lesions cause ominous-appearing periosteal reactions such as the sunburst pattern, spiculated pattern, onion-skinning, or Codman's triangle[3].

The matrix of a bone lesion can be either osseous, cartilaginous, fibrous, combinations of the above, or there can be no matrix, as in a simple cyst. Osseous matrices produce a typical blastic appearance on radiographs. Cartilaginous matrices are radiographically characterized by either a stippled or flocculated pattern, often described as "C's and O's" or an "alphabet-soup" appearance. Fibrous matrices appear radiographically as a hazy, soft density, often termed a ground-glass appearance[3].

The location of the lesion in the bone is of critical importance. Most bone lesions occur in the metaphysis because that is the area of most active growth of the bone. The only two lesions that commonly occur in the epiphysis are chondroblastomas (Codman's tumor) and giant-cell tumors. Chondroblastomas occur only in the epiphysis. Diaphyseal lesions are typically small round-cell tumors, such as Ewing's sarcoma, multiple myeloma, and lymphoma of bone, or metastases.

Finally, the above information must be interpreted in light of the patient's age, as different neoplasms are more common in different age groups. For example, in patients over 60 years old, it should be remembered that the most common cause of a bone lesion is a metastasis. Several of the references list the most common bone tumors and their age distributions in large series[4–6]. By using this information, and the above four radiographic parameters, it is often possible to be quite specific about the differential diagnosis of a bone lesion.

Frequently, the radiograph will be equivocal. Additional staging studies such as computed tomography, magnetic resonance imaging, bone scans, and arteriograms may better define the lesion, but often open or needle biopsy is necessary to establish the diagnosis. Biopsy of a bone lesion should not be undertaken lightly. Enneking has stressed that it is often more difficult to plan and perform the biopsy than it is to do the definitive operation. Because the incision and biopsy will contaminate all the intervening tissue planes, it must be planned carefully so that all contaminated tissue can be removed during the definitive procedure[7].

All staging studies should be done prior to performing a biopsy[7]. This is because bone tumors often bleed profusely and are difficult to control, even during biopsy. Performing the biopsy will often spread hematoma around the area of the tumor and make interpretation of the imaging studies almost impossible.

Further discussion of the details of biopsy and definitive tumor surgery is beyond the scope of this monograph. Interested readers are referred to Enneking's text for further study[7].

Stress Fractures

The treatment of stress fractures depends on the bone involved and the activity that caused the stress fracture. The classic stress fracture is a "march" fracture—the stress fracture of the second metatarsal shaft suffered by Army recruits on long marches. Other common sites are the femoral neck, tibial shaft, and tarsal navicular.

In all cases, treatment of the stress fracture should include removing the offending activity causing cyclic overload. For the above fractures, this includes an appropriate length cast (below-knee for the foot fractures and above-knee for the tibial fracture) and nonweight bearing as an activity. After the fracture is healed, the patients need to be advised about resuming the activity more gradually or in some way altering their biomechanics or environment to decrease the overloading.

BASICS OF FRACTURE MANAGEMENT

Fractures may be treated by either closed or open methods. There are advantages and disadvantages to both techniques, and there are also specific indications and contraindications for the use of both methods.

The advantage of open reduction is that it is often possible to achieve anatomic alignment of a fracture, and to rigidly stabilize it using internal fixation. If rigidly stabilized, it is often possible to begin weight bearing and/or early motion of adjacent joints. This prevents what the AO/ASIF group (Arbeitsgemeinschaft für Osteosynthesfragen/Association for the Study of Internal Fixation) calls "fracture disease"[8]. Fracture disease includes all the complications of immobilization and recumbency, including muscle atrophy, soft-tissue atrophy, loss of joint motion, joint contractures, decreased articular cartilage viability, and increased risk of pulmonary and thromboembolic complications.

The primary disadvantage of open reduction is that a closed fracture is converted to an open fracture, with the attendant higher risk of infection. In addition, surgical exposure causes disruption of the surrounding soft tissues and circulation, which may compromise healing of the fracture. Also, the scarring of surgery may later interfere with muscle function and limit motion in the adjacent joints.

The main advantage of closed reduction and immobilization is that a closed fracture remains closed, with no increased risk of infection. In addition, other complications of surgery are not risked, and usually hospital stay is shorter (if needed at all), and the cost of treatment is generally less.

The main disadvantage to closed treatment of fractures is that it is almost impossible to achieve exact anatomic reduction, and external stabilization by casts and splints can never be as rigid as properly applied internal fixation. In addition, casts and splints must often immobilize adjacent joints to be effective, and this can cause problems with loss of joint motion, especially in the elderly. Finally, in intraarticular fractures, the inability to achieve exact anatomic alignment predisposes to future problems with degenerative arthritis.

Absolute indications for open reduction are as follows[9]:

1. Displaced intraarticular fractures, in which the fragments are sufficiently large to allow internal fixation.
2. Unstable fractures failing an appropriate trial of nonoperative management.
3. Major avulsion fractures with significant disruption of an important muscle or ligament. Included in this group are displaced fractures of the greater tuberosity of the humerus, the greater trochanter, the olecranon, the patella, the intercondylar eminence of the tibia, and the tibial tubercle.
4. Displaced pathologic fractures in patients not imminently terminal.
5. Fractures for which nonoperative treatment has been shown to give poor results. Examples include femoral neck fractures and Galeazzi fracture-dislocations.
6. Certain displaced physeal injuries—mainly displaced Salter III and IV injuries.
7. Fractures associated with compartment syndromes that require fasciotomies.

8. Nonunion of a fracture that has not healed by prior methods.

Relative indications for open reduction are as follows[9]:

1. Multiple fractures. Although individual fractures may be treated acceptably by closed methods, the multitrauma patient with multiple fractures is usually better treated by open reduction/internal fixation (ORIF) of most of his or her major fractures. This allows early mobilization of the patient and helps prevent the complications of fracture disease.
2. Delayed union of a fracture that has received adequate treatment by a closed method.
3. Impending pathologic fractures.
4. Unstable open fractures.
5. Fractures with questionable soft-tissue coverage (open 3B fractures, burns, preexisting dermatitis).
6. Avoidance of the morbidity and mortality associated with recumbency and immobilization. This is especially true in brain-injured patients or the elderly, and allows for easier nursing care.
7. Fractures accompanied by neurologic or vascular disruption requiring repair. Stabilization of such fractures will allow better protection of the neurovascular repair.

Relative contraindications to open reduction are as follows[9]:

1. An active infection or osteomyelitis is often felt to be an absolute contraindication to the implantation of a foreign body in the form of an internal fixation device. However, infected fractures will heal better when rigidly stabilized if the infection can be kept under control until the fracture is healed. Perhaps the best treatment for situations that cannot be controlled with antibiotics are open debridement and external fixation.
2. Severely comminuted fractures or fractures in which the fragments are too small to accept placement of internal fixation devices.
3. Bone that is too osteoporotic to allow secure internal fixation.
4. Abnormal skin conditions or surrounding soft tissues that might greatly increase the risk of infection. These situations are best treated by external fixation.

5. General medical problems that contraindicate the use of anesthesia.
6. Nondisplaced, stable fractures that are not at risk to displace or angulate with weight bearing or early motion.

SPECIFIC FRACTURES/DISLOCATIONS

The following discussion concerns the most common types of skeletal injuries. It is not intended to be encyclopaedic. Emphasis will be placed on radiologic evaluation, classification schemes, the basics of treatment, and the most common complications. The decision of whether to treat open or closed is critical and will be discussed in some detail, although open methods of treatment will be mentioned only briefly. All fractures are assumed to be closed initially. Treatment of open fractures begins with debridement of the fracture. Further treatment then depends on the degree of soft-tissue trauma as discussed in the section on open fractures.

Adult Fractures

Phalangeal Fractures[10,11]

The treatment of phalangeal fractures depends on the amount of displacement, the phalanx involved, and whether the fracture is intraarticular or not. Distal phalanx fractures occur most frequently in the middle finger and thumb. Reduction is rarely necessary unless the articular surface is involved and splinting is primarily for pain and protection. Open and intraarticular injuries need additional treatment and often require K-wire stabilization. Nailbed injuries often occur with these fractures.

Extraarticular proximal and middle phalangeal fractures are complicated by the pull of adjacent flexor and extensor tendons and the intrinsic muscles that can cause angulation and rotation deformities. Rotation may be difficult to recognize but, if not corrected, can leave the patient with overlapping or underlapping fingers. Rotation can be evaluated clinically by flexing the digits and checking that fingernails all lie in approximately the same plane and that all fingers point toward the scaphoid.

Nondisplaced or impacted fractures may be splinted initially followed by buddy taping. Closed reduction, if required, may be followed by immobilization in a gutter splint or in a gauntlet cast with a metal outrigger. Most phalangeal fractures can be treated closed by immobilizing the hand in the "position of safety" (Fig. 6.14) in which the wrist is dorsiflexed 30–40 degrees, the MCP joints are immobilized in 70–90 degrees flexion, and the PIPJ and DIPJ are flexed 10–20 degrees. This decreases tension on the intrinsics and, to a degree, the flexor tendons. Additionally, this position helps to prevent flexion contractures of the PIPJ and extension contractures of the MCPJ. External fixation may be employed if there is marked comminution or bone loss. ORIF with K-wires or screws is indicated when articular displacement is >1 mm.

Many intraarticular phalangeal fractures are avulsion fractures at the sites of tendinous or ligamentous insertions. A bony mallet finger is an avulsion of the DP at the insertion of the dorsal hood. Typically, if the fragment involves 30%–40% or less of the articular surface of the DIPJ or if displacement is <2 mm, then the fracture can be treated closed. If it involves more of the articular surface, and/or volar subluxation of the distal phalanx is present, open treatment may be indicated. In either case, immobilization can be accomplished with the DIPJ in slight extension to diminish tension on the extensor tendon.

Another frequently seen entity is a volar DP fracture associated with avulsion of the deep flexor. This is known as a "jersey

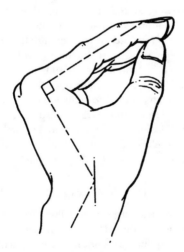

Figure 6.14.   "Safe" position for hand splinting.

finger" and it most frequently involves the ring finger. These injuries require ORIF of the fracture or tendon repair.

Metacarpal Fractures (Excluding the Thumb)[10,11]

Metacarpal fractures can occur through the head, the neck, the shaft, or the base of the metacarpal. Treatment varies according to the location of the fracture.

Metacarpal head fractures can be badly comminuted. If the comminution is distal to the origin of the collateral ligament, a short period of splinting followed by early, active motion should mold the articular surface. The early motion will also help to prevent a stiff joint, but loss of motion is common after this difficult type of fracture. ORIF is indicated if a collateral ligament avulsion injury is displaced and involves >20%–30% of the joint surface.

Fractures through the neck and shaft of the metacarpals usually angulate with the apex dorsal. This is not a great problem in fractures of the fourth and fifth metacarpals ("boxer's fracture") because the corresponding CMC joints are quite mobile and angulation up to 40–50 degrees is acceptable. However, the second and third CMC joints allow little motion, and residual angulation of >15 degrees in these metacarpals is generally unacceptable. Shortening of 2–3 mm is acceptable. Once again, one must carefully examine the patient to rule out any rotational deformity. ORIF is indicated if rotational deformity persists.

Closed treatment of these fractures involves reduction by longitudinal traction followed by the 90/90 technique. In this technique, the MCPJ and PIPJ are both flexed 90 degrees and the proximal phalanx is used to reduce the fracture by exerting a dorsally directed force on the fracture's distal fragment. Immobilization in this position, however, is not recommended, as the PIPJ will often develop a flexion contraction. Immobilization in the position of safety is usually adequate (Fig. 6.14).

Thumb Metacarpal[10,12]

Thumb metacarpal fractures can usually be treated closed if they are extraarticular. Owing to the wide range of motion of the thumb, anatomic reduction is not necessary to achieve adequate motion, strength, and function. Although reduction should be attempted, if it cannot be maintained, some degree of angulation/rotation is acceptable.

Intraarticular fractures at the trapeziometacarpal joint are usually one of two types. The most common fracture here is called a Bennett's fracture (2-part fx). In this fracture, the fracture line is oblique such that a triangular fragment at the ulnar base of the metacarpal remains attached to the trapezium with proximal displacement of the metacarpal. This fracture is unstable because of the pull of the abductor pollicis longus (APL) on the base of the metacarpal, and the pull of the adductor pollicis (AdP) on the proximal phalanx. These two forces tend to lever the metacarpal away from the triangular fragment, by adducting and shortening the metacarpal. Current management involves percutaneous pinning of the fracture to maintain reduction, or possibly ORIF of the fracture if fracture displacement is >3 mm.

The second type of trapeziometacarpal fracture is a Rolando's fracture (traditionally, a 3-part fx). This is a comminuted intraarticular fracture at the base of the thumb metacarpal that carries a worse prognosis than a Bennett's. The original description was for a T- or Y-shaped fracture pattern, but virtually all comminuted fractures in this location are now termed Rolando's fractures. Three-part fractures are often treated open using K-wire or screw/plate fixation. Comminuted fractures are treated with a distractor intraoperatively and finally K-wire or external fixation with bone graft to maintain reduction. Others think that these do as well if treated with a short period of immobilization, followed by early range of motion in an attempt to use the soft-tissue sleeve to restore articular integrity.

Scaphoid[10,12]

The scaphoid is the most commonly fractured carpal bone. The difficulty with the management of this fracture is the risk of nonunion and avascular necrosis. These complications are related to the peculiar blood supply of the scaphoid, which enters the bone dorsoradially and distally. Consequently, mid- or proximal scaphoid fractures will often be at least partially devascularized by the fracture, resulting in increased rates of nonunion or osteonecrosis.

In addition to an A-P, lateral, and oblique radiographs of the wrist, a scaphoid view is often obtained (an A-P view of the wrist in ulnar deviation). A clenched fist view demonstrating widening between the scaphoid and the lunate >3 mm is indicative of ligamentous injury.

Nondisplaced fractures of the scaphoid are usually treated closed in a long arm thumb spica, leaving the thumb IPJ free. A long arm cast is required for 4–6 weeks to prevent displacement. Then, a short arm thumb spica cast is used until the fracture is healed, about 10–12 weeks.

One problem in the treatment of scaphoid fractures is late diagnosis because of negative radiographs at the initial presentation. It is important that the physician have a high index of suspicion when treating a patient with history of a fall on outstretched hand, snuffbox tenderness, and negative films. If in doubt, it is acceptable to immobilize the extremity in a short arm thumb spica until repeat radiographs can be performed in 7–10 days when a fracture, if present, should be obvious. A poor prognosis is associated with delayed diagnosis, middle or proximal third location, and fracture displacement or angulation.

Displaced fractures require reduction, which is not easily done without opening the fracture. ORIF is typically performed using a volar approach and the Herbert screw. This screw has two sets of threads of differing pitch and width, connected by a smooth shaft. Advancing the screw causes compression of the fracture site, because of the differing pitches of the screw. A CT scan is often helpful preoperatively if the scaphoid is displaced and ORIF is indicated. If a CT is to be performed, short arm thumb spica immobilization should be used while the patient is in the scanner to allow some elbow motion to obtain optimal imaging. There have been several procedures described for treatment of nonunions, and many salvage procedures are documented in the literature.

Distal Radius[10,12,13]

Fractures of the distal radius are quite common, the classic example being the Colles' fracture, in which the distal fragment is dorsally angulated with the fracture apex volar. Prior to discussing these fractures, it is important to understand the normal radiographic appearance of the distal radius. The three measurements that have become well accepted in the literature are a volar tilt (palmar angle) of 11–12 degrees on the lateral radiograph, a radial inclination of 23 degrees on the A-P view, and a radial length of 11–12 mm describing the perpendicular distance between the radial styloid tip and the distal articular surface of the ulna. Several prospective studies have linked functional results with restoration of the normal anatomy of the distal radius. Patients with poor restoration had increased disability demonstrated by decreased grip strength and endurance. Additionally, impacted intraarticular fractures with >2 mm articular incongruity ("die punch injuries") lead to symptomatic osteoarthritis, especially in young adults. Older patients with osteoporotic bone often function adequately despite intraarticular fractures with less than anatomic results because of a low-demand lifestyle. Subsequently, a history including the patient's age, handedness, occupation, and hobbies is important in creating a treatment plan. One also needs to evaluate stepoff in the distal radioulnar joint (DRUJ), since incongruity there can lead to accelerated morbidity.

In addition to three views of the wrist, a CT scan can occasionally be helpful for visualizing articular stepoff and creating an operative plan. Fractures are typically unstable and require surgical intervention if prereduction radiographs demonstrate >20 degrees dorsal angulation, marked dorsal comminution, and >10 mm loss of radial length.

Many extraarticular Colles' fractures can be treated closed with cast immobilization. Undisplaced and minimally displaced fractures can often be treated with a short arm splint followed by a short arm cast. Above the elbow immobilization is required if there is any axial instability or intraarticular involvement. Many now prefer to cast the postreduction wrist in neutral while others prefer the more traditional Cotton-Loder position (volar flexion and ulnar deviation).

Percutaneous pinning of unstable extraarticular and some intraarticular fractures is becoming increasingly popular, as more aggressive interventions are not yielding better results. Typically, one K-wire is inserted in the radial styloid and is directed ulnar and proximal. The other wire is placed just ulnar to the 4th extensor compartment.

External fixators are placed dorsoradial to the wrist with two pins attached to the junction of the middle and distal radius and two pins attached to the index metacarpal. These devices are excellent for disimpacting the fracture and bringing it out to length. Many prefer to use external fixation alone (especially if there are soft-tissue problems) or in combination with pins and/ or plate fixation. External fixators are typically removed at 6 weeks postop in order to reduce the risk of permanent wrist stiffness.

ORIF using pins, screws, and buttress-type plates is still used by many on young patients with unstable, intraarticular fractures because of increased stability. Bone graft is often used for very comminuted or impacted fractures.

Two other types of distal radius fractures are Smith's and Barton's fractures. Smith's refers to volar angulation and proximal diplacement of the distal fragment. Barton's indicates a fracture-dislocation, in which the wrist subluxates volarly (most frequently) or dorsally owing to an intraarticular distal radius fracture. Barton's fractures are treated with buttress plating. Sometimes, an external fixator and percutaneous pins are also required.

Arthroscopic reduction and internal fixation (ARIF) is used by some hand surgeons in an effort to reduce articular incongruity. Articular stepoff >1 mm in young people is thought to accelerate arthritis.

Ulnar Shaft[12,13]

The isolated ulnar shaft fracture resulting from a direct blow is more commonly known as the "nightstick fracture." This fracture can be treated effectively in a well-molded short arm cast even if the shaft is displaced by as much as 50%. Angulation up to 15 degrees can be tolerated in the midshaft. In distal third fractures, the distal radio-ulnar articulation must be observed closely.

Monteggia/Galeazzi[12,14]

A Monteggia fracture is a fracture of the proximal ulna with a concomitant dislocation of the radial head. A Galeazzi (or Piedmont) fracture is a fracture of the radial shaft (usually distal third) with a concomitant subluxation or dislocation of the distal radio-ulnar joint (usually dorsal subluxation). If there are no contraindications, the recommended treatment in the adult for either fracture is closed reduction of the dislocation, with ORIF of the fracture. If the distal radio-ulnar joint is unstable following plating of the radius in a Galeazzi fracture, ORIF of the ulnar styloid fragment, if present, should be performed. If no such fragment is present, some physicians recommend maintaining the radio-ulnar reduction with a K-wire or pin despite the risk of synostosis formation. Often, the distal radio-ulnar joint will reduce with appropriate forearm pronation or supination. Pediatric Monteggia or Galeazzi fractures can often be treated with closed reduction.

It is imperative in forearm fractures that both the wrist and elbow be radiographed. Dislocation at one joint does not preclude concomitant dislocation at the other joint. Such a case would imply a complete disruption of the interosseous membrane and a severely unstable fracture.

Both-Bones Forearm[12,14]

Both-bone fractures of the forearm are concurrent fractures of the shafts of the radius and ulna. In the adult, treatment is ORIF of both fractures, usually with 3.5 mm plates and screws and six cortices on each side of the fracture on each bone.

The ulna is subcutaneous in the forearm and a plate can easily be applied beneath the ECU or FCU. Care must be taken to avoid injury to the dorsal cutaneous branch of the ulnar nerve in the distal third of the ulna.

The anterior (Henry) approach is best for proximal and distal third fractures of the radius. Proximally, one supinates the forearm and must initially look for the lateral antebrachial cutaneous nerve. One then passes medial to the brachioradialis and lateral to the biceps and brachialis. The lacertus fibrosis is divided and the radial nerve is visualized. The supinator muscle is then dissected off the proximal radius with the forearm completely supinated, in order to protect the posterior interosseous nerve.

Distally, one approaches the radius anteriorly between the brachioradialis and the FCR. One must then pronate the forearm and remove the origins of the pronator quadratus and the FPL from the lateral aspect of the radius. The superficial radial nerve runs with the brachioradialis just posterior to it.

The dorsolateral (Thompson) approach provides excellent exposure of the proximal and middle radius. The interval is between the mobile wad (ECRB) and the ECU. Proximally, the supinator must be carefully elevated off the radius in order to avoid damage to the posterior interosseus nerve.

Olecranon[12,13]

Olecranon fractures will often be displaced because of the pull of the triceps on the proximal fragment. Nondisplaced fractures (<2 mm displacement) with an intact extensor mechanism, although uncommon, can be treated closed in a long arm cast with the elbow in 90 degrees of flexion for 3–4 weeks, followed by functional bracing to allow elbow motion. The elbow cannot remain immobilized for more than a few weeks because of the risk of motion loss.

Simple transverse intraarticular fractures are treated with ORIF using tension-band wire techniques. Eighteen- or twenty-gauge wire is used with either two parallel K-wires or a pre-tapped 4.5 or a 6.5 cancellous intramedullary screw with a washer. The K-wires should penetrate the anterior cortex on their distal end for better fixation. The wire should pass anterior to the triceps proximally and form a figure-8 crossing over the posterior cortex of the ulna before looping through the posterior half of the ulna distally. This hardware often requires removal following fracture healing.

Two-part oblique fractures extending into the radial notch or the coronoid process are often best treated with a lag screw and compression or neutralization plating. Displaced comminuted fractures that extend to and include the coronoid process are not amenable to tension-band wiring. These challenging fractures are typically plated and often require bone grafting.

An alternative treatment for comminuted fractures of the olecranon is excision of the proximal fragment and triceps advancement. Some experts think that up to 50% of the olecranon can be excised without loss of elbow stability. This method is not appropriate for fractures associated with elbow instability, coronoid avulsion, and comminution extending to the distal part of the olecranon. This procedure is advised only for older patients with low functional demands.

Radial Head[12,13]

Radial head fractures are frequent injuries. These fractures often coexist with other injuries and are thought to occur during a fall on an outstretched hand with the forearm in pronation.

Radial head fractures with minimal or no displacement can be treated with early mobilization if they are stable and have a near normal ROM without an obvious mechanical block. A radial head fracture is stable if it involves <1/3 of the articular surface, is angulated <30 degrees, and is displaced <3 mm. If the injury meets these radiographic criteria, the physician must then aspirate the joint and then inject 2–3 cc of lidocaine in order to rule out a mechanical block to motion. If the patient has a near normal ROM, the elbow should be splinted for 1–2 weeks, followed by continued protection for a few weeks with range of motion exercises.

Displaced two-part fractures are preferably treated by ORIF through the ECU/anconeus interval using 2.0 or 2.7 mm screws (some suggest self-compressing Herbert screws). Cancellous bone graft is suggested if correction of an impacted articular fragment leaves a bony defect. If internal fixation is not possible, fragment excision is a possibility if the fragment involves less than one-third of the articular surface. If the displaced fragment is large or there is extensive comminution, using a minifragment plate is often preferable to prosthetic replacement of the head. The posterior interosseus nerve is at risk during plate fixation. If substantial comminution is present, prosthetic replacement of the radial head is probably the best option. If the medial collateral ligament has been injured, it needs to be repaired to stabilize the elbow.

Radial head excision has been associated with proximal migration of the radius and a reduction in grip strength. Excision is not a good option if medial collateral ligament instability or disruption of the distal radioulnar joint (Essex-Lopresti lesion) is noted. The DRUJ can often be reduced by splinting the forearm in a supinated position. Pinning the DRUJ is to be avoided, if possible, because of the risk of synostosis.

Distal Humerus (Intraarticular)[12]

Distal humerus fractures are relatively uncommon in the adult. Many surgeons have started to describe these injuries as single- or bicolumn fractures instead of the traditional condylar, transcondylar, and bicondylar fractures. Single-column injuries are divided into their medial and lateral locations. Bicolumn fractures are divided into T, Y, H, and lambda patterns. One should also look for capitellum and trochlear fractures in order to be complete. Fractures that are more distal tend to be more difficult to handle. These are complex fractures that are not infrequently associated with neurologic or vascular injuries. Bicolumn fractures are the most common fracture of the distal humerus. They are also the most complicated and are associated with the highest morbidity.

Nondisplaced fractures are treated with immobilization in a long arm cast for 3–4 weeks, followed by protected motion. If possible, displaced fractures should be treated by ORIF, followed by early motion postoperatively. If possible, the patient is placed prone and a posterior approach is used. An olecranon osteotomy that is later fixed with a 6.5 mm cancellous screw and a tension band is often used for improved exposure. Two 3.5 mm plates, a dynamic compression plate posterolaterally and a pelvic reconstruction plate medially, offer good fixation. One or two bicondylar screws are often necessary, depending on the fracture pattern. An anterior subcutaneous ulnar nerve transposition is frequently performed following skeletal fixation. Up to 20% of patients will have temporary ulnar nerve dysfunction postop. CPM (continuous passive motion) is not recommended postop; instead, passive and active assisted ROM exercises by a therapist are preferred. Heterotopic bone formation is associated with delayed fixation and closed head injuries. Treatment with Indocin should be considered in those circumstances.

If for some reason the patient is not able to tolerate a long, involved peripheral surgical procedure (e.g., polytrauma), closed reduction may be considered and the arm splinted with 90 degrees of elbow flexion. If closed reduction cannot be performed, overhead traction can be considered. This can be performed using skin traction or skeletal traction through the olecranon (pin placed medially and exits laterally).

Humeral Shaft[12,13,14]

Humeral shaft fractures can almost always be treated closed with an expected union rate of 90%–100%. The direction of angulation is variable depending on the anatomic location of the fracture and the muscular forces at work. The treating physician must decide if the fracture is above the insertion of the pectoralis major, between the pectoralis major and deltoid insertions, or distal to the deltoid insertion prior to reduction attempt. Studies have shown that the humerus can heal in 30 degrees of varus and 20 degrees of anterior angulation and be acceptable owing to the large range of motion of the shoulder. Additionally, up to 3 cm of shortening is tolerated without notable functional deficit. However, greater deformity indicates the need for operative intervention.

Immobilization can be of various types. Initial treatment in a coaptation splint is often adequate and keeps the patient comfortable for the first 7–10 days. After the swelling decreases, a prefabricated functional (Sarmiento) brace allows compression of the fracture by the soft-tissue envelope, maintaining the reduction and allowing elbow motion. The patient should perform triceps/brachialis isometric exercises and elbow and shoulder range-of-motion exercises as tolerated. Union typically occurs in 10–12 weeks.

Operative indications include failed closed reduction, concomitant intraarticular fractures, neurovascular injuries (see below), ipsilateral forearm fractures (''floating elbow''), impending fracture in pathologic bone, polytrauma, and segmental fractures. A transverse or oblique fracture in an active individual is a relative indication. Fractures associated with brachial plexus injuries tend to have higher rates of nonunion than normal when treated closed. Additionally, periprosthetic fractures or fractures with ipsilateral shoulder or elbow fusions require anatomic reduction and fixation. Fixation can be attained using an intramedullary rod, plates and screws, or an external fixation device.

Radial nerve palsy may occur in up to 18% of closed humeral shaft fractures and, of these, 90% will be because of a neuropraxia and will recover spontaneously. Therefore, the status of the radial nerve must always be evaluated and documented both before and after reduction of the fracture. A radial nerve palsy on presentation (as a consequence of the initial trauma) is not an indication to open the fracture and explore the nerve, since these virtually always resolve. However, normal radial nerve function prior to a reduction attempt followed by loss of radial nerve function after reduction is an indication to open the fracture site and explore the nerve.

If the radial nerve is out prior to a reduction attempt and a neuropraxia is suspected, one must immobilize the fracture appropriately and be sure to splint the wrist and thumb until nerve function returns for comfort and function. If there are no clinical signs of radial nerve recovery, either by physical examina-

tion or by electrodiagnostic studies, within 6 weeks, surgical exploration of the radial nerve is indicated.

Approaches for plating are anterolateral in the deltoid/bi-
ceps interval and then the biceps/brachialis interval in the proximal 2/3 of the shaft. In the distal 1/3 of the shaft, the interval
between the mobile wad and the triceps is used. Six cortices are
needed on each side of the fracture when plating an acute injury;
eight cortices are suggested if treating a nonunion. Intramedullary nails can be placed antegrade through the rotator cuff or
retrograde entering the bone 2.5 cm proximal to the olecranon fossa.

Proximal Humerus[12,13]

Proximal humerus fractures were classified by Neer in 1970 as
either nondisplaced, two-part, three-part, or four-part fractures.
The parts involved are the greater and lesser tuberosities, humeral
shaft, and humeral head. The fracture between the shaft and
head can occur either at the surgical or anatomic neck. The
classification originally required that a fragment be displaced
1 cm or angulated 45 degrees in order to be considered displaced.
Today, most shoulder surgeons recognize any fragment displacement in the grouping of these fractures. It is important to obtain
at least an A-P and an axillary lateral to evaluate the fracture and
to rule out a humeral head dislocation and a glenoid rim fracture.
A CT scan with reconstructed images is often very helpful in
planning operative fixation.

These injuries are often associated with avascular necrosis
because of blood vessel damage at the time of injury or during
operative intervention. The anterior and posterior humeral circumflex arteries supply the humeral head. The arcuate branch
of the anterior humeral circumflex supplies blood to the greater
tuberosity. Neurological injuries to the axillary, suprascapular,
and musculocutaneous nerves are typically neuropraxias and
should be treated conservatively unless the nerve deficit follows
a reduction attempt.

Nondisplaced fractures can be treated with a shoulder immobilizer, followed by early motion when the pain subsides. Two-
part fractures include: 1) fracture at the surgical neck; 2) fracture
at the anatomic neck; 3) avulsion of the greater tuberosity; and
4) avulsion of the lesser tuberosity (very rare as an isolated injury).

Fracture at the surgical neck can usually be treated by closed reduction, if needed, followed by placement in a shoulder immobilizer. Early motion should be started once the patient is able to tolerate it (around 3–4 weeks). If the fracture is unstable, closed reduction and percutaneous pinning with 2.5 mm pins is a good option. Polytrauma patients may be best treated with a 4.5 mm L-plate through a deltopectoral approach. This will allow the patient to use the extremity for support for ambulation with crutches or a walker sooner than other modalities.

Fracture of the anatomic neck is quite rare by itself but is difficult to treat and has a high risk of avascular necrosis of the humeral head. Adequate screw fixation is difficult to obtain, and many consider hemiarthroplasty to be a more reliable result in older patients.

Greater tuberosity fractures that are displaced more than 5 mm will usually cause problems with subacromial impingement, so this fracture is typically treated with internal fixation. The approach is usually through the deltoid (the axillary n. passes 5 cm inferior to the acromion), and screw fixation with a tension band of nonabsorbable suture is used. Some surgeons prefer a deltopectoral groove approach. Additionally, one should be aware that an isolated two-part fracture involving a tuberosity is often accompanied by a shoulder dislocation. In fact, in two-part fractures involving the lesser tuberosity, a posterior dislocation should be taken for granted until imaging studies can disprove it. Greater tuberosity fractures are typically associated with anterior dislocations.

Three-part fractures can include various combinations of any of the above four injuries. If significantly displaced, the age of the patient becomes critical. In a young patient, adequate closed reduction is usually not possible and ORIF of the fracture is indicated. The technique is similar to that mentioned for surgical neck fractures. It is important to tension band even minimally displaced tuberosity fractures to increase stability. In the elderly, a humeral head hemiarthroplasty is usually the procedure of choice.

Four-part fractures usually occur in very osteoporotic bone and are uncommon except in the elderly. Recommended treatment is insertion of a humeral head prosthesis. The greater and lesser tuberosities are attached to the prosthesis by wires and nonabsorbable suture in effort to create a functional rotator cuff.

ORIF may be attempted in younger patients, but the risk of AVN is great unless the surgical neck fracture is impacted in valgus. In those four-part fractures, the rate of AVN is reduced somewhat. Patients will normally have no functional deficit after union. Unfortunately, an unsightly bump or asymmetry of the clavicles may disturb some patients. Nonunions are treated with plating with or without bone graft.

Clavicle[14]

Clavicle fractures can be classified according to their location—medial third, middle third, or lateral third. Nearly all of the these fractures are treated by closed means. Even severely displaced fractures will usually heal. The traditionally recommended treatment was a figure-8 brace to depress the medial fragment, which is usually elevated by the pull of the sternocleidomastoid muscle. New studies are showing that treatment in a simple arm sling may improve outcome in adults. Some lateral third clavicle fractures will be unstable and require fixation (Rockwood screw or Mersilene tape). These fractures are typically just medial to the coracoclavicular ligaments.

Upper Cervical Spine[12,13]

Fractures of the upper cervical vertebrae can be of several types. Recognition of fracture stability is of critical importance because of possible disastrous neurologic complications.

A Jefferson fracture is a burst fracture of the ring of C1 (atlas) and is usually caused by an axial load to the top of the patient's head. Other types of atlas fractures include posterior arch, anterior arch, lateral mass, transverse process, and inferior tubercle avulsion fractures. These fractures do not impinge on the spinal canal and most patients are neurologically intact unless they are seen in association with an odontoid fracture or rupture of the transverse atlantal ligament. An atlantoaxial offset of >6.9 mm on an open mouth view or an atlantodental interval (ADI) of >3 mm in adults (or 5 mm in children) on lateral view indicates a likely rupture of the transverse ligaments. If the ADI is >5 mm, the accessory ligaments are also thought to be incompetent. Posterior arch fractures can sometimes be treated with a Philadelphia collar. The other injuries require halo immobilization for 2–3 months unless there is radiographic evidence of transverse ligament damage. An atlas fracture with transverse ligament damage usually requires C1–2 fusion. A "wink" sign on the open mouth (dens) view is indicative of rotary subluxation of the atlas on the odontoid. This injury requires C1–2 arthrodesis for stabilization.

Fractures of the odontoid (dens) make up 7%–14% of cervical fractures and are classified as follows (included in parentheses are the relative frequencies):

Type I (10%)—avulsion fracture of the superior tip
Type II (60%)—fracture through the isthmus of the odontoid
Type III (30%)— fracture extending into the body of C2

Type I fractures are usually stable and require only a brief period of collar immobilization. Larger displaced avulsion fractures could result in instability because of incompetence of the alar and transverse ligaments that may be attached to the fragment. Treatment of Type II and III fractures are more controversial because of relatively high rates of malunion or nonunion. Factors predisposing to these poor outcomes include displacement >4–5 mm, age >40, improper immobilization (halo immobilization is recommended), and angulation >10 degrees. Union rates for Type II and III fractures with halo immobilization have been reported between 66% and 80%. On the other hand, posterior fusion of C1 to C2 is successful 96%–100% of the time. Type III fractures were previously thought to do well with conservative therapy, but recent studies have shown them to be quite problematic, especially if displaced or angulated.

A Hangman's fracture is a fracture through the pedicles of C2. The patient, if alive, is usually neurologically intact. The fracture is usually produced by an axial load to the head with the neck in an extended position. Treatment is immobilization in halo collar and jacket.

Lower Cervical Spine[12,13]

Fractures in this region of the spine are caused by excessive flexion, flexion-rotation, axial load, and extension. A common injury mechanism in the lower cervical spine is axial compression with the neck flexed, causing what is known as a "teardrop fracture." Radiographically, the fracture is a small, triangular fragment at the antero-inferior margin of the vertebral body, similar in appearance to a teardrop. The name is also derived because the fracture is commonly associated with the devastating complication of immediate quadriplegia. Treatment is by halo collar and traction for closed reduction, if necessary, followed by immobilization in a halo jacket for 3 months.

Flexion-rotation injuries to the cervical spine can cause facet dislocation with or without fracture of the facet articular surface. In this injury, the facet joints dislocate (''jump'' over one another) and become locked. Consequently, the injury is often described as jump-locked facets. The dislocation may be either unilateral or bilateral. If the dislocation is not complete, the facets may be said to be ''perched'' upon one another. Unfortunately, as one might expect, neurologic injuries are common with this injury. Unilateral jump-locked facets have a better prognosis, since the vertebral body cannot subluxate forward more than 25% of the disk space, resulting in less cord impingement. Bilateral jump-locked facets usually cause at least 50% subluxation of the vertebral body. Severe damage to the cord results unless the patient has an unusually large spinal canal.

Treatment of jump-locked or perched facets is reduction by halo traction and then placement of a halo jacket. The patient must be admitted to an intensive care unit or at least a setting with one-to-one nursing care to monitor his neurologic status. Traction is applied using 10 pounds to counteract the weight of the head, and 5 pounds for each inter-space involved, starting with no more than 20 pounds. After placement of the weight, a STAT lateral cervical radiograph and full neurologic examination is mandatory. If reduction does not occur, weight is then added in 5-pound increments, in approximate half-hour intervals, being certain to repeat the lateral radiograph and the neurologic examination after each weight increase. One should obviously remove the recently applied weight if any further neurologic compromise is noted on physical examination.

If reduction does not occur after using 50–60 pounds (depending on the level), most spine surgeons recommend open reduction and fusion. If closed reduction is achieved, a halo vest is applied, traction is released and another radiograph and neurological examination are performed. This is followed by 3 months of immobilization if there is no fracture. If a facet fracture is present, most recommend posterior fusion because conservative treatment has been associated with late instability. Closed reduction of bilateral jumped facets should be performed on an emergency basis. This is generally easier than reduction of unilateral jumped facets because essentially all of the posterior ligamentous support has been disrupted. In unilateral injuries, a portion of the PLL remains intact. Following closed treatment of bilateral jumped facets, an MRI is performed emergently to rule out compression of the cord by anterior elements. If there is compression anteriorly, a discectomy with anterior decompression and fusion is required. If the MRI is negative, a posterior fusion is performed.

Burst fractures involve the middle column (see Denis three-column classification under thoracolumbar spine) and often result in some retropulsion of the vertebral body into the spinal canal. These injuries occur in the cervical spine during diving or athletic accidents that result in a large axial load while the neck is in slight flexion or extension. Retropulsion of all or part of the vertebral body into the spinal canal is common and must be evaluated by CT or MRI. If the posterior elements of the spine are stable and the patient is neurologically intact, treatment can be closed reduction and halo vest immobilization for 3 months. Associated nerve or spinal cord injuries require emergent attention and closed reduction using cervical traction. If the posterior elements are intact radiographically, corpectomy and strut graft fusion are indicated. If the posterior elements are unstable, posterior fusion should precede corpectomy/strut graft fusion.

Simple compression fractures (involving only the anterior half of the vertebral body) and isolated fractures of the lamina, posterolateral pillars, or spinous processes are thought to be stable fractures and can typically be treated with a Philadelphia collar. One should remember to obtain flexion extension views prior to discontinuing the collar in order to rule out ligamentous instability.

Penetrating injuries to the cervical spine can usually be treated with local wound care and a Philadelphia collar. However, if the penetrating trauma passed through the pharynx, aggressive debridement should be performed and intravenous antibiotics administered.

Caution in handling a patient with a suspected cervical spine injury is critical. This is discussed in Chapter 5. A full radiographic evaluation of the cervical spine includes A-P, lateral, obliques, and open-mouth odontoid views. It is mandatory that the lateral view visualize the top of the T1 vertebral body. Otherwise, fractures or dislocations of lower vertebrae may be missed. When one cervical fracture is identified, there is a 10%–20% incidence of a second fracture in the neck. The lateral radiograph must be closely inspected to rule out excessive translation (listhesis), kyphosis, angulation, and vertebral height loss. The anterior and posterior cortices, the spinolaminar junction, and the posterior spinous processes should all line up to form gentle curves without interruption. If the soft tissues anterior to C3–4 are >7 mm in width or the soft tissues anterior to C7 are >14 mm in the adult or >21 mm in the child, excessive swelling exists indicating significant trauma. Routine obliques are normally performed by rolling the patient on his side. Therefore, when obtaining oblique radiographs prior to C-spine clearance, be sure to keep the patient supine and have the radiologic technician angle the beam to obtain views that are termed "trauma obliques." If a fracture is discovered on plain films, a CT scan with three-dimensional reconstructions using 1.5 mm cuts is usually required to further identify the fracture anatomy.

Ligamentous instability of the cervical spine can be as dangerous as osseous instability. When no fracture is identified, translation of two adjacent vertebral bodies by more than 3.5 mm on the lateral radiograph is indicative of significant ligamentous instability. On the lateral radiograph, angulation between the inferior borders of two adjacent vertebral bodies of more than 11 degrees compared with adjacent levels is also consistent with ligamentous instability. This angulation must be compared with neighboring interspaces for correct interpretation because of the natural lordosis of the cervical spine. An example is shown in Figure 6.15. Ligamentous instability is treated with posterior fusion with interspinous wiring, since several series have demonstrated late displacement and/or painful instability following treatment with only cervical orthosis or halo immobilization.

Often, no fracture or ligamentous injury can be seen on the radiographs, but cervical spine pain persists. In these cases, lateral flexion-extension views of the cervical spine can be performed to rule out instability if the patient is neurologically intact, alert, and capable of cooperating. Under no circumstances should the physician or any health-care provider move the patient's neck for the patient. The neck motion must be an active movement by the patient only. If there is too much pain or spasm to allow

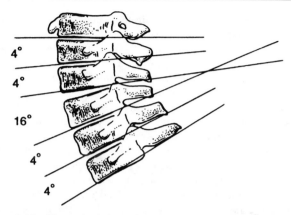

Figure 6.15. The method of evaluating ligamentous instability of the cervical spine by measuring the angle between the lower borders of adjacent cervical vertebrae.

these views, presumptive evidence of soft-tissue injury exists and the patient should be placed in a semirigid (Phiadelphia) collar until the pain has subsided enough to allow adequate flexion-extension views. This means that patients will often be sent home in a Philadelphia collar for 7–10 days prior to returning for repeat flexion-extension views.

Thoracolumbar Spine[12,15,16]

Thoracolumbar spine fractures are often discussed in terms of the three-column spine concept of Denis. In this classification, the anterior one-half of the vertebral body constitutes the anterior column, the posterior one-half of the vertebral body constitutes the middle column, and the posterior elements (lamina, pedicles, processes) constitute the posterior column.

Compression fractures involve only the anterior column and are, as the name implies, noted by seeing compression of the anterior margin (occasionally, the lateral margin) of the vertebral body. These are usually stable fractures and can be treated by bed rest and symptomatic treatment when there is no neurologic injury. A common complication of these fractures is an ileus, which should be watched for closely. These fractures are common in the elderly, with very osteoporotic bone. A compression fracture in a young, healthy person without significant trauma is highly suspicious of a pathologic fracture. One needs to be sure that the middle column is not involved in order to rule out a burst fracture. Sometimes this distinction is not clear on plain films, and a CT scan is required.

Burst fractures by definition involve the middle column. Radiographically, they are diagnosed by seeing either widening of the pedicles on the A-P radiograph, or posterior displacement of the posterior border of the vertebral body on the lateral radiograph. A CT scan is needed to further evaluate the fracture anatomy when plain films are suggestive of a burst fracture. These injuries are caused by a large axial load (often MVAs) and are often associated with neurologic injury. They are most common in the thoracolumbar region (L1 bursts are the most frequent), and usually require surgical stabilization. Surgical indications are canal compromise >40%–50%, kyphosis >25 degrees at the injury level, and/or neurological deficit. As little as 8–10 degrees of kyphosis is poorly tolerated in the lower lumbar spine (L3–5) and operative stabilization may be required to prevent disability. Fusion in adults is typically required from one level above the injury to two levels below. Nonoperative treatment includes wearing a TLSO for at least 3 months. Thoracic burst fractures are rare, but when they do occur, they are invariably accompanied by neurologic damage because of the relatively small size of the spinal canal in the thoracic spine.

Seat belt injuries are caused by flexion and distraction of the middle and posterior columns with the anterior column remaining intact and serving as a fulcrum for the forces. These forces may cause disruption of bone (Chance fracture), ligaments, or both. Chance fractures extending only through bone have an excellent prognosis and can often be treated with closed extension casting. Injuries involving only ligamentous damage are less predictable and typically require surgical stabilization.

Fracture-dislocation injuries involve a failure of all three columns owing to compression, rotation, tension, and shear forces. Surgery is required to at least stabilize these injuries. This type has the highest incidence of neurological deficit.

Acute spinal cord: injured patients who have complete or incomplete injuries should receive intravenous methylprednisolone if infusion can start within 8 hours of the injury and the patient meets exclusion criteria. Exclusion criteria include SCIs (spinal cord injuries) due to gunshot wounds, age <13, pregnancy, narcotic addiction, daily steroid use, associated life-threatening injury, and only nerve root or cauda equina involvement (use only on injuries above L2). Nearly all surgeons believe that steroids should be administered even if the patient uses narcotics or steroids. Many times, steroids will be given even if the injury was caused by a gunshot. A 30 mg/kg bolus is given initially and this is followed by 5.4 mg/kg maintenance for 23 hours.

Pelvic Fractures[12,14]

Pelvic fractures vary from the most innocuous of fractures to those possessing the highest mortality rates of any skeletal injury. Pelvic fractures are best classified as either stable or unstable. Features that make a pelvic fracture unstable are widening of the pubic symphysis by more than 2.5 cm, disruption of the posterior sacroiliac ligaments (the strongest ligaments in the body), or two breaks in the pelvic ring. Radiographically, an A-P pelvis is essential initially, and, when the patient is stable, specialized inlet-outlet views (assess pelvic ring), Judet views (iliac and obturator obliques to evaluate the anterior and posterior columns), and often CT imaging are needed for proper assessment and treatment planning. Unstable fractures generally require open reduction and internal fixation.

Unstable pelvic fractures are associated with high morbidity and mortality because the force necessary to create them also causes a significant amount of soft-tissue damage. These patients will frequently present with major head, chest, and abdominal trauma, as well as other extremity injuries. Pelvic hemorrhage (usually the venous plexus in the posterior pelvis) associated with a pelvic fracture can be life-threatening. Exploration to control bleeding is indicated only as a last resort for two reasons: 1) It is extremely difficult to find and ligate a single source of bleeding, and 2) exploration often makes the situation worse by disrupting the tamponade caused by the expanding hematoma in a somewhat limited space. In most cases, adequate control of bleeding can be achieved by application of an anterior or posterior external fixator to assist in reduction of the displaced fracture. This compresses the two hemipelves and decreases the intrapelvic volume, subsequently increasing the tamponade effect. In addition to hemorrhage, these patients often also sustain urogenital injuries, rectal tears, and damage to the lumbosacral plexus. Occasionally, a proctoscope or a retrograde urological study will need to be performed. Adequate radiographs should be obtained prior to these studies since residual dye can obscure bony detail.

Physical examination of the pelvis is extremely important. One must rule out obvious deformity or leg length discrepencies that may be caused by a pelvic fracture. One must carefully evaluate the skin both anteriorly and posteriorly. Some types of fractures may necessitate a rectal examination to ensure that a fracture is not exposed to rectal contents.

Following an A-P pelvis, inlet-outlet and Judet views are ordered. An inlet view is an A-P radiograph performed with the patient supine and the radiographic beam directed from the patient's head toward the pelvis. This view demonstrates any breaks in the pelvic brim and any A-P translation at the SI joints posteriorly or around the pubic rami anteriorly. The sacral ala and body are easily seen. Rotational and impaction deformities of the sacrum or ilium can also be visualized. The outlet view is another A-P radiograph taken with the beam angled cephalad from the feet. This view is useful for evaluating superior rotation or vertical displacement of a hemipelvis. The sacral foramina can also be seen. Judet views (iliac and obturator obliques) are A-P radiographs taken at 45-degree angles to the patient. The iliac oblique demonstrates a wide view of the ilium and also allows evaluation of the ipsilateral posterior column of the pelvis and the anterior lip of the acetabulum. The obturator oblique view is recognizable because it shows the obturator foramen at its widest angle. This radiograph allows assessment of the anterior column and the posterior lip of the acetabulum. CT scans allow for easy assessment of the sacrum, SI joints, and the acetabulum. Three-dimensional reconstructions are extremely valuable in preoperative planning.

There are several classification schemes for fractures of the pelvic ring. Anterior posterior compression injuries typically result from MVAs, while falls from heights tend to cause lateral compression and shear injuries. Tile's classification is the most frequently used. It combines injury mechanism and stability to determine treatment options and prognosis. Type A injuries are stable, and fractures are minimally displaced. Treatment is symptomatic, and prognosis is good. Type B fractures are rotationally unstable or displaced but are vertically stable. The sacrotuberous and the posterior longitudial ligaments remain intact. Type C injuries are vertically, posteriorly, and rotationally unstable and involve complete disruption of the posterior osseous and/or ligamentous structures. Most B and all C injuries will require ORIF or external fixation. These procedures are scheduled 2–3 days following the injury to allow for patient rescuscitation and preop planning.

Acetabular Fractures[12,14]

Acetabular fractures are typically seen in young adults involved in motor vehicle accidents. Virtually any displacement and subsequent incongruity in the articular surface can lead to increased cartilage breakdown and early posttraumatic arthritis. Surgical treatment of these fractures is nearly always indicated in effort to restore the articular surface unless the patient is elderly and would be better treated with a hip replacement if he or she developed posttraumatic osteoarthritis following union.

The fracture is usually noted on an A-P pelvis and is the further evaluated by obturator and iliac oblique views. A CT scan (1.5–3 mm cuts usually with three-dimensional reconstruction) is then performed to further elucidate the fracture pattern. Surgery is often performed 2–3 days following the injury, allowing time for intrapelvic bleeding to subside and giving time for adequate preoperative planning. During this preoperative interval, skeletal traction is usually employed, especially if there is any hip instability. Lateral traction through the greater trochanter is generally not indicated. Buck's traction is often used merely for patient comfort.

The five simple fracture types described by Letournel include fractures of the posterior wall, posterior column, anterior wall, anterior column, and transverse fractures. Other fracture patterns include associated posterior column and posterior wall, associated transverse and posterior wall, T-shaped, associated anterior column and posterior hemitransverse, and both column fractures.

In describing these fractures, one should know that the anterior column consists of the anterior border of the iliac wing, the entire pelvic brim, the anterior wall of the acetabulum, and the superior pubic ramus. The posterior column is the bony strut running from the posterior superior iliac spine to the ischial tuberosity and includes the posterior wall of the acetabulum.

Femoral Neck[12,13]

Femoral neck fractures generally occur in individuals >50 years old (>95%) and are associated with substantial rates of nonunion, avascular necrosis of the femoral head, and mortality. In two large series, the mortality rate in the month following femoral neck fracture was 13%–17% in males and 7%–10% in females. These fractures tend to occur more frequently in females than males (ratio of 3.4 to 1) and 90% of these fractures result from a fall from a standing position. It is important to know the patient's past medical history and the patient's preinjury ambulatory status. The physician should also ask if the patient experienced any pain in the days and weeks prior to the injury, as this can elucidate preexisting arthritis or possibly a pathologic lesion.

The bone density of the proximal femur declines with age, partially explaining why these low energy fractures occur primarily in the elderly. Other conditions such as surgical or biological menopause, steroids, barbiturates, and seizure medications have a detrimental effect on bone metabolism and likely decrease bone density. The Singh index grades proximal femoral osteopenia, with a normal appearing grade VI having well-defined primary and secondary tension and compression trabeculae. On the other end of the spectrum, a severely osteopenic grade I has only a few residual primary compression trabeculae.

The diagnosis is typically made with an A-P and cross-table lateral view of the hip. These fractures are best seen on an internal rotation A-P view of the hip. If the internal rotation view does not demonstrate a fracture in a patient who clinically appears to have one, an MRI should be obtained to rule out a nondisplaced fracture. Once the fracture is diagnosed, 5–10 pounds of Buck's traction will often decrease the patient's pain.

These fractures were previously grouped according to the Garden classification but are now generally classified as nondisplaced (Garden I and II) and displaced (Garden III and IV). Nondisplaced fractures include truly nondisplaced fractures and impacted valgus femoral neck fractures. Displaced fractures include all femoral neck fractures with any notable displacement.

Nonunion resulting in groin/thigh pain and frequently a Trendelenburg gait occurs 50%–60% of the time following treatment of a displaced fracture with traction or casting. Nonunion will occur in 15%–33% of these patients if treated with internal fixation (three threaded pins).

Femoral neck fractures can lead to avascular necrosis of the femoral head by causing an ischemic event. Revascularization follows, with consequent trabecular thinning and collapse. AVN occurs in 10%–15% of nondisplaced and 30%–35% of displaced fractures after pinning. AVN seems to be caused, in part, by arteriolar disruption secondary to fracture displacement and subsequent intracapsular tamponade. This happens frequently in the femoral head because of the tenuous blood supply to the region. The primary blood supply comes from the lateral epiphyseal artery, which is the terminal branch of the medial femoral circumflex artery. Blood is also supplied by the inferior metaphyseal artery, which is a branch of the lateral femoral circumflex artery. The third major blood supply of the femoral head is from the medial epiphyseal artery of the ligamentum teres that originates in the obturator arterial system. This artery typically flows into the lateral epiphyseal system. This anastomosis is thought to be responsible for head revascularization.

Treatment of nondisplaced (Garden I or II) femoral neck fractures is usually by fixation in situ using threaded pins. Three parallel pins are placed inferior to the greater trochanter into the femoral neck and advanced to within 5 mm of the articular surface of the femoral head. Most suggest fixing these fractures within 24 hours to reduce the likelihood of AVN. Internal fixation is recommended for all nondisplaced fractures of the femoral neck, and patients are mobilized on the day after surgery (touchdown weight bearing) to decrease mortality. Many laboratory papers support the concept of performing a capsulotomy to decrease intracapsular pressure and subsequently reduce the risk of AVN. Capsulotomy is not routinely performed at our institution. Treatment of displaced (Garden III or IV) femoral neck fractures depends, to a degree, on the age of the patient. In a relatively young patient, an attempt at closed reduction followed by pin fixation may be indicated. In older patients, treatment is usually insertion of a femoral head prosthesis. In patients with preexisting acetabular disease, primary total hip arthroplasty may be indicated. Deep venous thrombosis prophylaxis using medication (usually low molecular weight heparin) and intermittent compression devices, as well as early mobilization, are indicated for all femoral neck fractures.

Intertrochanteric Femur Fractures[12,13]

Intertrochanteric fractures occur with alarming frequency and, like femoral neck fractures, are typically seen in elderly women (2:1 compared with men) as a result of a fall. As in other hip fractures in the elderly, it is important to document preoperative ambulatory status and comorbidities. One should always look for pathologic fractures and make sure that the patient did not have a syncopal episode requiring medical workup. Physical examination frequently reveals the shortened, externally rotated lower extremity. A careful inspection of the skin is important in all patients but is essential in the elderly. A preoperative A-P pelvis and crosstable lateral usually demonstrate the fracture pattern sufficiently. If operative intervention is temporarily delayed, 5 pounds of Buck's traction will make the patient more comfortable.

These fractures are organized using the Evan's Classification system based on the presence or absence of displacement and the number of fragments. In this system, the primary fracture line runs between the lesser and greater trochanter. Increasing comminution involving either trochanteric region results in more instability and higher grade. Type I is an undisplaced two-part fracture, and type II is a displaced two-part fracture. These are both stable fractures. Type III refers to a displaced three-part fracture with posterolateral comminution. Type IV is a displaced three-part fracture with a large posteromedial comminuted fragment. Type V is a displaced four-part fracture with comminution involving both trochanters. Evan's placed reverse oblique intertrochanteric fractures in a special category. The precarious pattern of this fracture is not as stable with the fixation used for other fractures in this class.

Most intertrochanteric fractures are treated with closed reduction and internal fixation using a sliding compression screw system. These fractures are fixed on a fracture table and reduction involves longitudinal traction followed by varying amounts of internal rotation, depending on the fracture appearance using fluoroscopy. The implants available have neck shaft angles ranging from 130–150 degrees. The selection of an implant with a higher angle will fix the fracture in more valgus. This causes more compression and stability at the fracture site, but fixation can sometimes be difficult if too much valgus is selected. The compression screw enters the femur inferior to the greater trochanter and is threaded through a side plate, which is fixed to the proximal lateral femoral shaft. The compression screw works by its threads gaining purchase on the head and neck fragment, while being free to slide in the sleeve attached to the side plate. This allows compression at the fracture site while maintaining relative stability. Complete stability of the fracture depends on the quality of the cortical bone on the medial (especially posteromedial) aspect of the proximal femur. As in femoral neck fractures, the chance of fixation failure is increased with decreasing Singh grade. Patients are touchdown weight bearing on the day after surgery in effort to reduce morbidity.

Nonoperative treatment is sometimes recommended for nonambulatory demented patients who appear to be pain-free or for patients who are terminally ill (life expectancy <3 months).

Subtrochanteric Femur Fractures[12,13]

Subtrochanteric femur fractures account for 10%–34% of all hip fractures. They occur in a bimodal distribution, with a majority occurring in the elderly population as a result of low energy trauma (e.g., a fall from the standing position), but a large fraction (approximately $\frac{1}{4}$) result from high energy trauma (e.g., MVA) affecting people less than 50 years old. They are defined as any fracture occurring between the lesser trochanter and the isthmus of the femoral diaphysis.

Low energy fractures are often short, transverse, oblique, or spiral in appearance, while high energy injuries can be severely comminuted. The muscular attachments of the iliopsoas, gluteus medius and minimus, gluteus maximus and adductors all serve to displace and angulate the fracture fragments.

Several options for treatment exist including fixation with a sliding compression screw with a long side plate; a blade plate, which enters the femoral neck and attaches to a long side plate; flexible intramedullary nails; rigid intramedullary nails; and traction in the 90/90 degrees position. Another option is a rigid, crossed intramedullary nail device, the prototype of which is the Zickel nail.

The Russell-Taylor classification is relatively simple and provides an operative treatment algorithm. The A-P and lateral radiographs must be carefully evaluated to decide whether the fracture extends into the piriformis fossa and whether the lesser trochanter is fractured (i.e., is there excessive medial comminution?).

The piriformis fossa is intact in Type 1 fractures, and these can be treated with intramedullary nailing. If the lesser trochanter is intact (Type 1A), a conventional interlocking nail or a reconstruction nail may be used. If the lesser trochanter is not intact (Type 1B), a reconstruction nail is recommended.

The piriformis fossa is fractured in Type 2 fractures, and these must be treated with a hip compression screw and a long side plate. If the lesser trochanter is intact (Type 2A), no bone graft is required. If it is not (Type 2B), autogenous bone graft is recommended.

Femoral Shaft[12,13]

Femoral shaft fractures frequently result from high energy trauma. The Winquist classification describes the amount of comminution present at the fracture site.

0—no comminution
I—insignificant butterfly fragment, <25% shaft comminution
II—<50% shaft comminution
III—>50% shaft comminution
IV—comminuted, no continuous bone
V—segmental fracture with comminution

These fractures are typically treated with the insertion of a rigid intramedullary nail. This often allows for immediate mobilization of the patient and touchdown weight bearing on the injured extremity.

Preoperative evaluation includes a thorough trauma assessment. One must attempt to assess the stability of the knee to rule out a knee dislocation that was reduced in the field. Distal neurovascular status must also be documented. Radiographs should include an A-P and lateral of the femur and knee, an A-P pelvis, and an internally rotated A-P of the ipsilateral femoral neck to rule out a nondisplaced fracture. If the femur fracture is comminuted with resultant shortening, an A-P of the contralateral femur should be obtained to template the expected nail length. If surgery is to be delayed more than a few hours, balanced skeletal traction should be applied with a traction pin through the proximal tibia unless the knee is thought to be unstable. It is important to provide nail fixation within 24–48 hours for these fractures to reduce pulmonary complications. Many trauma surgeons are nailing grade 3B and 3C open fractures on the night of admission to reduce pulmonary complications.

These patients are usually positioned supine on a fracture table using either a tibial traction pin or a traction boot. Some surgeons prefer to nail these fractures in the lateral position on a normal OR table. Fluoroscopic guidance is essential for finding the starting hole in the piriformis fossa, reducing the fracture, and placing distal interlocking screws. Both proximal and two distal interlocking screws are recommended except when the fracture is middle $\frac{1}{3}$ of the shaft and transverse without comminution. Surgeons are currently debating whether the femoral shaft should be reamed prior to nail insertion. Unreamed nails are quicker and may disrupt the intramedullary blood supply less. Reamed nails offer greater stability, since a nail of typically greater diameter is placed down a reamed canal of known diameter, offering a better fit.

In adults, a uniaxial (standard) external fixator or an Ilizarov fixator is rarely chosen when there is a relative contraindication to insertion of an IM nail. These include some grade III open fractures that are too contaminated and cannot be adequately debrided. Additionally, a fracture entering the piriformis fossa is a contraindication to an intramedullary nail, though, in these cases, a retrograde nail inserted through the knee could be used.

Supracondylar Femur[12,13]

These fractures are located in the transition zone beween the distal diaphysis and the articular surface of the femoral condyles. They occur in young adults as a result of high energy trauma and in the elderly following low energy trauma. In both groups, the knee is usually in a flexed position and sustains direct trauma. Supracondylar fractures characteristically deform with femoral shortening because of the proximal pull of the quadriceps and the hamstrings. The distal fragment is posteriorly angulated and displaced owing to the force of the gastrocnemius muscles. These fractures, especially the high energy ones, are often intraarticular.

These fractures are often associated with acetabular fractures, hip dislocations, femoral neck and shaft fractures, and ligamentous damage to the knee. Tibial plateau and femoral shaft fractures (resulting in a "floating knee") are not infrequent. The house officer needs to rule out these injuries on examination and radiographically (always image joints above and below a fracture). A careful vascular examination (pulses, ankle-brachial indices) is imperative because of the proximity of the adductor canal and because of the relative frequency of knee dislocations. If there is a possible arterial injury, an arteriogram is indicated unless the extremity is obviously pale and without blood supply. In these cases, the patient should be taken urgently to the OR for revascularization.

The Muller classification (an updated AO classification) divides these fractures into extraarticular (Type A), unicondylar (Type B), and bicondylar (Type C) fractures. Each of these types is further broken down into three subdivisions according to fracture location for Type B and amount of comminution for Types A and C. Obviously, intraarticular and/or bicondylar involvement, and increased comminution are indicative of increased severity and poorer prognosis.

Oblique views of the fracture are often helpful, and, when there is metaphyseal comminution, an A-P and lateral with traction can help in fracture reduction. A CT scan can be beneficial when the fracture is intraarticular.

Except in the very elderly, all of these fractures are usually treated with internal fixation. Several methods of fixation exist for this fracture including a 95-degree condylar blade plate; a dynamic compression screw (DCS) and side plate; a condylar buttress plate; occasionally, a retrograde interlocked intramedullary nail; a Zickel supracondylar device, and flexible nails. External fixation is usually reserved for treatment of grade III open fractures.

A DCS with a 95-degree side plate through a lateral approach is a relatively simple, stable way to fix these fractures. If the fracture extends into the condyles, two partially threaded cancellous screws are placed prior to compression screw placement. The main advantage of this system over a blade plate is that is easier to adjust the flexion and extension of the plate while using the DCS. Additionally, placement of the screw is less traumatic, since the blade plate has to be hammered into position. If too much comminution exists, a condylar buttress plate offers adequate fixation though less ability to resist varus angulation than the DCS or the blade plate.

A retrograde (Seligson) nail is sometimes appropriate for extraarticular fractures and some bicondylar fractures that are stabilized with cancellous screws distally but that also have proximal extension. This fixation is also sometimes used for fixing periprosthetic fractures proximal to the femoral component of a total knee replacement. A medial parapatellar approach is utilized and the reamer is inserted in the intercondylar notch of the femur. These nails are also used when one has a "floating knee," so both the femoral and tibial fractures can be fixed through the same wound. Tibial and femoral nails have been used retrograde with success to treat fractures with extreme proximal extension. The Seligson nail is only 250 mm long.

Type B fractures are unicondylar and are usually treated with a partially threaded cancellous screw or a Herbert screw. One must be on the lookout for the Hoffa fracture, which is a unicondylar fracture in which the fracture line passes in the frontal plane and can be easily missed.

Massive comminution or severe osteopenia is sometimes an indication for skeletal traction followed by application of a cast brace with early motion. If surgery is to be delayed more than a few hours, a tibial traction pin should be inserted 10 cm distal to the tibial tubercle to avoid contamination of the operative field. The patient should then be placed in balanced skeletal traction.

Patella[14,17]

Simple patellar fractures can be stellate, transverse, and vertical in orientation. Stellate fractures are usually the result of a direct blow, while transverse ones are caused by a tensile stress applied to the extensor mechanism. The mechanism of vertical fractures is a little less clear. A-P, lateral, and (sometimes) sunrise views should be obtained. A bipartite patella should not be misdiagnosed as a fracture. Bipartite patellas are often bilateral, and the ossicles are typically in the superolateral corner of the patella. Bilateral radiographs and close scrutiny of the radiographs should make the diagnosis.

Nonoperative fractures may have no fragment displaced or translated more than 3 mm, and active knee extension must be intact. There may not be >2 mm articular stepoff on the lateral film. These can be treated in a cylinder cast or brace with the knee in extension for 4–6 weeks. Progressive active flexion is started at that time.

Displaced fractures are divided into noncomminuted and comminuted fractures. Noncomminuted fractures are further broken down into transverse (fracture is located at the patellar equator) and polar (referring to fractures occurring proximal or distal to the equator). Comminuted fractures are divided into stellate, transverse, polar, and a highly comminuted and displaced group. Most of these fractures are transverse and are repaired using some type of anterior tension band wiring with K-wires or screws with 18-gauge wire. In some of the polar fractures, a partial patellectomy may be performed, with direct repair of the tendon to remaining patella through drill holes using #2 or #5 nonabsorbable suture. In highly comminuted and displaced fractures, total patellectomy is sometimes the best option, though approximately $\frac{1}{3}$ of the quadriceps' strength is lost and an extension lag nearly always occurs. The goal of surgical intervention is to reconstruct the extensor mechanism and the articular surface. Fixation should be stable enough to allow early motion.

Tibial Plateau[12,13]

Tibial plateau fractures occur because of a medially directed, a laterally directed, or an axially compressive force, or a combination of a force from the side and an axial load. These fractures can be associated with collateral and cruciate ligament damage, peroneal nerve injury (especially laterally directed forces), vascular insult, and compartment syndromes. Arterial injuries are more frequent with the higher energy Type IV, V, and VI fractures. The soft tissues of the proximal tibia must be carefully examined, since they will certainly affect treatment. Normal A-P and lateral radiographs often need to be supplemented with oblique views that are angled 10 degrees caudad in effort to compensate for posterior slope. Traction radiographs are often helpful. Operative cases often need either tomograms or a CT scan with reconstructed images. Tibial plateau fractures are classified by Schatzker into six groups (Fig. 6.16).

Type I—split wedge fx of the lateral plateau
Type II —split depression fx of the lateral plateau

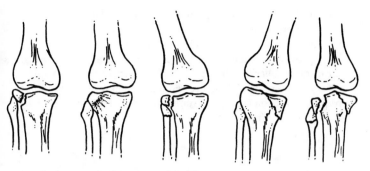

Figure 6.16. Tibial plateau fractures.

Type III—pure depression fx, varying location
Type IV— fx of the medial plateau
Type V—bicondylar fracture
Type VI—an additional metaphyeal fx separating the plateau fx
    and the shaft

Treatment of these fractures is not specifically related to the classification. Instead, the key factors are the age and functional level of the patient, the joint stability, the articular surface congruence, and the axial alignment. Depression of a portion of the articular surface of more than 4 mm is usually treated by open reduction with elevation of the fragments, bone grafting the resulting defect, and some form of fixation (usually T- or L-buttress plates and screws). Strong consideration for ORIF should be given if there is >10 degrees of varus/valgus instability. Intraoperative fracture distraction by an external fixator is often helpful. The approach is determined by the location of the fracture. The meniscus is also injured in nearly 50% of these fractures. The meniscus often has to be elevated during the arthrotomy for fracture exposure. One has to be careful to preserve and possibly repair the structure after fracture reduction.

When open reduction is indicated but has to be postponed or cannot be performed for whatever reason, the fracture should be treated with skeletal traction and early motion. Minimally displaced fractures are usually treated in a long leg cast with weight bearing delayed until fracture healing is present radiographically. In elderly patients, the fracture may be treated closed initially and a total knee replacement performed if posttraumatic osteoarthritis results.

Ring external fixators, including the new hybrid fixators, can often provide excellent stability for fractures that are too proximal for intramedullary nailing (proximal one-fifth of the tibia). Olive wires can be used for fracture reduction. These fixators do not require soft-tissue stripping (unlike plating) and are especially useful in open injuries.

Tibial Shaft[12–14]

Tibia fractures occur several times more frequently than femoral fractures. These fractures can be extremely serious because of the tibia's subcutaneous location and its proximity to neurovascular structures. Tibia fractures are frequently seen in polytrauma patients and are often open fractures. They are sometimes associated with ipsilateral femoral shaft fractures ("floating knee"), knee ligament damage, arterial injury above and below the popliteal trifurcation, and compartment syndromes. The most important factor in predicting problems with healing of these fractures is the extent of soft-tissue damage, with the amount of initial fracture displacement usually being of secondary importance.

Fractures that are open or associated with arterial injury or elevated compartment pressures require emergent operative intervention. After treatment of the limb-threatening emergency, these fractures are stabilized by an unreamed intramedullary nail or an external fixator. Depending on the time since the injury, the vascular surgeon may prefer that skeletal stabilization be performed prior to arterial repair.

Open fracture Types I, II, and IIIA are usually treated with intravenous antibiotics, irrigation, and debridement, followed by unreamed intramedullary nailing. Types IIIB and C are usually treated with a uniaxial or ring external fixator. Antibiotics include cefazolin and gentamicin, as well as penicillin, if the injury occurred in a barnyard. Soft-tissue coverage using a gastrocnemius (proximal $\frac{1}{3}$ fractures), soleus (middle $\frac{1}{3}$), or free flap (distal $\frac{1}{3}$) should be performed within 7–14 days. Osteocutaneous flaps (often free vascularized fibula grafts) can be used to treat soft tissue and segmental bone loss. Nonunions or delayed unions following intramedullary nailing are infrequent except for high energy, open fractures. These can be treated with nail dynamization (remove either proximal or distal interlocking screws and allow weight bearing), bone grafting, fibular osteotomy, or by nail exchange using a reamed nail.

After years of aggressive limb salvage efforts, many experts have come to the conclusion that there are some indications for primary amputation in Type IIIC open fractures of the tibia to minimize risk and hospital stays, and to allow patients to move on with their lives. Two absolute indications mentioned in the literature for open tibia fractures with arterial injuries include a crush injury with a warm ischemia time of >6 hours and anatomic division of the tibial nerve in adults. Relative indications include IIIC fractures with other life-threatening injuries or significant ipsilateral foot trauma. Patients with popliteal artery injuries tend to fare much better than those with injuries below the trifurcation. Increasing age worsens outcome. Extremity severity scores can assist in decision-making.

Relative indications for operative intervention include any articular involvement, segmental fractures, "floating knee," bilateral lower extremity fractures, and tibia fractures in polytrauma patients. A radiograph of the contralateral normal tibia can often be invaluable for preoperative planning for complex cases.

Most closed, stable, minimally displaced tibial shaft fractures can be treated by closed reduction, a long leg cast, and nonweight bearing. Usually, this is worn for 6 weeks, and if there is evidence of healing, the cast is then changed to a patellar tendon bearing (PTB) cast or brace and weight bearing as tolerated is started. Proximal tibia fractures should not be treated with a PTB, as fracture movement and loss of reduction can occur.

Predicting stability and judging the success of a closed reduction requires clinical experience. Basically, comminuted, segmental, spiral, and oblique fractures tend to be unstable, with a tendency to shorten, angulate, and/or rotate. These typically require operative stabilization. When treating tibal shaft fractures closed, frequent follow-up radiographs are needed to be certain the reduction is maintained. A-P and lateral radiographs of the tibia-fibula should include the knee and the ankle on the same cassette to assess angulation. Closed treatment is relatively contraindicated if there is comminution or displacement of $>\frac{1}{3}$ of the shaft diameter, >1 cm of shortening, or >5 degrees of angulation in the A-P or lateral planes.

Any tibial shaft fracture for which these requirements cannot be met by closed treatment probably warrants internal or external fixation. Further, any tibial shaft fracture that proves to be unstable on early follow-up radiographs and fails the aforementioned requirements should also be considered for closed intramedullary nailing. Intramedullary nails are less reliable when treating proximal $\frac{1}{3}$ or distal $\frac{1}{5}$ tibia fractures, since there is more room for the nail in these metaphyseal regions. Other less-used methods of treatment include plate fixation, calcaneal pin traction, pins and plaster, cerclage wiring, and pure lag screw fixation.

Pilon Fractures[12]

Pilon fractures refer to fractures involving the weight-bearing articular surface (tibial plafond) and the overlying metaphysis of the distal tibia. This challenging subset of ankle fractures results from shearing and compressive forces on the distal tibia frequently sustained in falls and motor vehicle accidents. The management of these complex injuries is often dictated by the condition of the thin soft-tissue envelope of the distal tibia. Radiographic evaluation of these fractures includes an ankle series and often a CT scan with sagital reconstructions. In operative cases, a contralateral ankle is often helpful for comparison.

The Ruedi and Allgower classification is the most frequently used. Type I injuries are essentially cleavage fractures without significant fragment separation and articular displacement. Type II fractures have notable articular displacement, but the joint itself is not crushed or comminuted. Type III fractures are crushed and comminuted in the metaphyseal and articular regions. Nondisplaced fractures do well with either operative or conservative therapy. Intraarticular fractures are best treated with open anatomic reduction, rigid internal fixation, and early motion. Type III fractures are associated with high energy and substantial soft-tissue trauma. ORIF of these fractures is associated with high complication rates and low rates of satisfactory results. Therefore, many surgeons have started to choose external fixation (uniaxial or ring) or hybrid fixation (minimal ORIF with supplementary external fixation). Primary ankle fusions are rarely performed, as they are associated with delayed healing and fusion rates.

One must carefully evaluate the soft tissues preoperatively and assess the risk of wound slough or infection that could lead to a chronic infection, nonunion, or possibly even amputation. The condition of the skin may often delay ORIF 7–14 days while swelling subsides. Other treatment options include closed reduction and casting or calcaneal pin traction.

Careful preop planning is critical with careful outlining of the fracture anatomy. ORIF is usually performed with a tourniquet, and incisions are just medial to the anterior tibialis and posterolateral to the fibula, taking care to leave a 7 cm skin bridge between the two. Generally, the associated fibula fracture (85% of the time) is plated first with a $\frac{1}{3}$ tubular plate to get the fracture out to length. This is followed by reconstruction of the articular surface of the tibia and bone grafting for any metaphyseal defect. Finally, a buttress plate is applied to the tibia. Wounds are closed primarily over drains if swelling allows. They are carefully inspected postoperatively. Serious consideration should be given to free flap coverage at the first sign of wound breakdown.

Ankle Fractures[12–14]

Ankle fractures vary in severity from closed, relatively low energy, stable unimalleolar fractures to open, high energy fracture-dislocations with massive soft-tissue destruction. The management and prognosis of the two extremes is obviously quite different. Initially, it is important to assess the perfusion of the foot and ankle. If it is poor, it may be improved by the immediate reduction of a fracture-dislocation that may be causing obvious deformity, tenting skin over bony prominences, and kinking vessels. A neurological deficit, especially damage or division of the tibial nerve, may affect the prognosis and, consequently, may have implications on patient management. Wounds should be evaluated as to whether they extend into the joint or the fracture. One should attempt to assess the integrity of the tendons and ligaments in the region. Radiographic assessment should begin with A-P, lateral, and mortise views of the ankle.

The classification of ankle fractures is quite complex. The most commonly used system is the Lauge-Hansen classification, which divides ankle fractures into four main types:

Supination-External Rotation (SER)
Supination-Adduction (SAD)
Pronation-External Rotation (PER)
Pronation-Abduction (PAB)

The first word in each of these types describes the position of the foot at the time of injury. The second word(s) describes the direction of the force causing the injury. These four fracture types are further divided into 13 subtypes, making this system quite complex. It is probably not necessary to memorize the many subtypes, but a working knowledge of the four main groups can be beneficial in ankle fracture reduction. Closed reduction of these fractures is performed by reversing the fracture mechanism. Closed reduction is followed by placement in a short or long leg splint. The four main groups can be distinguished by the pattern of the fibular fracture (Fig. 6.17).

SER—spiral fibular fracture, distal end at the level of the tibial plafond

PER—spiral fibular fracture, distal end usually 4–7 cm above the tibial plafond

SAD—transverse fibular fracture at or below the level of the tibial plafond; if accompanied by a medial malleolar fracture, it will have an oblique pattern

PAB—oblique fibular fracture with distal end at the level of the tibial plafond; if accompanied by a medial malleolar fracture, it will have a transverse pattern

With a greater emphasis on rigid internal fixation and early motion, it is much more important to be able to describe the actual fracture and assess its stability. It has become more important to describe fractures as unimalleolar, bimalleolar, and trimalleolar. A trimalleolar fracture refers to one involving the lateral and medial malleoli, as well as the posterior articular surface of the tibia, known as the posterior malleolus.

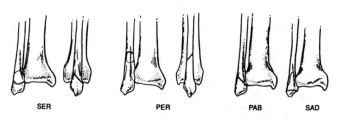

SER   PER   PAB   SAD

Figure 6.17. Lauge-Hansen classification.

Ankle stability is evaluated by examining the ankle mortise. The joint space between the talus and the tibial plafond and the distal fibula should vary by no more than 1 mm on any side on the A-P and mortise views of the ankle. A second method is to draw one line down the center of the tibia, and another line through the center of the talar dome on both the A-P and lateral radiographs. These lines should be coincident or nearly so within 1 mm. If either parameter is not met, this implies that the talus has shifted in the mortise, and the fracture is potentially unstable. It also implies that it may be difficult to hold in a cast without internal fixation.

Most unimalleolar fractures are stable. If the ligaments on the opposite side of the ankle or the syndesmotic ligaments have been damaged, the talus may be able to shift beneath the plafond. These are both unstable situations, and ORIF is required. Tenderness or bruising over the unfractured malleoli is assumed to indicate ligamentous damage. A common situation is a spiral fracture of the lateral malleolus with tenderness medially, indicating a likely deltoid injury. This requires ORIF of the fibula only. The deltoid does not need to be repaired unless it appears to be in the joint blocking reduction of the fibula. In that case, exploration of the medial side of the ankle is indicated.

Many unimalleolar fractures do not have associated ligament damage and can be handled in a closed manner. Closed treatment of a reduced fracture requires about 6 weeks of non-weight bearing in a cast followed by 2–3 weeks in a short leg walking cast or brace. These periods obviously vary according to fracture type, bone quality, and patient compliance. If a lateral malleolus fracture remains displaced >3 mm following reduction, ORIF needs to be performed, as this amount of displacement can lead to premature ankle arthrosis.

Most bimalleolar fractures are unstable, since nothing is holding the talus in the mortise. An exception to this rule is when the fibular fracture is below the level of the plafond, as it will block the talus and keep it centered in the mortise. Though these fractures may occasionally be treated in a cast, more often they require ORIF. ORIF usually consists of a $\frac{1}{3}$ tubular plate applied to the posterolateral aspect of the fibula and typically one or two 4.0 mm malleolar (or cancellous) screws placed into the medial malleolus. Occasionally, a small $\frac{1}{3}$ tubular plate or a tension band will offer superior fixation to screws. Laterally, care should be taken to avoid the sural nerve and branches of the superficial peroneal nerve. Medially, the saphenous vein is at risk.

Trimalleolar fractures imply severe soft-tissue damage or a rotational injury, and are invariably unstable. Open reduction and internal fixation are indicated unless there is a specific contraindication. Fixation of the posterior malleolar fragment is suggested if the articular fragment involves >25% of the articular surface and it remains unreduced after fixation of the medial malleolus and the fibula.

An injury to the syndesmosis is suspected when a patient has a high fibula fracture (>4.5 cm above the plafond) and deltoid tenderness or a medial malleolus fracture. A Maisonneuve fracture refers to a proximal one-third fibula fracture and a medial malleolus fracture. When one suspects a syndesmatic injury, the fibula is plated and pulled laterally (Cotton test). If the distal fibula moves >3–4 mm lateral from the talus, the syndesmosis is ruptured and fixation should be performed. One typically places one or two 4.5 mm fully threaded cortical screws through the fibula and into the tibia with the ankle dorsiflexed to neutral as the screw(s) is tightened. Some surgeons will also engage the far cortex of the tibia for additional fixation. This screw(s) is removed 12–16 weeks postop, since it will tend to break if left in position and normal activity is resumed.

Talus Fracture/Dislocations[12,13]

More than 60% of the surface of the talus is articular, and anatomic restoration of fractures of this bone is necessary for normal gait mechanics. The talus can be fractured in several areas but the most common injury is to the talar neck. The Hawkins' classification system is used to describe these fractures:

Type I— nondisplaced fracture of the talar neck without dislocation

Type II —displaced fracture of the talar neck with or without slight displacement of the ankle or subtalar joints

Type III—displaced fracture of the talar neck with subluxation or dislocation of the body of the talus from both the subtalar and ankle joints

Type IV—(added to Hawkins' original classification) subluxation of the head, dislocation of the body from the ankle and subtalar joints, extrusion of the body

Since the blood supply to the talar dome enters through the talar neck, one complication of this injury is avascular necrosis of the talar dome with secondary degenerative arthritis of the tibiotalar joint. The risk of avascular necrosis in the body increases with the severity of the injury. It is <10% in Hawkins' Type I, <40% in Type II, >90% in Type III, and nears 100% in Type IV injuries. Hawkins' sign refers to the radiographically evident osteolysis of the subchondral bone of the talar dome that occurs secondary to disuse and revascularization. This sign typically appears at 6 weeks if AVN has not occurred.

Type I fractures can be treated closed if a CT scan confirms that the fracture is truly nondisplaced. There is evidence suggesting that the risk of AVN can be reduced by compression fixation using cannulated screws and K-wires. Therefore, immediate reduction of the subtalar or ankle joint is followed by closed reduction and internal fixation or ORIF in effort to achieve anatomic reduction. Most surgeons recommend placing two partially threaded cancellous screws across the fracture site for compression. These screws are typically cannulated and placed posterior to anterior in order to get excellent fixation in the dense bone of the head of the talus.

Most surgeons think that talectomy, subtalar fusion, and ankle fusion should be avoided initially even in the most severe Type IV injuries. These salvage procedures do not improve the likelihood of revascularization and can always be performed at a later date. A pantalar fusion is often performed as a salvage procedure for the patient who develops painful, segmental collapse of the talus.

Fractures of the body and head of the talus should frequently be treated with ORIF if displaced. Small osteochondral fractures of the talar dome, often presenting as persistent ankle sprains, are often arthroscopically debrided, if possible, but they may also be anatomically repositioned and fixed with bioabsorbable pins or screws if they are large enough.

Calcaneus Fractures[12,13,17]

Calcaneus fractures are usually caused by an axial load on the heel sustained most often in motor vehicle accidents or falls from a height. These fractures are occasionally seen bilaterally and are commonly accompanied by a compression fracture of the lumbar spine (10%). One should be aware that 2%–5% of severe calcaneus fractures will develop a compartment syndrome in the sole of the foot secondary to hemorrhage. Foot compartment fasciotomies are rarely performed.

In addition to A-P and lateral views of the foot, a Harris heel view should be obtained. This is radiographed by angling the beam at 45 degrees from behind the leg and centering it on the posterior portion of the subtalar joint. The lateral view demonstrates subtalar joint involvement, posterior facet depression, and the loss of Böhler's angle (tuberosity-joint angle, normally 30–40 degrees). The A-P shows the calcaneocuboid articulation. The Harris view demonstrates the sustentaculum tali, the medial and lateral cortices of the tuberosity, and any varus/valgus angulation. A CT scan (coronal slices) with three-dimensional reconstruction images is often performed to fully evaluate the posterior articular facet and to assist in preoperative planning. The calcaneocuboid joint can also be assessed using the axial images. The opposite foot is included and serves as a reference.

It is important to visualize more than just the subtalar joint, since the articular surface of the calcaneocuboid joint is occasionally displaced. If either the subtalar or calcaneocuboid joint is allowed to heal incongruously, the foot and ankle may experience abnormal force loads leading to accelerated joint arthrosis. Deformity in the subtalar joint following calcaneous fracture can cause the heel and arch to flatten, the talus to dorsiflex in the ankle, and the body of the calcaneus to widen, making wearing shoes painful and problematic.

If the fracture is extraarticular and minimally displaced or if the fracture is deemed not reparable by open methods, it should be treated by nonweight bearing and immobilization. Minimally displaced, extraarticular fractures are treated with nonweight bearing in a short leg cast for at least 6–8 weeks until radiographic union is visible. Extraarticular fractures of the tuberosity, the sustentaculum tali, or the anterior process of the calcaneous have an excellent prognosis and should be treated closed. Avulsion fractures of the Achilles insertion can also be treated closed in some individuals if the are displaced <5 mm.

ORIF is indicated for posterior facet articular incongruity, depression of Böhler's angle, significant lateral subluxation of the posterior tuberosity (impinges on lateral malleolus), and significant varus deformity. ORIF is usually performed via a lateral approach using screws and plates. ORIF is occasionally postponed 7–14 days in order to let swelling subside following the injury. Careful handling of the soft tissues has decreased wound complications postoperatively. Elderly patients or those with osteopenia, diabetes, or significant comminution may be best treated closed in order to reduce the risk of wound problems. Bone graft is often incorporated to fill in the defect created when the joint line is elevated. Late complications of ORIF include subtalar arthritis, peroneal tendon or sural nerve entrapment, and a widened or varus hindfoot.

Midfoot/Forefoot Fractures[12,13,17]

Multiple fracture types can occur in this region, and several will be discussed. In the midfoot, a serious injury is a Lisfranc fracture-dislocation. This is a rare fracture-dislocation through Lisfranc's joint (the tarsometatarsal joint). Since the second metatarsal extends farthest proximally, it will often be fractured at its base, with the other metatarsals dislocated. A careful neurovascular examination should be performed, since the vascular supply to the forefoot can be interrupted, especially with complete forefoot dislocations. Compartment syndrome of the foot is frequently seen with Lisfranc fracture-dislocations.

Radiographic findings include a small fracture at the base of the second metatarsal, widening between the base of the first and second metatarsals, or dorsal displacement of the second or third metatarsal bases. On the A-P radiograph, one should pay close attention to the alignment of the medial aspect of the middle cuneiform and the medial border of the second MT base. The same is true of the medial surface of the cuboid and the medial aspect of the fourth MT base. Comparison radiographs are sometimes helpful. A compression fracture of the navicular or the cuboid is often noted with these injuries. If no fracture is visualized and there is a high index of suspicion, stress radiographs should be obtained using adequate anesthesia and operative treatment performed if displacement is >2 mm.

Treatment of this fracture-dislocation is ORIF using two or three cortical screws medially and often percutaneous K-wires across the fourth and fifth tarsometatarsal joints. One screw must pass between the medial cuneiform and the second MT base to reconstruct Lisfranc's ligament. These screws should probably not be lagged. One 4 cm incision is made between the first and second metatarsal and the other is made between the third and fourth. The anterior tibialis can often be caught between the first and second metatarsals preventing reduction. The patient is kept nonweight bearing for 10 weeks and fixation removed at 3 months. Many advocate starting range of motion exercises as soon as the wounds have sealed and swelling has declined.

The base of the fifth metatarsal is frequently fractured in one of two patterns. The first pattern, frequently seen in dancers, is an avulsion of the tip of the base formerly thought to be caused by pull from the peroneus brevis muscle. A recent study suggests that the avulsion is caused instead by the lateral planter aponeurosis. If displacement is <2 mm, it can be treated in a hard-sole cast shoe for comfort or, if the patient is in a great deal of pain, a short leg cast or splint until the pain subsides. If displacement is >2 mm, internal fixation may be considered.

The second pattern is a transverse fracture through the base of the fifth metatarsal, about 1–2 cm from the proximal tip, known as a Jones fracture. This fracture is usually treated in a short leg cast when caused by acute trauma. However, there is a relatively high incidence of nonunion, and primary intramedullary fixation using a partially threaded cancellous screw to avoid this complication may be preferred, especially in athletes or people whose jobs require them to be on their feet, and is indicated in the treatment of stress fractures. When placing an intramedullary screw across this fracture, the starting hole is very important, and one needs to countersink the screw. A stress fracture can be diagnosed by eliciting a history describing a prodrome of pain and insignificant trauma. Radiographically, a stress fracture will demonstrate relatively smooth sclerotic edges at the fracture site unlike an acute fracture.

Fractures of the metatarsals and phalanges of the foot can be treated with a hard, wooden-soled cast shoe and immediate weight bearing, as tolerated. For severely displaced metatarsal fractures, closed reduction and percutaneous pinning or ORIF with a plate and screws will occasionally be indicated to avoid a painful prominence on the plantar aspect of the foot or difficulty in shoe wear.

Adult Dislocations

Finger Dislocations[11,12]

Most finger dislocations involve the PIP joint and are dorsally displaced, disrupting the volar plate and usually damaging the collateral ligaments. These can be recognized easily and reduced by the standard method of exaggeration of the mechanism, longitudinal traction, and reduction using a digital block. Radiographs should be obtained prior to and following reduction to rule out a fracture. Active and passive range of motion should be checked following reduction to check stability. Instability may be caused by soft-tissue interposition, and open reduction may be required. If stable, the joint should be splinted dorsally with the PIP joint in slight flexion for 2 weeks, followed by buddy taping for another 2 weeks.

Shoulder Dislocations[12,14,17]

Shoulder dislocations are common injuries in adolescents and young adults. The humeral head may dislocate anteriorly, posteriorly, inferiorly, and superiorly. Anterior glenohumeral dislocation is most common (95%–98%). Posterior dislocations occur approximately 2% of the time, and the other dislocations are rarely seen.

Anterior glenohumeral dislocations usually occur when the arm is forcefully abducted and externally rotated. The axillary nerve and artery, as well as the musculocutaneous nerve, are occasionally injured, so a careful neurovascular examination should be documented both before and after reduction. Nerve injuries are nearly always neuropraxias and require no treatment.

Multiple methods of closed reduction exist, but all use some method of traction on the arm in varying degrees of flexion and/or abduction. Reduction is almost impossible when the muscles are in severe spasm, and intravenous narcotics and muscle relaxants are often needed to allow the person to relax enough to allow reduction. Of course, reduction of someone with recurrent instability is typically easier and can often be performed without much premedication. After reduction, radiographs should be obtained to document the reduction and detect any fractures. An axillary view and/or a scapular Y view are the most helpful to assess glenohumeral reduction. Neurovascular status should be documented, then the arm should be placed in a shoulder immobilizer with the forearm across the chest. The length of immobilization is very controversial, varying from 1–2 days (until pain subsides) up to 6 weeks. Rotator cuff tears should be suspected in the elderly.

Anterior glenohumeral dislocations frequently become recurrent because of the incompetence of the disrupted anterior inferior glenohumeral ligament and the anterior labral complex (Bankart lesion). This is especially so in the adolescent age group, for whom the incidence of recurrence is as high as 90%. Once a dislocation occurs a second time in this age group, the chance of recurrence is almost 100%. Therefore, in adolescents, a second dislocation is usually an indication for an open reconstructive procedure. Typically, we prefer an open capsular shift with anatomic repair of the Bankart lesion if it is present to prevent further recurrences. Some surgeons are now advocating arthroscopic reconstruction of the anterior inferior glenohumeral ligament-labral complex following a first-time dislocation in young active people because of data coming from West Point physicians treating cadets.

Posterior glenohumeral dislocations are rarely seen, but are commonly missed (>60%) because there is no striking deformity of the shoulder and because it is held in the traditional sling position. The diagnosis is also missed owing to failure to obtain a complete radiographic series of the shoulder. The two important views to document posterior dislocation, if suspected, are an axillary lateral and a scapular Y lateral. Without these views, this injury will often not be diagnosed, leading to considerable morbidity.

The posterior dislocation occurs by a mechanism of forceful adduction and internal rotation. These dislocations are often seen following seizures or electric shock because the internal rotators of the shoulder overpower the external rotators. The diagnosis should be suspected whenever a patient has injured his shoulder and cannot externally rotate his hand to the neutral position. In addition a mass will often be palpable posteriorly. These can be reduced using intravenous sedation and by pulling longitudinally in the line of the defect while gently pushing the humeral head into the glenoid fossa. Following reduction, the shoulder should be immobilized in a few degrees of external rotation.

Treatment of a chronic posterior shoulder dislocation depends on the amount of humeral head involvement by CT scan axial cuts. If 20%–45% of the head is involved, a McLaughlin procedure is performed, in which the subscapularis is advanced into the head defect (reverse Hill-Sachs) created by the glenoid rim. Prosthetic head replacement is suggested if >45% of the head is involved.

To evaluate chronic instability, the West Point view allows visualization of the anterior glenoid margin and the Stryker notch view gives one a plain view of a Hill-Sachs lesion. CT scans are frequently used to help visualize or quantify humeral head or glenoid defects following acute dislocations, chronic unreduced dislocations (usually posterior), or to see the effects of chronic instability. MRI, MRI arthrogram, and arthroscopy are being used to evaluate and treat chondral, labral, and ligamentous anomalies.

Acromioclavicular Dislocations[12,14,17]

An acromioclavicular (A-C) dislocation is commonly referred to as a shoulder separation. It is usually caused by a blow to the top of the shoulder and is often seen in contact sports. Radiographic evaluation includes an A-P view of the A-C joint to evaluate superior or inferior displacement and an axillary lateral to see if the clavicle is anteriorly or posteriorly displaced. A contralateral A-P of the A-C joint is often used for comparison if the clavicle appears to be elevated compared with the acromion.

The scapula is fixed to the clavicle by the acromioclavicular (A-C) and the coracoclavicular (CC) ligaments. A-C dislocations are graded by the amount of damage to these ligaments.

Type I A-C dislocations imply a sprain of the joint without a complete tear of either ligament. A Type II injury implies a tear of the acromioclavicular ligaments with the coracoclavicular ligaments intact. Since the coracoclavicular ligaments provide stability in the coronal plane, this injury will not show marked elevation of the lateral end of the clavicle. However, in a Type III injury, in which both sets of ligaments are torn, the distal clavicle will usually be elevated 25%–100%, compared with its normal position above the coracoid. The normal distance is typically measured from the contralateral side. In Type IV–VI dislocations, both the acromioclavicular and the coracoclavicular ligaments are also disrupted. Additionally, in Type IV dislocations, the distal clavicle is displaced posteriorly into or through the trapezius muscle. In Type V, the muscular attachments (deltoid, trapezius) are ruptured allowing the clavicle to rise 100%–300% relative to the coracoid. In Type VI (extremely rare), the distal clavicle dislocates inferior to the coracoid posterior to the biceps and coracobrachialis tendon.

If there is a question between a Type II and III dislocation, stress radiographs can be obtained. These are filmed with 10–15 pounds suspended from both wrists by a strap (not held in the hands). Both A-C joints must be seen on the same film. A major discrepancy in the coracoclavicular interval probably indicates complete disruption of the coracoclavicular ligaments (a Type III dislocation). Distinguishing between a Type II and III injury is currently not crucial since both injuries are usually treated nonoperatively.

Treatment of the Type I injury is symptomatic. The patient should be given a sling for comfort for 7–10 days but can usually begin exercising his shoulder in 1–2 days and should be encouraged to do so. Treatment of the Type II is 3–6 weeks in a sling. Most physicians no longer advocate the Kenny Howard brace. Type III injuries are occasionally controversial, with most favoring nonoperative care (sling), but with a few physicians recommending internal fixation in some situations (e.g., heavy laborer). Type IV–VI dislocations are treated operatively in an effort to create an anatomic relationship between the clavicle and the scapula.

Elbow Dislocations[12,17]

Elbow dislocations account for 20% of all dislocations, behind only the glenohumeral and finger joints. Most occur from a fall on an outstretched hand. Posterior or posterolateral dislocation (of the olecranon) is found in >80% of the cases. Complex dislocations have associated fractures, while simple dislocations do not.

The stability of the elbow is determined by the highly congruous anatomy and the ligamentous support. The medial collateral ligament (MCL) is the primary stabilizer of the elbow. It consists of an anterior oblique ligament (strongest), a posterior oblique ligament, and a small transverse ligament. The lateral collateral ligament (LCL) is primarily a capsular thickening.

Prior to reduction, a careful sensory and motor examination must be performed to document any deficits. Reduction should be performed under general or regional anesthesia to minimize the required force and subsequent trauma. Reduction begins with gentle longitudinal traction on the forearm with countertraction on the upper arm. This is followed by correction of lateral or medial displacement and then gentle flexion, resulting in palpable and occasionally audible reduction. Most prefer to perform the reduction with the patient in the prone position, while others prefer supine. The deformity should not be grossly exaggerated in effort to minimize trauma to the brachialis and the neurovascular structures anterior to the elbow. One should fully flex and extend the elbow to rule out a mechanical block to motion and to see if the elbow dislocates again with extension. Varus and valgus stability should also be checked. Radiographs should be obtained to ensure joint congruency and identify any previously unidentified fractures. A posterior splint with the elbow at 90 degrees and sling should be used for 2–3 weeks, but active motion should then be encouraged to prevent an elbow flexion contracture or any loss of motion. If no instability was noted postreduction, 7–10 days of immobilization is adequate. Recurrent instability is very uncommon with simple dislocations.

The patient and the house officer should both be aware of the possibility of neurovascular compromise postreduction. Splinting should allow adequate access to the hand and wrist to allow easy monitoring, and forearm compartment pressures should be obtained if there is doubt.

Elbow dislocations are often associated with fractures of the medial epicondyle, radial head, olecranon, and coronoid process. The results of dislocations with these injuries are less favorable than simple dislocations. Coronoid process fractures have been identified in 10%–15% of elbow dislocations. These are divided into Type I, which is a tip avulsion; Type II, which is a single or comminuted fracture involving <50% of the coronoid; and Type III, which involves >50% of the coronoid.

Operative treatment is indicated for open dislocations, locked fragments, persistent instability, Type III coronoid process fractures, and medial epicondyle fractures that are displaced >1 cm. Chronic dislocations or valgus instability is sometimes treated with the palmaris longus or the third toe extensor for reconstruction of the anterior band of the MCL. Varus instability usually requires surgical repair of the LCL.

Hip Dislocations[12,17]

Hip dislocations usually result from major trauma (70% MVAs) and are often associated with fractures of the femoral head, the femoral neck, and the acetabulum. A common mechanism of this injury is an automobile accident in which the passenger's flexed knee strikes the dashboard, driving the femoral head posteriorly and often fracturing the posterior acetabular wall. This injury is typically obvious because of the drastic leg length discrepancy, though an ipsilateral femoral shaft fracture can sometimes disguise it. After the ATLS protocol is completed, a careful neurovascular examination should be performed documenting sciatic nerve function (injured 8%–19% of the time). Reduction should be obtained as quickly as possible to decrease stretch on the nerve and to reduce the risk of femoral head osteonecrosis. Post-reduction, sciatic nerve function must be checked to make sure that the nerve is not incarcerated in the joint. The ipsilateral foot, ankle, and knee are also frequently injured, depending on their respective positions at the time of the accident. A stat A-P pelvis is often performed when patients involved in major trauma arrive at the ER. This should typically be repeated following reduction. The ipsilateral femoral head and neck, as well as the acetabulum, must be closely scrutinized for fractures. Judet views of the pelvis, as well as a CT scan with 1.5–3 mm axial cuts, can help evaluate the bony anatomy and help ensure anatomic reduction of the femoral head.

Posterior dislocation is the most common type, occurring in about 85% of the cases. These dislocations are generally classified in five groups (Epstein classification), depending on reducibility, stability, and associated fractures. General anesthesia is often required for reduction, though most surgeons will try initially in the ER using intravenous sedation. Reduction is usually achieved using the Allis method with the patient in the supine position. The surgeon must gain a mechanical advantage by standing on the stretcher and by using a tied sheet looped around the patient's flexed knee and around the surgeon's back. An assistant should stabilize the pelvis as the surgeon places the affected extremity in progressively increasing amounts of longitudinal traction while slowly flexing the hip to 70 degrees. Gentle internal and external hip rotation and slight adduction may help the hip clear the lip of the acetabulum. An audible "clunk" usually indicates successful reduction. After reduction, one can assess hip stability by flexing the hip to 90 degrees and allowing the weight of the leg to rest on the posterior aspect of the acetabulum. Instability is an indication for emergent open reduction and fixation of all fractures for some, while others will place the leg in longitudinal traction and get a CT scan prior to fixing the fractures. Emergent open reduction using a posterior approach is indicated following 2–3 closed attempts with the patient completely relaxed.

Anterior dislocations result from forced hip abduction and are quite rare and can often be reduced using the same technique. If closed reduction cannot be achieved, emergent open reduction must be performed by an anterior approach. Postreduction instability is very rare following anterior dislocations.

If there is no fracture or just a posterior lip fracture of the acetabulum, weight bearing as tolerated can begin after a few days of bed rest. Significant posterior wall fractures typically require ORIF using reconstruction plates or spring plates.

Following posttraumatic arthritis, the second most significant consequence of this injury is osteonecrosis of the femoral head (15%–17% of the time) owing to vascular embarrassment. The risk of osteonecrosis is thought to decrease if the hip is reduced within 6–8 hours, depending on the source cited. Osteonecrosis is evident radiographically about 18 months following the injury.

A special problem is dislocation of a hip hemiarthroplasty or total hip prostheses. The direction of dislocation will vary in these cases according to the surgical approach used and the relative positioning of the components. These dislocations can also cause neurologic problems and also stretch the joint capsule (predisposing to future dislocation) so reduction should be achieved quickly. If the dislocation is more than 1–2 days old, this will often require skeletal traction on the limb to decrease the contracture of the abductor musculature. After reduction, the patient is usually placed in an abduction pillow temporarily followed by placement in a Bledsoe brace or hip spica cast with the lower extremity flexed and abducted slightly. Recurrent dislocations of a total hip prosthesis may be an indication to revise the prosthesis.

Knee Dislocations[12]

Knee dislocations are an orthopaedic emergency because of the high incidence of popliteal artery damage. The dislocation can be in the anterior/posterior plane (50%–75% incidence) or the medial/lateral plane and occasionally has a rotational component. The diagnosis is usually obvious, and the knee should be reduced immediately, even before proceeding to radiology, to reduce pressure on the vascular supply to the lower leg. To perform a closed reduction, one should first document the neurovascular status of the extremity and then attempt to provide appropriate analgesia. The physician then places longitudinal traction on the extremity followed by the necessary translation of the femur and tibia. Above all, one must be careful not to place any force on the popliteal fossa, as this may further compromise the vasculature. The knee should then be splinted in 20–30 degrees of flexion in a bulky dressing. If the pedal pulses are intact, an arteriogram of the lower extremity is mandatory to rule out an intimal tear that may later precipitate a thrombus and subsequent arterial occlusion. If the arteriogram is normal, the leg should be placed in a knee immobilizer for stabilization and for easy access for frequent lower extremity compartment and neurovascular checks. If pedal pulses are absent after reduction, immediate exploration of the popliteal artery is indicated. If the surgeon elects to obtain an arteriogram, this should be done in the operating room. After a knee dislocation, delay of more than 6 hours in restoring the blood flow is associated with a very high incidence of above-knee amputations. Following repair of the popliteal artery, a four-compartment fasciotomy should be performed to decrease the risk of a compartment syndrome.

The house officer must be aware that many knee dislocations are reduced spontaneously at the scene of the accident. These injuries often carry the same risks of dislocations that arrive unreduced. Unfortunately, sometimes there are not many signs of significant knee injury. A hemarthrosis will often be absent because of the capsular damage that occurred, and the best clues available may be diffuse tenderness around the knee and ecchymosis in the popliteal fossa. The presence of varus and valgus instability in full extension implicating possible tears of the ACL and PCL is reason for suspicion, though this is often difficult to check because of pain. Ipsilateral femur and/or tibia fractures are frequently present and make examination of the knee difficult.

Peroneal nerve damage occurs in 14%–35% of knee dislocations, and these injuries carry a poor prognosis even with surgical
intervention. Ligament reconstruction following dislocation is
often performed on a delayed basis, depending on the condition
of the patient and the extremity. Acutely, the knee is immobilized
with an external fixator or a knee immobilizer to ensure reduction.

Knee dislocations are stabilized surgically within 6 weeks of
the injury. Bony avulsions are usually fixed within a week. Intrasubstance tears, on the other hand, are often repaired after swelling has decreased to reduce the risk of arthrofibrosis. The PCL
is repaired primarily if the tendon was avulsed from bone and
still has a bony fragment attached. If the tear is midsubstance, a
bone patellar tendon bone autograft is used to reconstruct this
ligament. The MCL and LCL are typically repaired primarily,
though the LCL is usually reinforced with semitendinosis and/
or gracilis. If the ACL was avulsed with a bony fragment, it should
be repaired primarily. Otherwise, ACL reconstruction is usually optional.

Pediatric Fractures

Pediatric Both Bones Forearm[18]

Unlike in adults, both bones fractures in children can be treated
with closed reduction and casting. These fractures are divided
into torus or buckle fractures, greenstick fractures, and complete
fractures. Torus or buckle fractures with minimal angulation typically do not need reduction and are treated with a short arm
cast for 3–4 weeks. Greenstick fractures (one cortex is fractured
while the other side remains intact) often have a rotational component that must be corrected by either supination or pronation
prior to reduction of the typical angulatory defect. This is usually
performed under intravenous sedation, though some physicians
prefer general anesthesia. The bicipital tuberosity is used to judge
the amount of rotation present in the fracture. The tuberosity
is supposed to be directed in the direction opposite the radial
aspect of the distal radial styloid. One can normally see the profile
of the tuberosity pointing medially when the forearm is fully
supinated (90 degrees), and it is usually not visible when the
forearm is in neutral (0 degrees).

Reduction of complete fractures is usually achieved by placing a hematoma block into both bones with intravenous sedation as necessary. Many suggest using fingertraps with 10–15 pounds of traction if the bones are overriding and reducing each bone individually using thumb pressure. An image intensifier, if available, is of great assistance. The arm should be placed in a long arm cast or splint with the elbow at 90 degrees of flexion and the forearm pronated or supinated in the position that reduces the fracture best (usually neutral or full supination). If the child is <10 years old, overlap of both bones is acceptable if rotation and angulation are correct, because remodeling will occur and this will not affect later pronation and supination. If the child is over 12 years old, the surgeon should worry about decreased forearm rotation and should not hesitate to perform ORIF, especially in females, who mature skeletally prior to males. There are many opinions as to what is an acceptable amount of angulation or rotation in these fractures, so the senior resident or the attending should be consulted. One should keep in mind that little useful correction occurs in the diaphysis of the radius and ulna when the child is >8 years old. It is probably safe to accept 15 degrees of angulation in children <6 years old and 10 degrees in children <10 years old. Little, if any, rotational remodeling occurs in children >8 years old. One should remember that 10 degrees of malrotation will equal 10 degrees of decreased rotation if remodeling fails to occur. Immobilization should be for 7–8 weeks. One should switch to a hinged brace or a short arm cast after 3–4 weeks.

Nursemaid's Elbow[18]

This eponym is used to describe a subluxation of the head of the radius. The typical patient is an infant who refuses to use his or her arm. A history of a sudden longitudinal pull on the affected upper extremity can usually be elicited from the caretaker. The child is usually not in distress at initial presentation but begins to cry with any attempt to flex the elbow or supinate the forearm. Radiographs are often normal. Reduction is performed by first extending and distracting the elbow, supinating the forearm, and then hyperflexing the elbow with the surgeon's thumb over the radial head in order to feel the reduction as it occurs. No postreduction films are needed, since success is usually demonstrated by the infant who has resumed use of the previously unused extremity.

Pediatric Condylar Elbow[17,18]

Lateral condyle fractures of the elbow in children are usually caused by a fall on the outstretched arm and involve the lateral condylar physis. These are generally Salter-Harris II fractures (Milch II) that begin in the lateral metaphysis and pass through the physis, entering the joint just medial to the lateral condyle epiphysis. Rarely, Salter-Harris IV fractures (Milch I) occur when the fracture begins in the lateral metaphysis and extends distally through the lateral epiphysis and into the joint. Nondisplaced fractures (<2 mm) can be treated by immobilization in a long arm cast for 3 weeks, but frequent radiographs are needed to be certain displacement does not occur. If the fracture is displaced (>2 mm) but the articular surface appears intact, flexion to >90 and maximal pronation will often reduce the fracture and a long arm splint or cast can be applied. These also require 3 weeks of immobilization and close radiographic observation.

If stability is in question or the articular surface is significantly displaced, the extremity should be examined using fluoroscopy with the patient under general anesthesia. Percutaneous pinning can be performed if closed anatomic reduction can be achieved. Open reduction using a lateral Kocher approach followed by K-wire fixation may be required for fractures that are >24–48 hours old or if closed reduction is unacceptable. Pin removal and early motion should begin at 3 weeks postop.

Some think that Milch II (SH-2) injuries can often be treated conservatively if the fracture is minimally displaced and the joint is stable. Milch I (SH-4) injuries, on the other hand, require anatomic reduction in order to the reduce the risk of bony bar formation and subsequent angular deformity. Arthrogram can be useful in distinguishing these two injuries in children <7–8 years old, since the trochlea is often not visible on plain film.

The order and timing of the appearance of the ossification centers around the elbow is often of interest and is difficult to remember. A helpful mnemonic to get a ballpark idea is "cars ruin many thousands of limbs" for capitellum (1 year old), radial head (3 years old), medial epicondyle (5 years old), trochlea (7 years old), olecranon (9 years old), and lateral epicondyle (11 years old).

Nonunions can be treated with bone graft and pinning through a lateral (Kocher) approach. Valgus deformity can be treated successfully with an osteotomy.

Pediatric Supracondylar Elbow[13,18]

This fracture is fairly common in the pediatric population, often resulting from a fall on an outstretched extremity. These can be very difficult to treat because neurovascular structures are often involved and complications such as ischemic contractures occur not infrequently.

Supracondylar fractures are divided into three types, depending on the amount of A-P tilt, rotation, and displacement present. In Type I, the fracture line is difficult to visualize, there is no varus/valgus angulation, and A-P tilt is <15–20 degrees. Oblique views are often helpful for identifying nondisplaced fractures. Type II refers to fractures that are clearly displaced but the posterior cortex is intact. Type III fractures are completely displaced with no cortical contact between the two fragments. Type III fractures are usually displaced posteromedially or posterolaterally.

Prior to any treatment or manipulation, one must document the function of the radial, median, ulnar, anterior interosseous, and posterior interosseous nerves and quantify peripheral pulses and capillary refill. Nondisplaced fractures can be treated by immobilization in a long arm splint with the elbow flexed at 90 degrees for 3 weeks. One may choose to admit the child for observation if there is excessive pain or swelling and there is risk of compartment syndrome or other neurovascular compromise.

Type II fractures are hyperextension greenstick fractures that can be reduced by completely relaxing the patient (using intravenous sedation or general anesthesia), fully pronating the forearm, and hyperflexing the arm beyond the resistance that is typically felt just beyond 90 degrees. The arm is then placed in a long arm posterior splint with the elbow flexed to 90–100 degrees. Elbow flexion greater than 90–100 degrees offers greater stability but can predispose to neurovascular compromise. After application of a splint, the postreduction radiographs and neurovascular status of the arm must be evaluated. If neurovascular compromise has occurred, the arm must be extended until the neurovascular status of the limb returns to normal. *Postreduction radiographs*

*should again be checked, and if the reduction is lost, closed reduction
and percutaneous pinning under general anesthesia is indicated.* Most
surgeons prefer to treat this type of fracture with closed reduction
and smooth K-wires from the start in order to immobilize the
elbow at 90 degrees of flexion without fear of instability.

Grossly displaced fractures usually require percutaneous pinning of the fracture or open reduction and smooth K-wire fixation
under fluoroscopic guidance. Closed reduction is performed by
applying longitudinal traction with the elbow in extension and
forearm in supination to regain length. The fracture is then
hyperextended to obtain bony apposition as varus or valgus angulation is corrected. The elbow is then flexed with the forearm
remaining in supination and pressure being applied over the
olecranon. Soft-tissue interposition often prevents adequate reduction, necessitating opening the fracture. Once reduction is
achieved, a K-wire is placed in the lateral condyle and advanced
until it captures the medial cortex proximal to the fracture site.
The reduction can now be reviewed more critically prior to placement of the medial pin. Before the cross pin is placed in the
medial condyle, the elbow should be extended somewhat to limit
the risk of the ulnar nerve subluxating anteriorly over the medial
condyle. A miniopen incision with blunt dissection down to the
bone should be performed prior to pin placement and advancement to the lateral cortex. Some surgeons prefer the placement
of two parallel pins from the lateral side to eliminate the risk to
the ulnar nerve, but this has been shown to be biomechanically
inferior to cross pins. Any decline in the child's neurovascular
examination during or following closed manipulation is an indication for open exploration of the fracture site.

Alternative treatments include Dunlap's sidearm skin traction or overhead traction using an olecranon pin to achieve
reduction followed by a long arm cast. These are rarely used.

A common complication following this injury is development
of a cubitus varus or valgus deformity or a hyperextension deformity at the elbow. These are cosmetic deformities that are usually
not of functional significance. Parents should be warned about
the seriousness of these fractures and should be informed about
the potential complications before treatment begins.

Neurological injuries occur about 7% of the time, with the
radial nerve being affected most. The radial nerve is injured most
because posteromedial displacement of the distal fragment (most

common) leaves the nerve vulnerable to the lateral spike from the proximal fragment. Median nerve injuries tend to occur with posterolateral displacement and are sometimes present with brachial artery injuries. Anterior interosseus nerve injuries are rare but are easily missed. Vascular compromise is seen approximately 5% of the time, with a full blown Volkmann's ischemic contracture occurring in 20% of those cases in one series.

Fat pad signs are often indicative of a nondisplaced fracture. The anterior and posterior fat pads overlie the capsule and only become "signs" when the capsule is intact and an intraarticular effusion has developed. The anterior fat pad is more visible with small effusions and is associated with more false negatives. Posterior fat pads, when present, are more commonly associated with fractures.

Baumann's angle measured off the A-P radiograph correlates well with the "carrying angle"of the elbow and is helpful in determining the presence of a fracture or the adequacy of a reduction. This angle is formed by the line passing through the superior physeal line of the capitellum and the line that is perpendicular to the long axis of the humerus. Baumann's angle should be 10–20 degrees and, more important, should not be more than 5 degrees different from the normal side. Especially in Type III fractures, a contralateral A-P of the elbow should be obtained as part of the preop workup so it can be re-created on the injured side. On the lateral view, the anterior border of the humerus (anterior humeral line) should be in line with the middle third of the ossification center of the capitellum. Additionally, the angle between the humeral shaft and the capitellum should be 35–40 degrees on lateral radiograph on a normal elbow.

Proximal Humeral Physeal Injuries[18]

Eighty percent of the longitudinal growth of the humerus occurs in the proximal humeral physis. Consequently, an injury to this physis is of great clinical significance. However, this large percentage of growth allows tremendous remodeling of the proximal humerus if not reduced perfectly. Additionally, a malunion because of varus or valgus alignment is rarely problematic because of the large range of motion of the shoulder.

Most of these injuries are either Salter I fractures (more frequent in neonates) or Salter II injuries (more common in adolescents). Operative treatment is almost never indicated. In neonates <1 year old, the diagnosis is made clinically, with ultrasound sometimes providing confirmation. Radiographs are rarely helpful, since the proximal humeral physis is not ossified at birth. The neonate often presents with pseudoparalysis of the arm. The differential diagnosis includes clavicle fracture, brachial plexus injury, and infection. With significantly displaced fractures, reduction should be attempted under general anesthesia by longitudinal traction and gentle manipulation with the arm flexed and abducted at 90 degrees. The arm is kept in sling and swathe for 10–14 days until the shoulder becomes more comfortable.

In children 1–5 years old, any apposition and angulation up to 70 degrees is acceptable. In the 5–12-year-old age group, 50% apposition and 50 degrees of angulation are acceptable. Reductions in these two groups can be performed in a similar manner to the neonatal group, and placement in a shoulder immobilizer is usually adequate for stable fractures. For unstable fractures, a shoulder spica cast in the "salute position" should be applied. Older children may be best treated with percutaneous pinning.

In the adolescent group, displacement must be less than $\frac{1}{3}$ the width of the shaft, since there is less time remaining for remodeling. Fractures should be opened if an adequate closed reduction cannot be performed. If instability is present in this age group, serious consideration should be given to percutaneous pinning to allow earlier rehabilitation. Percutaneous pinning also allows the patient to be maintained in a sling with the arm at the side.

Pediatric Hip Fractures[17,18]

Pediatric hip fractures are quite rare and usually occur from major trauma. Though infrequent, these injuries deserve mention because of the high likelihood of complications despite appropriate treatment. Typical complications include avascular necrosis (most notably), coxa vara, malunion, nonunion, and premature physeal closure. These fractures are divided into four classes: transepiphyseal separations, transcervical fractures, cervicotrochanteric fractures, and intertrochanteric fractures.

Transepiphyseal fractures occur through the growth plate of the capital femoral epiphysis and may be associated with or without the dislocation of the femoral head from the acetabulum.

These account for only 8% of pediatric hip fractures but are associated with a nearly 100% incidence of AVN. These fractures must be treated with immediate closed reduction and threaded pin fixation. If closed reduction cannot be achieved, open reduction is indicated. Other complications include leg length discrepency and degenerative arthritis.

Transcervical fractures account for 45%–50% of pediatric hip fractures and are complicated by AVN 40%–45% of the time. Treatment for displaced and nondisplaced fractures is closed reduction and fixation with threaded pins, with care taken not to cross the epiphyseal plate, if possible. Nonunion, premature physeal closure, and coxa vara are less frequent complications.

Cervicotrochanteric fractures occur just proximal to the anterior intertrochanteric line and account for 30%–40% of pediatric hip fractures. Nondisplaced fractures are treated in an abduction spica cast, and displaced ones are closed reduced and fixed with threaded pins avoiding the physis. AVN occurs 20%–30% of the time, nearly exclusively in displaced fractures.

Intertrochanteric fractures account for 10%–20% of pediatric hip fractures and are associated with substantially lower rates of complications. AVN occurs 14% of the time. Treatment is skin or skeletal traction followed by an abduction spica cast. Fixation is used only if reduction cannot be maintained in a cast.

Pediatric Femoral Shaft[17,18]

Treatment of pediatric femoral shaft fractures varies depending on the age of the patient, other injuries, and family dynamics. Infants under 2 years old with isolated femur fractures can usually be treated with immediate fiberglass hip spica cast application. The child should be sedated and the infant's hip should be flexed and externally rotated as longitudinal traction is applied in effort to decrease angulation and shortening. Shortening of 1 cm and angulation of 30 degrees are acceptable in this group. Union occurs in about 2 weeks, and the cast is removed after 4–6 weeks. If there is any question of child abuse or of the family's ability to manage the spica cast, it is appropriate to admit the child temporarily for split Russell's traction.

In the 2–10-year-old age group, the patient can be treated with temporary oblique or horizontal skin traction overnight followed by $1\frac{1}{2}$ hip spica casting in the morning. Shortening of up to 2 cm, angulation of 20–30 degrees in the sagittal plane, and 15–20 degrees in the frontal plane are acceptable in this age group. Obviously, angulation is more acceptable in the younger patients. Union occurs at about about 4–8 weeks (the child's age in years plus 2 is the approximate number of weeks to union). Split Russell's traction is suggested if the child has multiple injuries or if the fracture has a propensity to shorten because of substantial swelling or because of shortening of >2 cm at initial presentation. Traction weight can be adjusted so shortening is optimal at 1–1.5 cm (to allow for some overgrowth at the fracture site). Many practitioners treat 5–14-year-olds with an external fixator to gain better reduction and to avoid the morbidity and inconvenience of traction and/or spica casting. This is especially true in the multitrauma setting.

Femoral shaft fractures in children >10 years old behave more like these fractures in adults. Shortening is more often a problem because of the increased muscular forces of this age group and because the propensity for growth acceleration at the fracture site has decreased. There is less time for remodeling to occur, and union takes about 6–12 weeks, with the period of immobilization lasting for 8–12 weeks if traction and casting are used. Treatment is placement of an external fixator for children <13–14 years old. Unreamed intramedullary nailings are now being used in some children as young as 11–12 years old.

Distal Femoral Physeal Injuries[17,18]

Injury to the distal femoral physis can cause a number of complications. Most of these fractures will be Salter I or Salter II types. The most common mechanism is hyperextension causing the epiphysis to be displaced anteriorly, placing the neurovascular structures at risk. Varus or valgus injuries to the physeal plate are also frequent, and these require an anatomic reduction, since normal growth is unlikely if the epiphysis is displaced at an angle to the plane of knee motion.

Treatment for the Salter I or Salter II injury is closed reduction and application of a well- molded $1\frac{1}{2}$ hip spica to maintain reduction. The knee should be flexed in the cast. One should perform neurovascular checks before and after reduction. Aspiration of a tense hemarthrosis may make the manipulation easier. Intravenous sedation is usually adequate. The reduction begins first with longitudinal traction followed by attempted replacement of the epiphysis on the metaphysis. Fluoroscopy is useful to ensure that reduction is adequate, and it is helpful in deciding how much knee flexion is appropriate following reduction of an anterior displaced fracture. The amount of flexion is determined by placing the knee in the "safe zone" between too much flexion, risking vascular compression, and too little flexion, risking redisplacement. Percutaneous pinning is recommended for unstable Salter II fractures or for undisplaced Salter III or IV injuries. Open reduction is used for displaced Salter III or IV injuries.

Although nearly a third of these patients sustain damage to the growth plate, they are typically close enough to physeal closure that any shortening or angulation is insignificant. Other possible complications include popliteal artery injury (1%), peroneal nerve neuropraxia (3%), and ligamentous damage around the knee.

OTHER MUSCULOSKELETAL INJURIES

Nearly all acute soft-tissue injuries can initially be treated by protection, rest, immobilization, compression, and elevation (PRICE). Treatment is important to prevent further injury to the area, and to decrease the swelling, which lengthens the rehabilitation period.

Carpal Instability[11,12,19]

The wrist is a complex composite of structures whose job it is to provide motion and transmit force between the wrist and the forearm. The wrist consists of seven bones (the pisiform is merely a sesamoid for the FCU) that are divided into two rows. The scaphoid, lunate, and triquetrum make up the proximal row, and the trapezium, trapezoid, capitate, and hamate make up the distal row. The carpal bones are stabilized by both intrinsic and extrinsic ligaments. The most notable volar ligaments include the radioscapholunate, the radiolunate, the radioscaphocapitate, the ulnolunate, and the ulnocarpal meniscus homologue. It is also important to know that the scapholunate interosseous and the lunate-triquetral interosseous ligaments are responsible for stabilizing the proximal row.

Carpal instability is defined as the acute or chronic loss of normal carpal alignment as a result of acute or repetitive trauma.

The instability can be severe and easily diagnosed or subtle and difficult to identify. Static radiographs are frequently negative. The patient may or may not complain of pain. The patient may or may not report a fall on an outstretched hand. Sometimes "clicks" or "clunks" are present. Identification of the painful region, various stress tests, ROM measurements, and grip stress measurement are all important on examination.

Mayfield's biomechanical studies indicate that the mechanism of injury is extension, ulnar deviation, and intercarpal supination. The resulting sequence of injury from this mechanism is described as a progressive pattern of perilunar instability that is divided into four stages. Stage I is scaphoid instability with respect to the lunate (scapholunate diastasis). Stage II is scaphoid and capitate instability with respect to the lunate. Stage III adds triquetral instability with regard to the lunate in addition to Stage II. Stage IV refers to lunate dislocation.

A-P, lateral, and oblique views of the wrist will sometimes demonstrate findings consistent with carpal instability. Other helpful views include an A-P "clenched fist" or ulnar- deviated view. One should first look at the lateral and confirm that the radius, lunate, and capitate all have a colinear existence. If the lunate is angled dorsally, a dorsal intercalated segment instability (DISI) pattern may be present. Conversely, if the lunate is angled volarly, a VISI pattern may be present. DISI and VISI patterns are frequently seen in clinically important instabilities. While inspecting the lateral view, one should measure the angle between the long axis of the scaphoid and the longitudinal axis of the lunate. This angle (scapholunate angle) averages around 47 degrees and the normal range is 30–60 degrees. On the A-P view, a foreshortened scaphoid with a "ring" bicortical density indicates that the scaphoid is excessively perpendicular with respect to the radius. This often occurs in scapholunate dissociation and in VISI patterns. A scapholunate interval greater than 3 mm (compare with other side) suggests a chronic diastasis. Another important number is the carpal height ratio, which is the height of the two rows of carpal bones divided by the length of the third metacarpal. This number is normally $0.54+/-0.03$, and a decreased value indicates longitudinal collapse of the carpal bones as is seen in some wrist instabilities and some degenerative conditions.

Other modalities are becoming increasingly useful for the diagnosis of carpal instability. Fluoroscopy can be performed in the office and can often reveal abnormal motion in patients with normal static films. Arthrography is used to identify scapholunate and triquetrolunate interosseous tears, as well as tears in the triangular fibrocartilage complex (TFCC). MRI has become an increasingly useful tool in the diagnosis of ligament tears, chondral defects, occult ganglia, and synovitis. Wrist arthroscopy is becoming increasingly useful in the diagnosis of obscure wrist pain and in the treatment of some disease entities.

Scapholunate and triquetrolunate dissociation, as well as midcarpal instability, are frequently diagnosed. Acutely, realignment and stabilization should be performed to prevent chronic problems. Chronic carpal instability should be treated aggressively with dorsal and/or volar ligamentous reconstruction to avoid posttraumatic osteoarthritic changes such as scapholunate advanced collapse (SLAC wrist). Salvage procedures including four corner fusions and proximal row carpectomy are indicated after degenerative changes have occurred.

Triangular Fibrocartilage Complex Tears (TFCC)[20]

Triangular fibrocartilage complex tears have received increasing attention in the literature as a cause of ulnar-sided wrist pain. The TFCC overlies the distal ulna and is interposed between the distal radioulnar joint and the radiocarpal joint. This complex refers to a central articular disk overlying the distal ulna that originates from the hyaline cartilage of the distal radiolunate fossa, the dorsal and palmar radioulnar ligaments, the meniscus homologue, and the sheath of the extensor carpi ulnaris.

Injuries to the TFCC can result in pain and/or instability. Injuries to the central (avascular) portion of the articular disk are usually treated by arthroscopic debridement without sacrificing distal radioulnar joint stability. Injuries to the vascular periphery of the articular disk are often repaired open. Degenerative changes in the TFCC are associated with ulnocarpal impaction syndrome, which is seen in individuals with positive ulnar variance (relatively long ulna). If conservative measures fail to relieve discomfort, the correction of the length disparity between the radius and ulna is usually treated by ulnar shortening.

DeQuervain's Stenosing Tenosynovitis[10,11]

DeQuervain's stenosing tenosynovitis is the only frequently encountered tendonitis on the dorsal side of the wrist. It is diagnosed by inflammation, tenderness and often thickening over the extensor tendons of the first extensor compartment (AbPL and EPB) and a positive *Finkelstein's test*. Finkelstein's test is performed by asking the patient to make a fist over a flexed thumb and ulnarly deviating the wrist. Pain experienced over the radial styloid indicates a positive test. Often, the thumb-in-fist position is itself acutely painful in this condition and the patient refuses to ulnarly deviate the wrist. Patients will often complain of pain in this region when they use their thumb.

DeQuervain's tenosynovitis must be differentiated from degenerative arthritis at the trapeziometacarpal joint, especially in older age groups. The test to differentiate the two is the *grind test*. This test is usually negative in DeQuervain's and positive in degenerative arthritis. It is performed by holding the thumb proximal phalanx and MCPJ in the examiner's hands and placing an axial load on the trapeziometacarpal joint. The examiner should also rotate the thumb metacarpal to cause a grinding motion.

Initial treatment of DeQuervain's begins with nonsteroidal antiinflammatories and immobilizing the thumb in a thumb spica splint. If this fails, injections in the tendon sheath with corticosteroids will usually provide relief. Rarely, conservative measures will fail and surgical release of the tendon sheath will be required. Care must be taken to identify the radial sensory nerve and its branches to prevent injury.

First Carpometacarpal Joint Arthritis[10,11]

One of the first sites of degenerative joint disease is the thumb basal joint. Patients will typically present complaining of pain in the thumb with use. A positive ''grind test'' helps to distinguish it from DeQuervain's tenosynovitis (see above). This physical examination finding combined with a radiograph showing degeneration of the articular surface of the trapezium, and often subluxation of the metacarpal off the trapezium, makes the diagnosis. Advanced chronic arthritis of the trapeziometacarpal joint occasionally will require a fusion, trapezial prosthesis, or by resection of the trapezium and replacement with a rolled tendon. The latter of these procedures is referred to as an *"anchovie procedure"* or LRTI (ligamentous reconstruction and tendon interposition). Usually, the entire trapezium is removed (sometimes only $\frac{1}{2}$ is removed in young patients or golfers) and the void is filled by a rolled ipsilateral tendon. Usually, $\frac{1}{2}$ of the FCR, all of the FCR, or the palmaris longus is used.

Compression Neuropathies[10,11]

Compression neuropathies have similar presentations and occur in anatomically predictable areas. Low levels of compression of brief duration cause intermittent symptoms that are probably caused by changes in intraneural circulation. These changes and the resultant symptoms are rapidly reversible following decompression. Higher levels of compression or compression that has been present for a longer period of time causes structural changes in the peripheral nerve and nerve body that resolves much more slowly with decompression.

The most common compression neuropathy is *carpal tunnel syndrome (CTS)*. This is a compression of the median nerve at the wrist by the transverse carpal ligament. The most common cause of nerve compression is inflammation within the carpal tunnel. Typical symptoms include pain at the wrist or hand and numbness or paraesthesias in the median nerve distribution (the radial $3\frac{1}{2}$ digits). Examination often reveals a positive Phalen's or Tinel's test (Percussion test), increased two-point distance discrimination (>6 mm), decreased sudomotor activity, and, in chronic cases, thenar atrophy and a weakened APB. Phalen's test involves holding the wrist in volar flexion for up to a minute. Often this will reproduce the paraesthesias in the radial three and one-half digits. Tinel's test is performed by gentle tapping over the median nerve at the wrist; a positive test will also elicit the paraesthesias in the median nerve distribution of the hand. The carpal compression test causes parasthesias in a median nerve distribution with compression on the palmar side of the wrist over the median nerve. The diagnosis can be confirmed by nerve conduction studies.

Treatment of carpal tunnel syndrome begins with nonsteroidal medication and wrist splinting. If unsuccessful, this is followed by injecting the carpal tunnel with a lidocaine-steroid preparation. This should be repeated no more than three times because of the risk of tendon rupture. Care should be taken not to inject the median nerve. Resistant or advanced cases should be treated surgically by dividing the transverse carpal ligament to decompress the median nerve. Care must be taken to fully release the ligament while not injuring the palmar cutaneous branch of the median nerve. Endoscopic release should be performed only by surgeons experienced in the procedure because of the high risk of complications (incomplete release, damage to neurovascular or tendinous structures).

Pronator syndrome refers to compression of the median nerve at the elbow by the supracondylar ligament of Struthers, the lacertus fibrosis (fibrous band extending medially off the biceps tendon to insert on the proximal ulna), the pronator teres, and the proximal arch of the FDS. Symptoms are similar to carpal tunnel syndrome except that the patient may report pain in the volar forearm that increases with activity. Physical examination is similar to CTS except that Tinel's test is positive in the forearm and negative at the wrist and Phalen's test is usually negative. Pain may be notable on resistance to pronation and/or on resistance to isolated flexion to the PIP joint of the long and ring fingers. Electrodiagnostic studies should be performed for confirmation. Conservative therapy consists of rest with 4–6 weeks of splinting. If unsuccessful, exploratory surgery is indicated for decompression of the nerve as needed.

Anterior interosseous syndrome refers to entrapment of this branch of the median nerve 4–6 cm distal to the elbow usually by the deep head of the pronator teres but also the origin of the FDS, the origin of the FCR, and also by accessory muscles running between the FDS and FDP and by Gantzer's muscle, which is an accessory head to the FPL. Thrombosis of the ulnar collateral arteries and an aberrant radial artery can also produce this syndrome. The anterior interosseous nerve innervates the FPL, the FDP to the index and middle, and the pronator quadratus, but it provides no sensory innervation. The patient typically presents complaining of forearm pain followed by paresis or paralysis of the previously mentioned muscles causing the patient to have decreased precise pinch strength. The differential diagnosis includes Mannerfelt syndrome, which is an attrition rupture of the FPL. Treatment of anterior interosseous syndrome is exploration and decompression of the offending structures.

Ulnar tunnel syndrome refers to compression of the ulnar nerve within Guyon's canal at the wrist. Etiologies include ulnar artery aneurysm or thrombosis, ganglia, anomalous muscle bellies or ligaments, idiopathic fascial thickening, and hypertrophy of the palmaris brevis. Patients present complaining of ulnar-sided pain and paraesthesias and sometimes cold intolerance. Examination reveals decreased sensation in the ulnar $1\frac{1}{2}$ digits, intrinsic muscle weakness, possible hypothenar atrophy, positive wrist flexion (Phalen's) or Tinel's tests, and occasionally delayed ulnar artery filling demonstrated by a positive Allen's test. Conservative therapy includes rest, immobilization, and limited steroid injections. Surgical intervention includes release of the volar carpal ligament and decompression of the ulnar nerve.

Cubital tunnel syndrome refers to compression of the ulnar nerve around the elbow usually between the ulnar and humeral origins of the FCU or at the proximal border of the cubital tunnel by an enlarged medial head of the triceps muscle. Other sites of compression include the arcade of Struthers (8 cm proximal to the elbow) and the intermuscular septum. Patients with a history of trauma with resultant cubitus valgus are at increased risk. These patients may complain of vague pain and may report ulnar-sided paraesthesias and numbness. On physical examination, they often have weakness of the intrinsics and, less frequently, they have some decreased FDP (ulnar digits) and FCU strength. Patients may also have a positive elbow flexion test and a positive Tinel's test at the elbow. One must carefully evaluate the patient to rule out thoracic outlet syndrome, C8–T1 root compression and Guyon's canal (ulnar tunnel) syndrome, and electrodiagnostic studies are nearly always needed. Conservative therapy includes night extension splinting and avoidance of provocative activities. Operative interventions include release of the FCU aponeurosis between the humeral and ulnar origins, anterior transposition (subcutaneous, intramuscular, and submuscular), and/or medial epicondylectomy.

Radial tunnel syndrome results from radial nerve entrapment around the elbow caused by fibrous bands from the radiocapitellar articulation, radial recurrent vessels (Leash of Henry), the tendinous origin of the ECRB, the tendinous origin of the supinator (Arcade of Frohse), and the distal edge of the supinator. There are no motor or sensory deficits. Electrodiagnostic tests are usually very normal. There is pain over the extensor origin that is most notable 5 cm distal to the lateral epicondyle. This is exacerbated with resistance to supination and with resistance to middle finger extension with the elbow at 45 degrees of flexion and the wrist in neutral position. This is often confused with "tennis elbow" (lateral epicondylitis). Conservative therapy involves rest and splinting of the extremity with the wrist dorsiflexed and the forearm supinated. If this fails, exploration and decompression are indicated.

Posterior interosseous syndrome is caused by compression of the posterior interosseous nerve as it passes through the arcade of Frohse causing pain, as well as weakness of the brachioradialis, ECRB/ECRL, and the supinator. There is no cutaneous sensory deficit. The syndrome often resolves spontaneously with activity alteration. If symptoms persist, surgical decompression is indicated.

Thoracic outlet syndrome and *cervical root compression* must always be considered when evaluating an upper extremity compression neuropathy. These entities can mimic other previously mentioned syndromes and can also present with them as part of a "double crush" syndrome.

Gamekeeper's Thumb[10,11]

Gamekeeper's thumb is an injury to the ulnar collateral ligament of the thumb MCP joint, causing instability at that joint. It was formerly seen in British gamekeepers who stretched out the ligament by wringing off the heads of rabbits, but today it is most commonly seen in skiers and basketball players who sustain forced radial deviation (abduction) at the thumb MCP. These injuries are frequently accompanied by injuries to the dorsal capsule and volar plate, as well as avulsion fractures of the volar base of the proximal phalanx, so radiographs should be closely inspected to rule out subluxation or fracture.

The stability of the MCP joint should be tested by applying a radially directed force to the joint with the joint fully extended and then flexed 30 degrees. Comparison with the opposite thumb is necessary because people have varying amounts of ligamentous laxity. A joint that opens up less than 30 degrees more than the opposite thumb and that has a definite endpoint has probably not sustained a complete rupture of the ligament. In this case, treatment would be a short arm cast with a thumb spica for 4 weeks. Care should be taken to apply a gentle ulnar deviating stress to the MCP joint to promote healing and prevent laxity.

If radial stress to the injured MCP demonstrates less than a 30-degree difference from the other side but one cannot appreciate a clear endpoint, a median and radial nerve block must be applied and the patient re-examined when he or she is more comfortable. This should prevent a false-negative because of patient discomfort.

A joint that deviates 30 degrees more than the opposite thumb because of a radially directed stress indicates a complete rupture of the ulnar collateral ligament. Most hand surgeons recommend open repair of the ligament in those cases to prevent chronic laxity.

The main complication of closed treatment is failure of the ligament to heal, resulting instability of the joint. In a complete rupture, this will often be caused by a Stener lesion, which is the interposition of the adductor aponeurosis between the distally avulsed ligament and its insertion on the proximal phalanx. Adductor interposition cannot occur in partial ruptures. This makes it critical to distinguish between partial and complete ruptures of the ulnar collateral ligament. Many physicians operate when they believe a complete rupture of the ligament exists, because of the high frequency of Stener lesions associated with complete ruptures.

Rotator Cuff Disease[21]

The pathogenesis of rotator cuff disease appears to be multifactorial, as both intrinsic and extrinsic factors have been implicated. Extrinsic factors are thought to contribute to impingement demonstrated by pain in the subacromial space when the humerus is elevated or internally rotated. This causes compression of the rotator cuff against the undersurface of the acromion and coracoacromial ligament, resulting in a subacromial bursitis and mechanical wear and degeneration of the cuff (especially the supraspinatus m.). More recently, intrinsic factors have received more attention, focusing on a hypovascular region of the supraspinatus tendon near its insertion on the greater tuberosity. This vascular "critical zone" is the site of anastomoses between the osseous and tendinous vessels. The rotator cuff musculature is normally supplied by the anterior humeral circumflex, the suprascapular, and the subscapular arteries. As the patient ages and vascular supply becomes more tenuous, intrinsic changes in the tendons are thought to occur, resulting in intrasubstance tears. These degenerative changes create a muscular imbalance, and the humeral head tends to migrate superiorly under the influence of the deltoid. This leads to a decrease in the subacromial space, further exacerbating extrinsic factors.

The patient will often complain of pain with both forward flexion and abduction. Pain is usually associated with overhead activities. The pain will often become worse at night, as the subacromial bursa becomes hyperemic after a day of activity. On physical examination, the physician should note any abnormal masses, bony prominences, and tender regions, as well the stability of the shoulder, since instability can cause impingement secondarily. Diagnosis is confirmed by the Neer and Hawkins impingement signs. Pain that is elicited when the arm is brought to maximum forward flexion while the examiner stabilizes the scapula is known as the Neer impingement sign. Pain that occurs with forward flexion of the arm to 90 degrees and internal rotation of the shoulder is known as the Hawkins impingement sign. If a patient has a positive impingement sign, one may confirm the finding by performing the impingement test. The *impingement test* is performed by first eliciting a positive impingement sign. Ten to fifteen milliliters of xylocaine is then injected into the subacromial space. If the impingement sign is then negative, the impingement test is positive, confirming that the subacromial space was the source of pain. The examiner should also document the active and passive range of motion of the shoulder and also check the relative strengths of the rotator cuff muscles.

Extrinsic causes of rotator cuff disease resulting in primary impingement include abnormalities in the bony architecture of the acromion and the acromioclavicular joint. Acromial shape has been described as Type I (flat), Type II (gently curved), and Type III (hooked). Type III decreases the space available for the rotator cuff to clear and has been associated with a higher incidence of impingement and rotator cuff tears. It is not clear whether a hooked acromion predisposes to rotator cuff disease or vice versa. A-C joint arthritis and osteophytes extending inferiorly from the A-C joint can also cause mechanical irritation to the tendons of the rotator cuff.

Secondary impingement may be caused by muscle imbalance, resulting in proximal migration of the humeral head. Another cause may be crowding of the subacromial space with a thickened, calcified bursa. Instability and proximal humerous malunions are other sources of secondary impingement. Subclinical istability can cause impingement in younger, more active patients by placing the tendons of the cuff under an abnormal amount of stretch, resulting in a tendinitis. Greater tuberosity fractures that are allowed to migrate superiorly in healing can cause impingement. Similarly, a fracture of the surgical neck that heals in varus may cause impingement as the patient attempts to use the extremity for overhead activity.

Rotator cuff disease is classified into three stages. Stage I is typified by edema and hemorrhage in the subacromial space caused by both intrinsic and extrinsic factors working together. These factors often exacerbate one another and may cause progression to Stage II, rotator cuff tendinitis, unless an appropriate intervention is performed. Stage III is a partial or complete tear, and some subscribe to a Stage IV describing a cuff-tear arthropathy.

Routine radiographic examination includes a true A-P view, an outlet (Bigliani) view, and an axillary lateral view. In chronic rotator cuff disease, sclerosis and sometimes spurring are noted around the greater tuberosity. Additionally, an acromiohumeral interval <7 mm (normal is 10–15 mm) is often associated with a significant tear, since the deltoid overpowers the weakened cuff, pulling the head proximally. Frequently radiographs will be normal despite the presence of cuff pathology. Recent studies indicate that a reduction of the acromiohumeral space to <2 mm on the active abduction view (A-P while arm is abducted at 90 degrees) may be helpful for diagnosing cuff tears.

Single- and double-contrast arthrography have a sensitivity and specificity of >85% for complete tears but are much less reliable in the diagnosis of intrasubstance and partial tears. MRI has become the most sensitive and comprehensive method of imaging the shoulder, though it remains very expensive. MRI is 100% specific and 95% sensitive in the diagnosis of full thickness tears. Currently, MRI still has difficulty distinguishing tendinitis from both degeneration and partial thickness tears and can only do so about 80%–85% of the time. Ultrasonography is much less expensive and is used in many centers instead of MRI in order to evaluate the rotator cuff.

Rotator cuff disease often begins as an overuse syndrome, which is exacerbated by certain anatomic variations in the acromion, A-C joint, and the rotator cuff. Initial treatment consists of activity modification and NSAIDs. These patients should avoid overhead activities and may benefit from cuff strengthening exercises and stretches to help restore motion lost because of pain and disuse.

Chronic cases are often treated by injection of a preparation consisting of a steroid and a long-acting local anesthetic. It is important to inject only into the subacromial space and not the tendons of the rotator cuff, because of the risk of tendon rupture. Using sterile technique, the lateral surface of the acromion is palpated and the needle inserted through the skin until it strikes the acromion. The needle is then "walked-down" the acromion until the needle passes under the acromion. It will then be in the subacromial space and the solution should then be injected with minimal, if any, resistance.

The subacromial space usually should not be injected with steroids more than 2–3 times because of the risk of tendon rupture. Cases that do not respond to the above conservative measures after 6 months of treatment are candidates for surgery. The procedure of choice is an anteroinferior acromioplasty combined with division of the coracoacromial ligament. Resection of the distal clavicle (Mumford procedure) is sometimes performed in addition to acromioplasty if the patient has pain localized to the A-C joint. Chronic rotator cuff tears are the end stage of impingement syndrome and are caused by continued mechanical irritation resulting in progressive tendon damage. These are typically treated by debridement in the older population. In younger patients (<60 years old), primary repair is typically attempted. The repair should not be under undue stress with the arm hanging at the side or it will not heal. Repair with autogenous fascial graft is rarely performed.

Tennis Elbow[10]

Tennis elbow is the term popularly used to describe tendinitis about the origin of the extensor muscles from the lateral epicondyle of the humerus (lateral epicondylitis). It also refers to inflammation of the origin of the flexor muscles from the medial epicondyle (medial epicondylitis), though this is usually termed "golfer's elbow."

The name originated because lateral epicondylitis is often seen in tennis players. It is an overuse syndrome seen primarily in individuals in their fourth and fifth decades of life, and it can be caused by many other activities besides tennis. Since the condition occurs on the lateral side 7–10 times more frequently than on the medial side, that will be the focus of this section. Though the conjoined tendon originating from the lateral epicondyle consists of fibers of the ECRB, EDC, EDM (minimi), ECU, and part of the supinator, the tears and degenerative tissue are nearly always present in the ECRB.

As mentioned earlier in discussing compression neuropathies, this problem can be difficult to distinguish from radial tunnel syndrome and, occasionally, the two conditions will co-exist. Patients with lateral epicondylitis report that the point of maximal tenderness is the lateral epicondyle, while in radial tunnel syndrome, the most tender region is the mobile muscle mass just distal to the radial head. In lateral epicondylitis, pain is reproduced with passive flexion of the wrist and fingers while the elbow is fully extended. In radial tunnel syndrome, pain is created by extending the elbow and resisting long finger extension or forearm supination.

Treatment is initially directed at decreasing the frequency of the activity causing the problem, and this is often supplemented with NSAIDs. After the condition resolves, the patient may resume the activity, but should be advised to limit the frequency and attempt to alter the biomechanics of the activity. For tennis players, this often involves lessons to improve the mechanics of the patient's/player's strokes or a change in the racket size or weight. Ice packs to the elbow after performing the exacerbating activity and/or a forearm support brace that compresses the extensor musculature just distal to the elbow often provides relief in difficult cases. Corticosteroid injections are controversial since they frequently provide relief but may put the muscle origins at risk for degeneration and possible rupture. Surgery is reserved for only the most recalcitrant cases and involves debridement of the damaged tendon fibers, partial excision of the epicondyle, and then replacement of healthy tissue over exposed bone.

Ankle Sprains[22]

Ankle sprains are common orthopaedic injuries and often occur with inversion of the ankle causing damage to the lateral structures of the ankle. In general, an ankle is sprained if an injury has caused pain about the ankle and radiographs are negative.

The orthopaedic surgeon must be careful to perform an accurate history and physical examination so another, more serious diagnosis is not missed. In history taking, it is important to identify the force that was placed on the foot and ankle at the time of the injury. With an inversion mechanism, the anterior talofibular ligament (ATFL) is the most likely to be injured. If the foot was dorsiflexed when the injury occurred, the calcaneofibular ligament (CFL) is the most likely to be injured. In more severe injuries, both of these ligaments may be involved. The posterior talofibular ligament (PTFL) is also on the lateral aspect of the foot but is rarely severely injured. If the foot happened to have been externally rotated or everted, the injury may involve the tibiofibular syndesmosis and possibly the deltoid ligament.

Physical examination is often difficult because of the swelling and pain in the region. Even so, it is important for the orthopaedic surgeon to palpate the ankle to identify the region of greatest injury. The inaccurate diagnosis of an ankle sprain can often delay the diagnosis of a ruptured Achilles tendon, subluxated or dislocated peroneal tendons, an osteochondral lesion of the lateral or medial talar dome, a fracture of the lateral process of the talus, a fracture of the anterior process of the calcaneus or an avulsion fracture of the base of the fifth metatarsal. Swelling about the lateral malleolus with tenderness about the anterior talofibular ligament indicates at least a Grade I ankle sprain, implying slight stretching of the ligament without disruption. Grade II ankle sprains imply partial tearing of a ligament, while a Grade III sprain is consistent with complete rupture of a ligament, usually the anterior talofibular ligament.

With an anterior talofibular ligament tear, the ankle drawer test should be increased compared with the contralateral side. To perform this test, place one hand around the heel, with the thumb on the talus. The other hand is placed just above the ankle joint to stabilize the tibia. While the tibia is stabilized, place the foot in slight plantar flexion and internal rotation, and then pull forward with the hand behind the heel. If damage is suspected to the calcaneofibular ligament, the drawer with the ankle dorsiflexed should be increased. Less than 3 mm translation is normal, while >5 mm is considered pathologic. These drawer tests should not be performed acutely since the patient will be guarding, often resulting in a false negative examination.

Diagnosis of these injuries is sometimes assisted by stress radiographs. These rarely need to be performed in the ER, since the patient is likely going to be treated in the same manner, regardless of the diagnosis. These radiographs are more typically used in the office when patients present later on complaining of persistent instability. The amount of talar tilt can be quantified using an A-P radiograph in both plantar flexion and dorsiflexion to test the competence of the ATFL and the CFL, respectively. Talar tilt >10 degrees more than the contralateral side is considered pathologic. To perform these stress films, the examiner simply grasps the patient's hindfoot with one hand and the distal tibia with the other and applies the appropriate stress.

Mild ankle sprains are typically treated with rest, ice, elevation, an air cast, and restricted activity for 7–10 days. Moderate to severe ankle sprains often require immobilization for a few days in a cast, followed by several weeks of an air cast and rehabilitation. Rehabilitation stresses range of motion, strengthening of muscles around the ankle, and peroneal muscular strengthening. A brace is often helpful because it increases proprioception about the ankle. Of course, NSAIDs and ice are the cornerstone for controlling inflammation. Chronic ankle instability is sometimes treated by ligamentous reconstruction of the structures on the lateral side of the ankle. These procedures often cause decreased ankle flexibility postoperatively.

Knee Injuries[23]

Many times a patient will sustain what appears to be a significant knee injury, but no fracture or dislocation will be seen. It is important in these cases to document the size of the knee effusion (mild, moderate, or large) and the chronologic development of the effusion (i.e., how quickly it developed).

When no fracture is present, most (85%) significant acute knee effusions are indicative of acute rupture of the anterior cruciate ligament. These effusions develop quickly (within a few hours) because of the vascularity of the anterior cruciate. Effusions that develop more slowly (over a few hours) are usually indicative of meniscal or osteochondral injuries. Effusions from meniscal injuries take up to 24 hours to form and will often not be significantly bloody, unlike ACL or osteochondral injuries. Though rarely performed, aspiration of the joint can be helpful diagnostically. Another less common knee injury is rupture of the patellar tendon, so the integrity of the extensor mechanism must be examined carefully.

Swelling about the knee does not necessarily indicate an effusion. Localized swelling with local tenderness can be seen with isolated injuries to the collateral ligaments. Collateral ligament injuries can be graded by varus or valgus laxity examination. In the pediatric population, varus/valgus instability can be because of a physeal injury (usually distal femoral physis). This injury can be ruled out by an examination under fluoroscopy.

Documentation of an acute knee effusion is quite important because it usually implies anterior cruciate ligament damage. Attempting to examine the knee for anterior instability is often impossible in the acute situation, because of pain and spasm. The injured knee should be placed in a compressive dressing and a knee immobilizer. The patient's extremity should initially be treated with ice, elevation, and NSAIDs. Weight bearing as tolerated with crutches is allowed. The patient should be instructed to follow up with an orthopaedic surgeon in 5–7 days. At that time, a repeat examination may yield an accurate diagnosis, and physical therapy, if needed, can be initiated.

If the ACL is torn, reconstruction is typically performed in young, active individuals who have complaints consistent with instability while participating in activities that they cannot or will not give up. The ACL is usually reconstructed using a bone patellar tendon bone autograft (central $\frac{1}{3}$ of the patellar tendon). Surgery is performed when the patient has regained a full range of motion following injury.

Meniscal injuries can prevent regaining adequate motion and can result in pain and swelling. These are treated with arthroscopic repair or debridement depending on the patient's age and activity level and the size and appearance of the meniscal tear. Chondral injuries tend to result in pain and recurrent effusion. These are treated arthroscopically with abrasion of the exposed bone and debridement of unhealthy cartilage in effort to stimulate fibrocartilage production (abrasion chondroplasty).

Adult Low Back Pain[23,24]

Adult low back pain is a very common complaint, striking 90% of people over their lifetimes. This musculoskeletal problem ranks third behind only arthritis and cardiac disease as causes for disability in the working class population. It is important to note that of the estimated $16 billion to $46 billion spent annually treating this condition, 90% of that sum is spent treating individuals with chronic low back pain (symptoms for >3 months).

Low back pain is typically a self-limited process, with nearly 70% of people recovering within 30 days, and 90% being fully recovered by 60 days. During the initial visit, the physician should attempt to understand the length of symptoms and the pain distribution. Additionally, the clinician needs to rule out the rare but serious causes of LBP (infection, cancer, or spondyloarthropathy). The physician must ask about pain at rest with no positional relief, night pain, fever, weight loss, history of malignancy, and morning stiffness. Positive responses to any of these questions should raise a "red flag." Radiographs are not indicated at the initial visit unless there is a positive "red flag," or symptoms have been going on for >1 month, or the patient is greater than 50 years of age.

Acute low back pain should be treated with a maximum of 2–3 days of bed rest, NSAIDs, and acetaminophen (Tylenol). Muscle relaxants and opioid analgesics may be helpful, but they have not shown any additional benefit, and they do have the increased risk of side effects. Some practitioners favor manipulation of the back, which refers to the manual loading of the spine using leverage. These techniques have no proven efficacy, though some patients appear to benefit from them. Others prescribe back school, in which patients are given techniques to allow them to take better care of their backs. At back school, patients learn how to lift and move more appropriately. Additionally, patients are taught stretches and abdominal exercises and are encouraged to participate in aerobic exercises and water aerobics.

Patients who don't get better after 3 months are referred to as having chronic low back pain. This may be the correct time for referral to the spine specialist. If not, the clinician must reconsider the "serious" causes of low back pain. Radiographs should have been performed after about a month of pain and, subsequently, eliminated the possibilities of degenerative disc disease, scoliosis, and spondylolisthesis. Seronegative arthropathies and metabolic bone diseases should be considered at this point. Another physical examination is indicated at this time. One must palpate the back to try to identify a source of discomfort. The range of motion of the back needs to be checked. The distribution of pain and/or lack of sensation needs to be properly delineated. The practitioner needs to check if the patient has a limp or stretch signs, and muscle atrophy or altered reflexes.

The practitioner needs to be cautious in using imaging techniques. One study demonstrated that 50% of the subjects >60 years old had positive MRI findings, with 21% having spinal stenosis and 36% having a herniated disc. The practitioner needs to confirm that MRI and imaging findings are consistent with the physical examination and history. MRI is very sensitive for evaluating suspected herniated discs, tumors, or infections. CT myelogram with contrast is considered better for evaluating central and root spinal stenosis.

Conservative therapy is indicated initially for herniated discs, as fewer than 10% of patients with symptoms ultimately require surgery. Lumbar discectomy, when performed, is successful 90% to 95% of the time, with leg pain typically better relieved than back pain. Open microdiscectomy is the gold standard for treatment of a herniated disc. Percutaneous lumbar discectomy is gaining favor owing to less postoperative pain and shorter hospital stays. Unfortunately, the success rate still lags behind the open discectomy. Chemonucleolysis is rarely used in the United States because of complications. Weight control is an important part of therapy. Braces are utilized only for patient comfort.

References

1. Carter DR. Biomechanics of bone fracture. Orthopaedic Update Series 1982;1.
2. Charnley JS. The closed treatment of common fractures. Edinburgh: E&S Livingston,1968.
3. Madewell JE, et al. Radiologic and pathologic analysis of solitary bone lesions. Part I: internal margins. Part II: periosteal reactions. Part III: matrix patterns. Radiol Clin North Am 1981;19:750–785,715–748,749–784.
4. Dahlin DC, Unni KK. Bone tumors. 4th ed. Champaign, IL: Charles C. Thomas, 1986.
5. Huvos, AG. Bone tumors: diagnosis, treatment and prognosis. Philadelphia: WB Saunders, 1979.
6. Scajowicz F. Tumors and tumorlike lesions of bone and joints. New York: Springer- Verlag,1981.
7. Enneking WF. Musculoskeletal tumor surgery. 2 vols. New York: Churchill-Livingstone, 1983.

8. Mueller ME, Allgoewer M, Schneider R, et al. Manual of internal fixation. Berlin: Springer- Verlag,1979.

9. Crenshaw AH, ed. Campbell's operative orthopaedics. 8th ed. 5 vols. St. Louis: CV Mosby, 1987.

10. Green DP, ed. Operative hand surgery. 3rd ed. 2 vols. New York: Churchill-Livingstone, 1993.

11. Regional Review Courses in Hand Surgery. American Society for the Hand. Durham, NC, 1994.

12. Browner BD, Jupiter JB, Levine AM, Trafton PG, eds. Skeletal trauma. 2 vols. Philadelphia: WB Saunders, 1992.

13. Residents' meeting. Orthopaedic Trauma Association. Tampa, FL, 1995.

14. Rockwood CA, Green DP, eds. Fractures in adults. 3rd ed. 2 vols. Philadelphia: JB Lippincott, 1991.

15. Denis F. The three column spine and its significance in the classification of acute thoracolumbar spinal injuries. Spine 1983;8(8): 817–831.

16. Bracken MB, et al. A randomized, controlled trial of methylprednisolone or nalaxone in the treatment of acute spinal cord injury. N Engl J Med 1990;322(20):1405–1411.

17. Southwestern Orthopaedic Surgery Board Review. Dallas, TX, 1997.

18. Rockwood CA, Green DP, eds. Fractures in children. 3rd ed. 2 vols. Philadelphia: JB Lippincott, 1991.

19. Taleisnik J. Post-traumatic carpal instability. Clin Orthop 1980; 149:73–82.

20. Chidgey LK. The distal radioulnar joint: problems and solutions. J Am Acad Orthop Surg 1995;3:95–109.

21. Rockwood CA, Matsen FA. The shoulder. Philadelphia: WB Saunders, 1990.

22. Review course. American Orthopaedic Foot and Ankle Society. Charlotte, NC, 1995.

23. Orthopaedic knowledge update 4. Home study syllabus. Chicago: American Academy of Orthopaedic Surgeons, 1993.

24. Bendo JA, Neuwirth M. Treatment of low back pain in adults. Orthop Spec Ed 1995;I:54–57.

Chapter 7

Casting and Splinting Techniques

The primary goals of casting and splinting are to immobilize the injured extremity for comfort and to maintain adequate alignment of fractures and/or ligamentous structures for healing to occur. Additionally, casts and splints are sometimes used to protect postoperative wounds or to relieve pressure from sores (e.g., diabetic ulcer).

Splinting is a useful method of immobilization in the acute injury period. A satisfactory mold can be applied to the splint to hold the fracture alignment while the splint allows for swelling to occur. Using a splint instead of a cast reduces the risk of an iatrogenic compartment syndrome resulting in ischemic contractures. The disadvantage of the splint is that the construct is not as stable as a circumferential cast and that it will loosen with time. Careful follow-up is necessary to prevent a loss of reduction when using a splint.

It is important to immobilize a joint above and below the level of a fracture to adequately stabilize the injury in all planes. One must remember to immobilize joints in the appropriate position, because many joints will stiffen permanently with prolonged casting despite appropriate physical therapy after cast removal. For example, immobilization of the metacarpophalangeal joints in extension for as briefly as 3 weeks can result in motion loss. If the metacarpophalangeal joints must be immobilized for extended periods, they should be immobilized in 90 degrees of flexion, if possible. Flexion maintains the length of the collateral ligaments and allows for recovery of range of motion after cast removal.

CASTING AND SPLINTING MATERIALS[1]

Casts are usually made from plaster of Paris. The plaster of Paris bandage consists of a roll of fabric (originally crinoline, now a fabric called leno) that is impregnated with plaster of Paris. The addition of water to calcium sulfate causes it to be transformed into its crystalline form (gypsum). This is described by the chemical equation $CaSO_4\ H_2O + H_2O = CaSO_4\ 2H_2O + heat$. This is an exothermic reaction in which the powdered plaster of Paris becomes a rocklike mass.

Plaster is available as rolls in a variety of widths (2-, 3-, 4-, and 6-inch-wide rolls) and as splints (3×15 inches, 4×15 inches, and 5×30 inches). The setting time of the plaster decreases when it is dipped in warmer water. Lukewarm water is typically used in order to give time for adequate molding. Gloves should be worn when rolling plaster, as it is difficult to remove from the skin once it is hard. Sugar water is helpful in removing hardened plaster from the skin.

Fiberglass casting material is becoming increasingly popular because it is strong, lightweight, waterproof, and sets very quickly. Disadvantages of fiberglass are that it requires skill to handle, is more difficult to mold, and is significantly more expensive than plaster. It is best used for long-term casts, and in patients who are particularly "hard" on casts. This material has little use in the acute injury setting in which molding is important and casts are changed frequently. Fiberglass is also available in varying sizes of splints and rolls.

Most casts and splints are applied over a layer of cast padding with or without stockinette. Several types of padding are available including sheet cotton, Webril, and synthetic polypropolene (for fiberglass casts). This material is also available in a number of widths (2-, 3-, 4-, and 6-inch-wide rolls). A stockinette is not necessary for cast application. It does, however, improve the overall appearance of the finished product and can prevent children from reaching down into the cast and pulling out padding.

CASTING AND SPLINTING TECHNIQUES[1,2]

Prior to the reduction of a fracture or application of a splint or cast, one must carefully examine the extremity. This examination should include a full neurovascular assessment, a description of the appearance of the extremity, a grading of the amount of swelling, and the skin condition. The range of motion of all joints to be immobilized should be documented if possible.

All materials for the cast or splint should be assembled prior to a reduction attempt. This should include sufficient padding, plaster or fiberglass, stockinette, and Ace wrap (or bias wrap) and tape, if needed. A bucket of lukewarm water should be available for dipping the casting material. Water should be changed after each application as the temperature and residual plaster in the water will alter setting time.

Padding is rolled onto the extremity to be immobilized, over-lapping each turn by 50%. In general, 3–4 layers of padding are adequate unless one is using the synthetic padding (for fiberglass casts), which is much thinner. Additional padding should be applied to bony prominences such as the heel, the malleoli, the fibular head, the patella, and the epicondyles of the humerus. The proximal and distal ends of the cast or splint should also be well padded (about 5 layers thick) to prevent impingement on the skin by a sharp edge. Cast padding should be rolled snugly onto the extremity such that it is free of wrinkles and folds. Care must also be taken not to "clump" padding over joints, specifically the dorsum of the ankle joint and the elbow crease. To prevent anterior "clumping" at the ankle and the elbow, one should apply 2–3 additional strips of padding to the bony prominences in these regions. Except for a few areas requiring extra padding, the thickness should be uniform.

Splints are typically made out of plaster. Prepackaged, easy to use fiberglass splints are becoming increasingly popular in the acute setting, though they are more expensive. Plaster splints are dipped in water, squeezed dry and usually applied 8–10 sheets thick over cast padding. The splints are held in place with bias-cut stockinette or elastic bandages (Ace wrap). If Ace wraps are to be used to hold splints, care must be taken not to wrap the extremity too tightly. During splint application, it is important to make sure that the individual slabs do not come together to form a circumferential ring of plaster that would disallow swelling. In treating fractures, splints are usually converted to casts after the swelling has receded. Splints, like casts, must immobilize the joint above and below the fracture to be effective. It is usually a good idea to place a stockinette over the wrapped splint for cosmesis unless the splint will be removed prior to the patient leaving the hospital.

Casting is performed by dipping a roll of plaster or fiberglass in water, squeezing it dry, and applying it over cast padding. One usually starts at the distal end of the cast and proceeds proximally, overwrapping the previous layer by about 50%. It is important to "push" plaster onto the extremity, gently smoothing the plaster as one applies each layer. One must never "pull" plaster because this can result in a cast that is too tight. Ultimately, the cast will be 4–5 layers thick. Splints that are 2–3 sheets thick should be used to strengthen the cast in particular regions (when crossing joints, the heel). It is important to reinforce the proximal and distal ends of the cast since they are exposed to higher stresses.

The cast should be molded as it is being applied. Fracture reductions are maintained with three-point fixation. A rule of thumb for molding of a cast is that the cast should look like the extremity that was casted. Specific molds should be made about the wrist and hand to ensure full range of motion of nonimmobilized digits. The epicondyles of the humerus should be molded, as well as the triceps in long arm casts. In lower extremity casts, the arches of the foot, malleoli, tendo-Achilles, and anterior crest of the tibia should be molded. The patella, femoral condyles, and quadriceps must be molded to obtain a well-fitting long leg or cylinder cast. Once again, the joints above and below the fracture need to be incorporated in the splint or cast.

Caution must be exercised when casting or splinting an extremity that has recently been injured, manipulated, or operated on because of the risk of creating an iatrogenic compartment syndrome when the extremity swells in a limited space. Casts should be split and splints should be carefully wrapped using Ace or bias wrap to prevent this complication.

Cast saws are used to trim and remove casts. These saws work by vibration of the blade and tend to become hot during use. It is very easy to "burn" a patient with the hot, vibrating blade. This is especially true when patients are anaesthetized or are not able to communicate well (infancy or mental retardation). One should be instructed in safe cast saw use by a senior resident prior to removing a cast without supervision.

UPPER EXTREMITY SPLINTS[1,2,3]

Sugar-tong Splints[3]

In the upper extremity, the sugar-tong splint gives excellent immobilization while allowing for significant swelling. A short arm sugar-tong does not completely immobilize the elbow. It allows for some flexion and extension of the elbow but prohibits forearm supination-pronation. These splints are generally suitable for stable distal radius fractures. In fractures in which flexion-extension of the elbow must be controlled, the sugar-tong can be supplemented above the elbow with an additional layer of plaster applied posteriorly with the elbow flexed 90 degrees. A long arm sugar-tong (or double sugar-tong) also immobilizes the elbow.

To apply a single sugar-tong splint, cast padding is placed from the metacarpophalangeal joints to above the elbow. The splint is a continuous slab of plaster extending from the distal palmar crease to and around the elbow and over the dorsal surface of the forearm to end over the dorsum of the metacarpophalangeal joints. Unroll a 3- or 4-inch roll of plaster to make a single slab that will reach the above distance. Since the injured extremity is usually painful, it is wise to measure the desired length by using the opposite (uninjured) limb. To obtain the desired thickness (7–10 thicknesses), often two or three rolls of plaster are necessary. While the patient's arm is held in the desired position by an assistant, the plaster slab is dipped, squeezed, applied to the extremity, and held on with a layer of elastic bandage or bias cut stockinette. The splint is molded to the extremity, and held until it is hard (Fig. 7.1). In the upper extremity, particular attention must be paid to the hand to avoid contractures (especially extension contractures of the MCPJ, adduc-

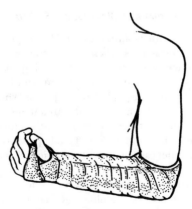

Figure 7.1. Sugar-tong splint.

tion contractures of the thumb, and flexion contractures of the wrist and PIPJ). Once the cast has hardened, the patient should be checked to ensure that full motion of the digits is present. This splint is typically used for distal radius (Colles') fractures. When immobilizing forearm fractures or fractures around the elbow, the sugar-tong may be extended onto the upper arm with an additional slab of plaster that runs from the lateral aspect of the upper arm around the posterior aspect of the elbow and up into the axilla. This completely immobilizes the elbow.

Coaptation Splints[3]

This splint is useful for the immobilization of fractures of the humerus. This splint is an adaptation of the double sugar-tong splint of the upper extremity. The patient's arm is padded from shoulder to the wrist. The splint is prepared similarly to the double sugar-tong except that the upper sugar-tong should extend from above the acromion, over the lateral aspect of the arm to the elbow, and incorporating the elbow, it should extend into the axilla. The axilla needs to be well padded with an ABD pad. This splint should also be 7–12 thicknesses of plaster. The lower sugar-tong is prepared in the usual manner, but it does not need to extend onto the hand. The splints are then overwrapped with Ace or bias-cut stockinette. When this splint is used, the shoulder is placed into adduction and internal rotation. The forearm is immobilized with a commercially available shoulder immobilizer or with a sling and swathe.

Radial and Ulnar Gutter Splints

Radial and ulnar gutter splints are useful for metacarpal fractures and some carpal fractures. These splints consist of a single slab (7–8 sheets thick) applied with cast padding to the radial or ulnar aspects of the forearm. These splints can be fashioned to extend over the metacarpophalangeal joints. When the splints are extended onto the hand for the treatment of metacarpal fracture, care must be taken to obtain a satisfactory mold. If the slab is too thick, the mold may not be adequate to maintain the reduction. Gauntlet casts are usually superior for metacarpal and proximal phalangeal fractures.

Ulnar gutter splints, in particular, are useful for the treatment of nightstick fractures of the ulna and fractures of the neck of the fourth and fifth metacarpals (boxer's fractures). The mold of this splint is important to obtain immobilization.

Aluminum Splints

Malleable aluminum splints are available in several sizes. They can be contoured by hand and cut with tin snips to the appropriate size. The splints are held in position by a durable tape. These splints are used to immobilize phalangeal fractures and dislocations, volar plate injuries at the PIP joints, and bony mallet fingers. The PIP joint should be immobilized in 10 degrees of flexion or less to reduce the risk of motion loss since the accessory collateral ligaments tighten with the PIPJ held in flexion. These splints can also be incorporated into casts and dorsal splints to obtain immobilization of metacarpal fractures. When incorporating the MCP joint in these splints, care must be taken to immobilize the MCPJ in 70–90 degrees of flexion, to avoid extension contractures from shortening of the collateral ligaments.

LOWER EXTREMITY SPLINTS[1,2,3]

Posterior Splints

This splint immobilizes the ankle. It has applications for isolated distal fibula fractures, fractures of the talus and calcaneous, metatarsal fractures, and ankle sprains. It should be noted that unstable ankle fractures and tibia fractures require long leg immobilization in order to control rotation.

Short leg posterior splints can be applied without assistance if the patient is able to cooperate. The patient should be positioned in the prone position with the knee flexed 90 degrees. The lower extremity is then padded from toe to knee, with additional padding placed over the malleoli, the heel, and the proximal/distal ends of the splint. In adults, the splint can be easily constructed from three sets of 5×30-inch splints (5–10 thicknesses each). These splints are applied over the padding. A 5-sheet thick medial slab begins 4 cm below the medial joint line of the knee and extends distally to encompass the heel and the lateral malleolus. A 5-sheet thick lateral slab is then applied distal to the fibular head and extends distally to overlap the medial slab at the heel and the medial malleolus. This forms a sugar-tong around the ankle. The splint is completed by bringing a third 10-thick slab from just distal to the knee over the heel and out over the toes.

Excess material is folded back on itself to form a footplate. The splint is wrapped into place with bias-cut stockinette. Do not allow the plaster slabs to overlap over the anterior aspect of the leg and come into contact with one another, as this will harden and not allow swelling. The splint is completed by molding the ankle into neutral (i.e., no plantar flexion).

Long Leg Posterior Splints

This splint is useful for the treatment of unstable ankle fractures or tibia fractures in which severe swelling is expected. The posterior splint is not as stable a construct as a bivalved or split cast, but it allows for greater swelling without the development of a compartment syndrome. A long leg splint is applied in the same fashion as a short leg splint initially. It is then extended above the knee with additional 5×30 inch plaster slabs (each 8–10 sheets thick) placed along the medial, lateral, and posterior aspects of the thigh. In addition to the mold of the splint at the malleolus, the splint can be molded at the supracondylar region and at the thigh.

UPPER EXTREMITY CASTS[1,2]

Upper extremity casting can be divided into short and long arm casts. Gauntlet casts are a type of short arm cast that is used for some phalangeal and metacarpal fractures. Short arm casts are used for carpal fractures, stable distal radius fractures, and nightstick fractures (ulna) in the acute phase. They are also used for protection of all distal radius fractures during the late phases of healing or after ORIF. Long arm casts are used for less stable fractures of the ulna, radius and distal humerus.

Short Arm Casts

The short arm cast extends from just proximal to the distal palmar crease to just distal to the elbow. In adults, rolls of 3- and 4-inch cast padding and plaster allow for easy application and a good finish. The cast is most easily applied with the patient lying supine with the shoulder abducted 90 degrees, elbow flexed 90 degrees, and the forearm and hand directed toward the ceiling. The wrist should be immobilized in 30–40 degrees of dorsiflexion unless the cast is being placed for a distal radius fracture and volar flexion and ulnar deviation help in maintenance of the reduction.

In this position, the short arm cast can be applied without assistance if the patient is able to cooperate. Cast padding is placed first in the manner previously described. Padding can be 2–3 layers thick with an additional layer or two at the proximal and distal edges. Plaster is rolled onto the extremity beginning at the hand. Several turns are taken through the palm. The plaster should be gathered through the web space to avoid interfering with thumb motion. The cast is then extended down the forearm to stop just distal to the elbow. Since a cross-section of the forearm has an oval shape, the cast should be molded in this manner rather than circular. This can be achieved by molding with the flat of both palms and gently pressing between the radius and ulna both dorsally and volarly to spread the interosseus membrane. The cast should extend as far proximally as posssible without interfering with elbow range of motion.

After the cast has set, the patient should have 90 degrees of flexion at the metacarpophalangeal joints. The thumb should have full extension and be able to oppose with the little finger. If the cast limits this motion, it should be carefully trimmed with a cast knife or power saw (Fig. 7.2).

Thumb Spica Casts

This modification of the short or long arm cast is used for scaphoid fractures, gamekeeper's thumb, Bennett's fractures (fractures of the base of the thumb metacarpal), and some thumb phalangeal fractures. This cast usually extends to the distal part of the thumb and should always immobilize the thumb MCPJ. For phalangeal fractures, the cast should be extended distal to the thumb IPJ. The difficulty with this cast is to obtain adequate thicknesses

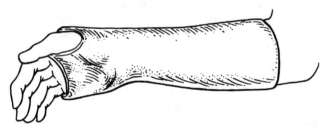

Figure 7.2.   Short arm cast.

of plaster to immobilize the thumb without wadding cast material into the palm and inhibiting motion of the MCP joints of the other digits. One method is to use 2-inch splints one thickness at a time, and apply them longitudinally and circumferentially to the thumb. The splints need only be long enough (about 6 inches) to extend to the base of the wrist, where they can be captured with a roll of plaster. The thumb can also be strengthened by an additional splint (2–3 thicknesses) on the radial aspect of the thumb and extending proximally onto the wrist. For scaphoid fractures, some advocate a long arm thumb spica cast.

Long Arm Casts

The long arm cast is an extension of the short arm cast, and it is used when forearm rotation or elbow flexion and extension must be controlled. The cast is applied to the forearm and arm over a layer of cast padding. Sufficient padding must be applied at the elbow to protect the ulnar nerve as it passes behind the medial epicondyle in the ulnar groove of humerus. The bony condyles and olecranon should be well padded using torn strips of padding that do not pass circumferentially around the elbow. One must be careful not to gather cast padding in the elbow crease, since this is constricting and can cause pressure problems.

Four-inch rolls of plaster are used to extend casts to the upper arm. In the upper arm and thigh, there is enough soft tissue present that the cast material can be "pulled" to obtain a well- fitting cast. In applying casts to the foot, ankle, leg, and forearm, plaster and fiberglass should be pushed onto the extremity and never stretched or "pulled."

A long arm cast then is made by first applying a short arm cast and then extending it above the elbow. To reinforce the elbow, 3×15- or 4×15-inch splints should be placed on the medial, lateral, and posterior sides. This creates a strong cast at the elbow without the need for additional circumferential layers of plaster. Gathering of the cast padding and the plaster in the antecubital fossa can be avoided by taking a figure-8 turn around the elbow.

Finally, the cast is then molded with attention paid to mold the upper arm over the humeral condyles and biceps muscle. The upper arm should be molded into a quadrilateral shape that is wide and flat posteriorly. Anteriorly, the medial and lateral aspects of the biceps should be well molded. Although it is possible to apply this cast without assistance, patients find it difficult to maintain their elbow at 90 degrees while the plaster is setting (Fig. 7.3).

LOWER EXTREMITY CASTS[1,2]

Lower extremity casts are divided into three general types: the short leg cast (SLC), which ends below the knee; the long leg cast (LLC), which extends above the knee; and the patellar-tendon bearing cast (PTB). The SLC protects stable ankle fractures but does not control rotation of the tibia. A well-molded PTB or LLC will control lower leg rotation.

The development of the cast shoe has simplified the conversion of nonweight-bearing casts to walking casts. The cast boot allows for better weight distribution over a greater surface area than the rubber walking heel. Casts used for weight bearing are subjected to greater stress than nonweight-bearing casts, and these casts warrant reinforcement over the heel, ankle, knee, and the proximal and distal aspects of the cast.

Short Leg Casts

The short leg cast replaces a posterior splint when the swelling has subsided from grade III ankle sprains, stable ankle fractures,

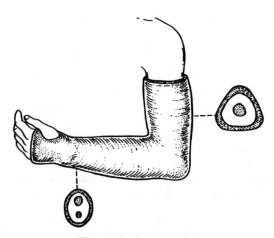

Figure 7.3. Long arm cast.

and fractures of the talus and calcaneous. Short leg "walking casts" are reinforced with a footplate and additional material around the ankle so patients can safely bear weight on the extremity in the later stages of healing.

The short leg cast is applied over 3–4 layers of cast padding. More layers are required if the thin, synthetic cast padding is used. Before applying plaster, make certain that the malleoli, heel and fibular head are well padded. One should also reinforce the padding under the proximal and distal edges of the cast to protect the skin from sharp cast edges. Four-inch rolls of padding and plaster are usually best for adults. When applying the casting material, make certain that enough material has been applied to the heel, since this is a common site of breakdown. If the cast is to be used for weight bearing, then three or four 4×15 splints applied anteriorly, medially, and laterally around the ankle and a footplate will reinforce the cast. The cast should also be reinforced at its proximal and distal edges, since these areas are subject to increased stress.

The cast should end just distal to the fibular head. After the first two rolls of plaster have been applied, the foot and ankle should be molded. Special attention should be paid to the transverse and longitudinal arches of the foot, the malleoli, and the heelcord. The crest of the tibia and the gastroc/soleus musculature should be molded, as well, to ensure a good fit. While applying the cast, several figure-8 turns should be taken around the calf musculature to "lock" the cast in position. One must continue to "push" the plaster and resist the temptation to "pull" the plaster in this situation. The ankle should be immobilized in neutral flexion. Plantar flexion at the ankle can result in contracture and diminished ankle dorsiflexion. If the cast is to be used for weight bearing, some think that gait is improved by molding the ankle into slight dorsiflexion (5 degrees).

When the cast is nearly complete, a footplate should be placed if the extremity is going to bear weight. A footplate that covers the heel and extends past the ends of the toes is easily fashioned out of 4×15 splints (8–10 thicknesses). This is easily incorporated into the cast by rolling additional plaster over the splints (Fig. 7.4).

When the cast is complete, the dorsum of the foot should be trimmed so that all toes are visible. Trimming can be done

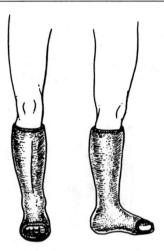

Figure 7.4.   Short leg cast.

with a cast knife, scalpel, or oscillating saw. If care is taken while applying the footplate, excessive trimming is not necessary.

Long Leg Casts

Most applications of the long leg cast are for the closed treatment of tibia fractures or ankle fractures. The short leg cast is applied first as previously described. The knee and thigh are then padded. The patella and the medial and lateral condyles require additional padding. The leg must be held by an assistant in the desired amount of knee flexion until the plaster has set. Though the roll of plaster should be "pushed" as it is applied to the knee, leg, and the foot and ankle, it may be "pulled" around the upper thigh to obtain a snug fit. The cast should be carried proximally to within inches of the groin on the medial side. Splints (5 × 30 inch slabs) should be used to reinforce the knee, and these are best applied medially, laterally, and anteriorly. In the application of the long leg cast, 6-inch plaster rolls should be used above the ankle, as this will allow for a faster application and a better finish (Fig. 7.5).

The mold of the thigh and knee are crucial to the efficacy of this cast. The cast must be molded around the condyles of the

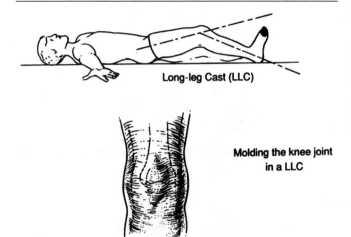

Figure 7.5.   Molding around the knee in a long leg cast.

femur so as not to slide down the leg. A quadrilateral thigh mold is applied manually by placing the heels of the palms just above the knee on the medial and lateral sides. The anterior aspect of the quadrilateral figure should reflect the medial and lateral borders of the quadriceps musculature. When the patient walks, the cast position will be maintained by the supracondylar mold (Fig. 7.5).

Cylinder Casts

This cast is often used to immobilize the knee following injuries or surgery. It is most often used to protect a surgical repair of the extensor mechanism of the knee (ORIF of the patella or surgical repair of the quadriceps or patellar tendon). This cast runs from within inches of the groin proximally to just above the medial and lateral malleoli distally. As in the application of the long leg cast, it is important to apply the cast material relatively tightly to the thigh and then to carefully mold the supracondylar region. If an excellent mold is not obtained, the cast will slide down the leg, allowing the knee to bend and painfully impinging on the malleoli.

Patellar-tendon Bearing Casts

This cast was first developed by Sarmiento for the treatment of tibia fractures without immobilizing the knee. Sarmiento's initial description calls for no cast padding to be used, with the cast material to be applied directly onto stockinette.

The patellar-tendon bearing cast is frequently used to allow early ambulation and weight bearing in patients with stable mid-shaft and distal one-third tibia fractures who are receiving nonoperative treatment. Most authors recommend cast padding in the application of these casts.

This cast is essentially applied as a long leg cast with the knee flexed at 30–45 degrees, and the ankle in neutral. Extra material must be applied over the tibial condyles laterally and medially, as well as over the patellar tendon anteriorly. The cast is well molded around the proximal tibial flare, and the patellar tendon is molded horizontally. After the plaster has set, the cast is cut down to allow for flexion at the knee, while the condylar "wings" prevent rotation, and the patella tendon and the tibial flare bear a majority of the weight (Fig. 7.6).

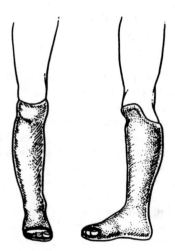

Figure 7.6.   Patellar-tendon bearing (PTB) cast.

Spica Casts[4]

Body casts are rarely used for the immobilization of fractures of the upper extremity. Lower extremity spica casts are often used in pediatrics for closed treatment of femoral shaft fractures and for maintenance of a hip reduction following closed or open hip reduction in infants with developmental dysplasia of the hip (DDH). In adults, spica casts are occasionally used to maintain a hip in reduced position after dislocation and closed reduction in patients with total hip arthroplasties.

This cast requires several assistants to apply expeditiously and correctly. Infants and small children should be placed on a spica table. Older children and adults can be standing during cast application. Stockinette should be applied over the entire surface to be casted. Depending on the intention of the cast, the cast can include one thigh (single pantaloon), two thighs (pantaloon), one entire leg (single-hip spica), and both legs (double-hip spica).

Padding should consist of multiple layers of cast padding and felt strips applied to bony prominences (the anterior superior iliac spines, the spine and sacrum, and the costal margins). Additional felt should be placed at the superior edge and on the inner groin under the cast for additional comfort. A few ABDs should be placed on top of the abdomen so they can be removed when cast application is complete in order to allow room for abdominal expansion within the cast. It is difficult to apply too much padding.

In infants and small children, the cast is applied circumferentially with 3- and 4-inch rolls of cast material starting on the abdomen. One then moves down to the lower extremities. After a layer of cast material is applied, the cast should be reinforced with multiple 3×15- and 4×15-inch splints, which are applied in layers of 3–5 thicknesses. When applying the splints, particular attention must be paid to the area where the cast crosses the hip joint (intern's angle). This is the area most susceptible to breakdown from stress, as the cast is not supported circumferentially at that point. Additional rolls are applied following splint application to give a smooth, finished appearance.

When the cast has set, it can be trimmed. A circular hole should be made in the abdomen to allow room for expansion. The cast should be trimmed around the perineal area. A spreader

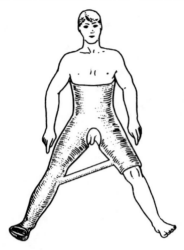

Figure 7.7.   Hip spica cast.

bar made of wood or plaster should be placed between the two legs to further stabilize and strengthen the cast. Finally, when the cast has dried completely, small areas of irritation can be padded with moleskin for comfort. An example of a spica cast is shown in Figure 7.7.

References

1. Lewis RC Jr. Handbook of traction, casting, and splinting techniques. Philadelphia: JB Lippincott, 1972.
2. Schneider FR. Handbook for the orthopaedic assistant. St. Louis: CV Mosby, 1976.
3. Charnley JA. The closed treatment of common fractures. Edinburgh: Churchill-Livingstone, 1972.
4. Rockwood CA, Green DP. Fractures in adults. Vol. 1. 2nd ed. Philadelphia: JB Lippincott, 1984.

Traction Techniques

As techniques for internal and external fracture fixation continue to improve, there are increasingly fewer indications for traction. In the pediatric population, traction is still widely employed in the treatment of femur fractures in the preadolescent age group, in the treatment of congenital hip dislocation, and occasionally in treating Legg-Calvé-Perthes disease. In this population, traction is usually the initial treatment, followed by plaster immobilization or bracing. Traction is rarely used as the definitive treatment of adult fractures, but it is sometimes useful if there is a delay in taking the patient to the operating room.

The purpose of traction in the treatment of fractures is to obtain satisfactory alignment of the fracture. This is performed by aligning the distal fragment with the proximal fragment through the use of continuous applied distraction. This continuous force is often able to overcome distracting forces (e.g., muscle spasm) and obtain excellent alignment, especially if the periosteum and soft-tissue envelope are not too severely disrupted. The deforming forces acting across the fracture must be known so the traction can be positioned to overcome these forces. For instance, in a distal femur fracture, the distal fragment is flexed by the gastrocnemius and pulled medially by the adductors. When a patient with this fracture is placed in traction, the knee is flexed to remove the effect of the gastrocnemius, and traction on the tibial pin would be placed such that the lower leg is slightly abducted. To adequately use traction, the physician must understand the force vectors of the local musculature and counteract those with the traction apparatus.

Traction requires constant vigilance by the health-care team. In the course of moving patients for linen changes or imaging studies, the traction will often be disconnected or malaligned. A responsible member of the team must check the patient at least daily to assess the adequacy of the traction. Frequent radiographs must be obtained to ensure the adequacy of the reduction.

This chapter is intended as an introduction to the many types of traction. Traction should never be applied without the supervision of an experienced orthopaedic surgeon. The patient can be significantly harmed by the misuse of traction with complications including full thickness skin loss and neurovascular injury.

TRACTION SETUP

Prior to initiating traction, the bed must be outfitted with the proper equipment. This usually includes an overhead frame with multiple outrigger bars for the attachment of pulleys. The overhead frame usually has a trapeze handle so the patient may move in bed. If the patient is unconscious or is to be treated for an extended period of time in bed, the mattress of the bed should be supplemented with an egg crate for the prevention of decubitus ulcers. In addition, special air mattresses and rotation beds exist for patients who will be recumbent for long periods of time. These special beds should be considered for any patient who is at high risk for the formation of decubiti.

TYPES OF TRACTION[1,2]

Traction can be divided into two general types by the method of application of the force: skin or skeletal. In skin traction, the pull of the weights is applied to the skin. The amount of force that can be applied by this type of traction is limited by the risk of injury to the skin. Skin is very susceptible to shear forces, and all skin traction should be removed and reapplied whenever the patient has a complaint, or at least every 48 hours. Additionally, skin traction does not allow for precise rotational control of fractures. The use of skin traction is limited to situations in which the maximum traction force needed is less than 5–10 pounds. Additionally, it should not be used when precise rotational control is necessary.

Skeletal traction uses pins placed into or through bone to apply the traction force. The advantage of skeletal traction is that greater forces can be applied with good rotational control. Moreover, skeletal traction can be maintained for a long period of time (8–12 weeks) with appropriate pin care. The disadvantages of skeletal traction are related to the pins. Pins can pull out and pin tracts can become infected. Occasionally, pin tract infections can lead to osteomyelitis. There is also some risk of neurovascular injury in the placement of the pins. In the adolescent population, the pin can be improperly placed into the physis and cause a growth disturbance. Placement of traction pins is discussed in Chapter 5.

SPECIFIC TYPES OF TRACTION

Buck's Traction[1,2,3,4]

The goal of Buck's traction is to maintain the lower extremity in extension. This traction is most commonly used in the temporary treatment of intertrochanteric and femoral neck fractures prior to fracture fixation. The traction pulls the hip and knee into extension in order to make the patient comfortable until more definitive treatment can be performed. The traction does not serve to reduce or align the fracture, it merely reduces the pain.

The traction is applied to the leg by a foam boot that fits the foot and calf. This boot is then connected to a traction rope and weight pan as shown in Figure 8.1. Five to 10 pounds of weight are typically applied while the patient is waitng to go to the operating room for fixation. This is a skin traction system, and the traction boot must be removed frequently to check the condition of the skin.

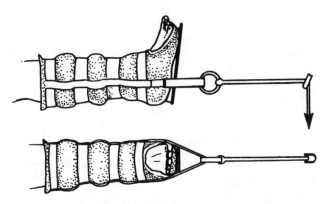

Figure 8.1. Buck's traction.

Bryant's Traction[1,2,3,4]

Bryant's traction is often used in the first stage of the reduction (1–2 weeks) of a subluxated or dislocated hip in an infant with developmental dislocation of the hip (6–18 months). The goal of traction in developmentally dislocated hips (DDH) is to stretch the surrounding musculature and gently bring the femoral head into alignment with the triradiate cartilage of the developing acetabulum. Prereduction traction allows gentle reduction of the femoral head and lessens the risk of avascular necrosis of the femoral head as a complication of overzealous reduction maneuvers. Bryant's traction is also rarely used for femur fractures in children up to 2 years old. It should not be used on patients weighing more than 30 pounds.

Bryant's traction is skin traction that consists of felt or moleskin strips applied to both lower extremities and held in place with elastic wraps (Coban and ace wraps). Both extremities are incorporated in the traction even if the pathology is unilateral, in order to provide more stability and control. The felt strips are connected to a traction cord that runs straight up to a pulley and then continues overhead to the edge of the bed. This is shown in Figure 8.2.

The hips are maintained in 90 degrees of flexion and 30 degrees of abduction. Some knee flexion is permitted to relax the hamstrings. The amount of weight applied is just enough to lift the buttocks off the bed (the ''just clear'' position) but should not exceed 5 pounds. If additional traction is necessary, Russell's or split Russell's traction may be used.

Bryant's traction is a **dangerous** method of traction that can cause vascular compromise to the lower leg. It is subsequently contraindicated in children over 2 years of age, who are at even higher risk for this complication. Neurovascular checks should be performed every 2 hours. The most frequent sites of excessive pressure is the skin over the fibular head and neck, the dorsum of the foot, and the Achilles tendon.

Split Russell's[1,2,3]

Split Russell's traction can be used in some femur fractures, as well as in hip traction for patients with Legg-Calvé-Perthes disease, or for an older patient with DDH (>18–24 months old). This system is usually employed when the patient is too large or old

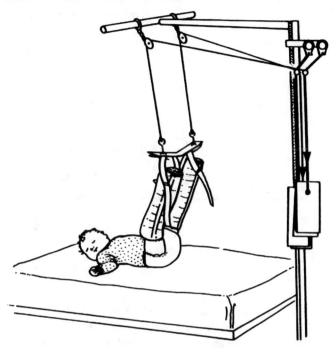

Figure 8.2. Bryant's traction.

for Bryant's traction. The application of force in two planes increases the resultant force vector on the hip.

In split Russell's traction, the leg is placed in skin traction, and a sling is applied to the proximal tibia with an upward force. The sling must be free of sharp edges so the skin is not injured. Weights should be balanced in order to keep the knee flexed 30–45 degrees and keep the foot off the bed. This traction is shown in Figure 8.3. A portable radiograph is often used to determine whether alignment is satisfactory. When this traction is used for DDH, the hips are kept moderately flexed (60 degrees), abducted 30–40 degrees, and the knees are flexed 60 degrees. If this traction is being used for long-term treatment of Legg-Calvé-Perthes disease, the patient should be taken out of traction for brief periods each day to examine the skin.

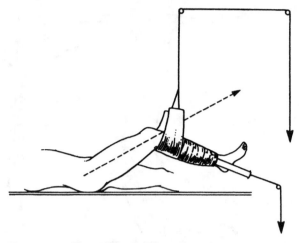

Figure 8.3. Split Russell's traction.

Russell's traction is similar to split Russell's in that it applies all the same forces to the leg in the same directions, but it differs in that it uses a single traction cord and weight. This tends to keep the leg in slightly more extension. Russell's and split Russell's traction are rarely used in the treatment of adult fractures.

90/90 Upper Arm Traction and Side-arm Traction[2,3,4]

90/90 and side-arm tractions are only rarely used to treat fractures of the humerus. Most of these fractures can be treated more effectively with functional bracing, plating, intramedullary rodding, or external fixation. This type of traction can be performed with an olecranon pin or skin traction on the upper arm. The olecranon pin must be placed carefully to avoid the ulnar nerve on the medial side of the elbow (see Chapter 5 for technique).

The purpose of 90/90 and side-arm traction is to obtain longitudinal traction of the humerus while supporting the forearm in the proper rotation. When treated in this fashion, the humerus will unite quickly even in the adult patient. Once early union has been obtained, the patient can be converted to another form of immobilization that is less confining.

In side-arm traction, skin traction or olecranon pin traction is placed on the arm with the patient supine in bed, and the arm abducted 90 degrees. This traction pulls perpendicular to the long axis of the body. Additional skin traction is applied to the forearm with the elbow flexed 90 degrees and the wrist in neutral. The forearm traction supports the weight of the forearm perpendicular to the coronal plane of the body. This is shown in Figure 8.4.

In 90/90 traction, the shoulder is positioned in 90 degrees of forward flexion and the arm traction is placed directly anterior to the patient, who is supine. The forearm is then positioned in the same plane as the bed and is supported by a sling.

90/90 Femoral Traction[1,2,3]

90/90 femoral traction is a form of traction devised specifically for the closed management of subtrochanteric femur fractures in adults. Again, it is rarely used because of improved results with operative fixation. In addition, it can be used to manage some high femoral shaft fractures in children. In 90/90 femoral traction, a pin is placed through the distal femur passing from medial to lateral (see Chapter 5). The leg is then suspended by skeletal traction through this pin such that the femur is flexed 90 degrees at the hip and aimed directly at the ceiling. The knee is also

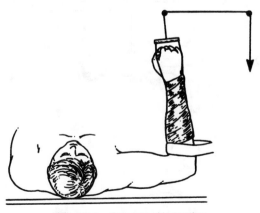

Figure 8.4.   Side-arm skin traction.

flexed 90 degrees, hence the name 90/90 traction. The lower leg is attached to a splint or a Buck's traction boot that has two traction cords attached to it. One is pulling directly upward on an attachment on the anterior aspect of the midshaft of the tibia. The other traction cord pulls toward the foot of the bed in a manner similar to Buck's traction. This prevents rotation of the leg at the hip and provides for greater fracture stability and patient comfort (Fig. 8.5).

90/90 traction is effective in subtrochanteric fractures because, by flexing the hip 90 degrees, the distal fracture fragments are made to align with the proximal fragment, which is usually flexed acutely by the pull of the iliopsoas. The pull of the short external rotators and the hip abductors make this a difficult fracture to treat nonoperatively.

Balanced Skeletal Traction[1,2,3,4]

Balanced skeletal traction is most commonly used in the temporary treatment of femur fractures. This traction uses a skeletal traction pin placed in the proximal tibia or distal femur connected to a traction bow. The use of traction pins allows for greater forces to be applied for fracture reduction. The remainder of the leg is then supported on a splint or frame that is well

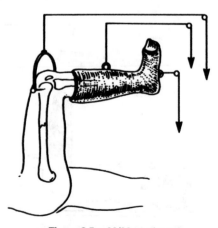

Figure 8.5. 90/90 traction.

padded. The amount of knee flexion can be varied to assist in the reduction of the fracture when the gastrocnemius is a major deforming factor. In addition, the splint and leg can be abducted to compensate for the deforming force of the hip abductors. Typically, the hip and knee are each in about 30 degrees of flexion. The amount of force pulling directly on the traction pin is approximately equal to the sum of the force pulling on the other two traction cords.

It is important to pad the ischial ring well with sheepskin and check the sacrum frequently for decubiti. Neurovascular checks should be performed every 2 hours. The leg should not be allowed to roll externally, as this may place undue pressure on the peroneal nerve. Skin checks over the fibular head, Achilles tendon, and heel should be performed at least daily.

Traction pins should be carefully placed with the surgeon conscious of the nearby neurovascular structures. A femoral traction pin is preferred in skeletally immature patients because the proximal tibial physis is more susceptible to injury. If more definitive treatment of the femur fracture is planned, a tibial pin should be placed rather than femoral pin. Hypothetically, a femoral pin will contaminate the intramedullary canal. Before the tibial pin is placed, an accurate examination of the knee must be made to ensure its stability. *Do not apply traction through an unstable knee!*

The Thomas splint with Pearson attachment is the most common splint system used in balanced skeletal traction. In using this splint, a common mistake is the selection of too large a splint for the patient. Subsequently, the Pearson attachment is well below the knee. This traction is demonstrated in Figure 8.6.

Cervical Traction

Cervical traction is used in the conservative treatment of cervical spondylosis. The purpose is to allow for some decompression of the facet joints and temporary relief of pain. This is usually prescribed as a home program in which the patient uses the traction intermittently several times per day.

Cervical traction is available in two configurations: 1) traction applied with the patient sitting, and 2) traction applied with the patient in the supine position. The patient uses a head halter that runs beneath the chin and occiput and is then connected to a spreader bar. Weight is then applied for traction as shown in Figure 8.7. In the sitting position, 12–15 pounds of traction are used, and in the supine position 5–7 pounds are applied. The forces should be directed to pull the neck in slight flexion to widen the foramina and the posterior disk space.

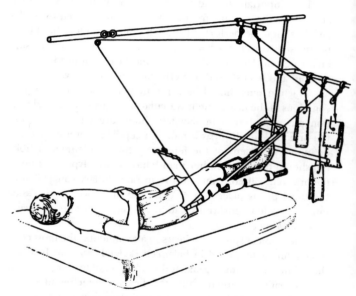

Figure 8.6. Balanced skeletal traction.

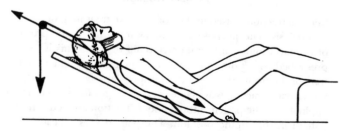

Figure 8.7. Cervical traction.

Halo and Gardner-Wells Tong Traction[1,2,3,4]

This form of traction is used in the reduction and stabilization of cervical spine subluxations, dislocations, and fractures. Only experienced physicians should apply or adjust this traction. Many cervical injuries can be reduced by closed traction. This is facilitated by the application of either Gardner-Wells tongs or a halo ring. When the halo ring is used in reduction maneuvers, the pins must be tightened to 8 kg/cm prior to the application of traction. The halo ring gives slightly better rotational control of the head than the Gardner-Wells tongs.

Traction is performed by connecting the tongs or ring to a traction cord at the head of the bed. To obtain direct longitudinal traction, some hospital beds will require an additional mattress to allow the traction cord to clear the head of the bed. The amount of flexion and extension of the cervical spine is controlled by the amount of elevation of the head of the bed or by the presence of a pillow beneath the patient's shoulders. Any movement of the bed will change the direction of the traction. All electric beds should be turned off once they are in the desired position.

Traction can then be applied gradually. The general rule of thumb is that 10 pounds of weight should be used to overcome the weight of the head, and an additional 5 pounds for each level of the cervical spine through which traction need be applied. For instance, in a fracture or dislocation at the C-5 level, 35 pounds of weight would be used—10 pounds for the head, and 25 pounds to overcome the pull of the five levels of the cervical spine. It is usually recommended to start by applying about 20 pounds of traction initially and then increase it in 5-pound increments. *After the initial placement of weight and after any change in the traction or weight, the position of the cervical fracture should be immediately checked with a lateral view of the cervical spine. Careful documentation of the neurologic status of the patient is mandatory after each change in weight or position. Any deterioration in neurologic status is an indication to immediately return to the previous level or position of traction.* The patient must be maintained in an intensive care or at least a step-down care setting while the fracture or dislocation is being reduced.

If the halo ring is employed in the reduction, the halo jacket can be applied to stabilize the cervical spine after the reduced position is achieved. *In applying traction through the halo ring, do not use the screw holes that will later be needed for halo jacket application. Otherwise, the risk of losing reduction during halo jacket application increases.*

References

1. Lewis RC Jr. Handbook of traction, casting, and splinting techniques. Philadelphia: JB Lippincott, 1977.
2. Schmeisser G Jr. A clinical manual of orthopaedic traction techniques. Philadelphia: WB Saunders, 1963.
3. Schneider FR. Handbook for the orthopaedic assistant. 2nd ed. St. Louis: CV Mosby, 1976.
4. The traction handbook. Warsaw, IN: Zimmer, 1991.

Chapter 9

Perioperative Management

PREOPERATIVE EVALUATION AND SCREENING[1,2,3,4]

Candidates for orthopaedic procedures represent a highly diverse group, ranging from healthy pediatric and adolescent athletes to elderly, debilitated individuals with multiple medical problems. Preoperative assessment is important in all groups but must be individualized, as the healthy young athlete will have a significantly different medical profile than the geriatric hip fracture patient. Blindly ordering a full battery of laboratory tests on both groups is cost prohibitive and unnecessary. The preoperative evaluation begins with a thorough history and physical examination, which should direct the physician to ordering specific lab tests for each individual.

The preoperative evaluation for the orthopaedic patient includes but is not limited to the following:

History and physical examination
Vital signs
CBC (complete blood count)
Serum chemistries/electrolytes
Coagulation profile
Urinalysis
Chest radiograph
Electrocardiogram (ECG)
Informed consent

One must be selective about ordering these tests, as a healthy individual will not need this entire battery while an individual with multiple medical problems may need all of these tests plus additional ones. Those considered to be at increased risk of perioperative complications independent of medical condition include patients greater than 70 years of age and those undergoing emergency procedures.

Vital signs must be assessed on all patients in their initial preoperative evaluation and just prior to surgery, and any identified abnormalities should be further investigated. Blood pressure should be under relatively good control prior to any elective procedure, as patients with uncontrolled hypertension are at increased risk of perioperative hyper- and hypotension. Also, newly diagnosed or labile hypertension should be evaluated further and treated prior to performing any elective procedures. Abnormal pulses should be evaluated with an ECG, and arrythymias should be further evaluated by a cardiologist. An elevated temperature immediately preoperatively is suggestive of occult infection and is a good indication to postpone surgery until the underlying cause is identified and eliminated.

Laboratory studies should be ordered for specific indications only. The complete blood count (CBC) will provide information on hemoglobin/hematocrit levels, platelet levels, and leukocyte (WBC) count. This test is indicated in procedures with predicted substantial blood loss (arthroplasty, spinal fusion), patients undergoing initial outpatient evaluation without any baseline values, pregnant patients, patients with malignancies, patients with chronic renal insufficiency or known anemia and patients with histories of a bleeding diathesis. Patients undergoing procedures with a high predicted blood loss should have packed red blood cells (autologous or banked blood) available in case transfusion is needed.

Thrombocytopenia (platelets <100K) places patients at increased risk of bleeding, especially at counts <50K, and thrombocytosis can cause an increased propensity for thrombosis. Newly diagnosed platelet abnormalities should preclude elective surgery until further evaluated by a hematologist. Leuckocytosis may indicate infection and should be further evaluated prior to elective surgery.

Serum electrolytes and chemistries commonly tested include sodium, potassium, chloride, CO_2, blood urea nitrogen (BUN), creatinine and glucose. Electrolyte evaluation is not necessary in healthy patients under the age of 60. Indications for evaluation are age >60, history of diabetes, renal disease, diuretic use, corticosteroid use, and underlying fluid/electrolyte abnormalities. Chemistry evaluation will help determine a patient's volume status and can identify those at risk for perioperative medical complications. Complications are increased in hypo- (K+ <3.0) or hyperkalemia (K+ >5.0), diabetes (cardiac, infection), renal insufficiency (creatinine >3.0), and uremia (BUN >50).

Coagulation studies include measurement of prothrombin time (PT) and activated partial thromboplastin time (APTT). These help identify coagulopathies, but they are not indicated as a screening test in patients without histories of bleeding disorders. History is perhaps the most important clue for identifying a coagulopathy, and patients should be asked about excess bleeding with any previous procedures or injuries. Family history is also an essential component for identifying a potential coagulopathy. A coagulation profile is indicated in patients with a history of a bleeding disorder, liver disease, malabsorption syndromes, malnutrition, and those on anticoagulation therapy. Those with elevated PTs should have consideration for preoperative vitamin K and should have fresh frozen plasma (FFP) available intra- and postoperatively.

Urinalysis (UA) is performed to evaluate for urinary tract infection (UTI) and renal problems. Abnormalities are commonly found and are frequently insignificant. This test is ordered too frequently and should probably be performed only to rule out UTI in cases of prosthetic implantation and in febrile patients. Another potential indication is a procedure involving urinary instrumentation. UTIs should be treated and if identified preoperatively in a patient undergoing joint replacement, should probably lead to cancellation of the case until the infection is eradicated. Clean catch specimens are often contaminated and should be followed by specimens obtained by catheterization if contamination is suspected.

Routine preoperative chest radiographs (CXRs) are not indicated on all orthopaedic patients. Asymptomatic abnormalities are common and do not necessarily require treatment. In addition, most abnormalities do not adversely affect surgical outcome. Chest radiographs are indicated for any intrathoracic procedure (anterior spinal decompression/corpectomy), or for patients with signs or symptoms of active chest disease. This includes patients with preoperative fevers and respiratory symptoms. The necessity of preoperative screening radiographs in elderly individuals is controversial.

The electrocardiogram (EKG, ECG) is another controversial preoperative screening test. Asymptomatic insignificant abnormalities are often identified in low-risk groups. Abnormalities identified on careful history and physical examination often provide the best clues to cardiac disease and can help dictate the need for ECG. An ECG is indicated for intrathoracic and intraperitoneal procedures, for men >45 and women >55, for emergency procedures, for patients on cardiac medications, and for patients with systemic diseases with potential cardiac involvement.

Informed consent is a crucial portion of the preoperative preparation and education of the patient. The physician should explain the nature of the procedure and all potential risks and complications associated with it. This will allow the patient to make an educated decision on whether to proceed with the surgery and is also necessary from a medicolegal standpoint. In emergent procedures when the patient cannot give informed consent (unconcious, demented), immediate family members (preferably legal guardian), should be contacted for consent and if not available or nonexistent, then at least two physicians should agree that the problem requires emergent attention prior to proceeding.

The preoperative evaluation should thus be tailored to meet the individual needs of each patient. The healthy young patient undergoing an elective ambulatory procedure may not need anything more than a history and physical examination, while the elderly, debilitated patient with multiple medical problems may require further lab evaluation and consultation with medical colleagues. Patients who require special attention perioperatively include those with chronic renal insufficiency, pulmonary disease, diabetes mellitus, cardiac disease, and those on systemic corticosteroids.

Patients with chronic renal insufficiency can generally undergo most orthopaedic procedures without difficulty as long as diligent attention is paid to their volume status. Volume overload should be avoided with judicious use of diuretics or dialysis, and volume depletion should be addressed with careful saline hydration. These patients need close attention paid to their potassium, calcium, and BUN/creatinine levels. Hyperkalemia is a constant threat, and the potassium level should be maintained between 3 and 5. If symptomatic and not responsive to medications, then hyperkalemia should be treated with dialysis.

Patients with chronic renal insufficiency are often also anemic and can generally tolerate hematocrits in the low 20% range if they do not have coexistent coronary disease. Anemia should be treated with erythropoietin, and transfusion should be reserved for symptomatic anemia. These patients also often require adjusted dosages of antibiotics, especially aminoglycosides, and should have decreased dosages of narcotics compared with similar weight non-renal patients. These patients often are malnourished and may require enteral or parenteral nutritional supplements.

Renal patients can also have wound healing problems especially if their electrolytes are uncontrolled. It is often prudent to have a nephrologist participate in the perioperative care of the patient with chronic renal insufficiency, especially if they are dialysis dependent or transplant recipients.

Patients with known or suspected pulmonary disease are at increased risk of medical complications in the perioperative period. Factors contributing to postoperative pulmonary morbidity and mortality include chronic lung disease, increased age, obesity, smoking, malnutrition, recent pulmonary infection, type of anesthetic (general worse than regional), and surgical/incisional site (upper abdominal and thoracic worst). Patients with these risk factors often require thorough preoperative evaluation and preparation, often with the aid of their primary physician or pulmonologist.

Chest radiographs are indicated in patients with known lung disease or with new pulmonary symptoms. ABGs (arterial blood gases) are also performed in the setting of COPD or for significant new pulmonary processes. PFTs (pulmonary function tests) are recommended in patients undergoing major procedures with greater than 20 pack/year smoking histories, unexplained cough, unexplained dyspnea, chronic lung disease, and planned lung resection. These additional studies can identify the high-risk pulmonary patient to allow for adequate preoperative preparation. High-risk patients often receive preoperative bronchodilators and steroids. Smoking cessation and weight loss should be strongly emphasized prior to elective procedures, and procedures should be performed under regional anesthesia if possible for these high-risk patients.

Postoperatively, a key factor in preventing pulmonary complications is early mobilization. This will require adequate analgesia in the immediate postoperative period. Oxygenation should be monitored with a continuous pulseoximeter in high-risk patients, and oxygen supplementation should be used to maintain saturations greater than 90%–92%. Excess oxygen should be avoided in patients with COPD, as they often require CO_2 retention to serve as a respiratory drive.Additionally, patients with sleep apnea may require a CPAP mask while sleeping.

Chest expansion exercises are essential in the postoperative period for all patients, and a standard part of postoperative orders should read: "Turn, cough, and breathe deeply every 2 hours," and "Incentive spirometer to bedside for use every hour." An incentive spirometer is a device that allows for lung hyperinflation by exhaling under pressure into a tube. The incentive spirometer should be ordered in cases in which the patient may have delayed mobilization and should not be ordered on every patient. DVT prophylaxis is important in pulmonary patients, as they have less reserve to tolerate even minor pulmonary emboli. Aerosolized bronchodilators are important measures to continue in the postoperative period to treat wheezing and prevent atelectasis and pneumonia. Prophylactic antibiotics greater than 24 hours postoperatively are not indicated in these patients and should be used only to treat known infections.

Patients with diabetes mellitus have perioperative mortality rates 1.5 to 2 times higher than nondiabetics. Myocardial ischemia and infection are the two most common problems. Tight glucose control (levels <180–200) in the perioperative period decreases the likelihood of wound healing complications and infection. Patients with differing degrees of diabetes will have significantly different perioperative requirements.

Those with diet controlled NIDDM usually do not require insulin or glucose infusion but should be monitored. Those on oral hypoglycemic agents should discontinue their use on the day prior to surgery or two days prior if long acting agents. They generally can be controlled with a sliding scale insulin regimen in the first day or two postoperatively until they can resume their oral agents. Those patients with IDDM or NIDDM on insulin present the greatest difficulty in perioperative management.

Surgical procedures make glucose control more difficult secondary to the stress of surgery (increased glucose), decreased fluid intake (dehydration can exacerbate ketosis) and NPO status on the day of surgery. Insulin dosage is adjusted on the morning of surgery by giving one-half the usual morning dose and starting an intravenous infusion of dextrose (D5W or D51/2NS) to prevent hypoglycemia and associated ketosis. Continuous insulin drips are not indicated unless the patient is in a state of diabetic ketoacidosis.

Postoperatively, the goals are returning the patient back to his or her usual insulin regimen and maintaining glucose levels in a range of 100–200. Depending on the type of procedure, it may take several days for the patient to begin eating and resume his usual dosage. In the interim, the glucose level should be monitored with fingerstick checks every 6 hours until tolerating a regular (diabetic) diet, then before every meal (qAc) and at bedtime (qHs) once on a regular diet. Patients may require a basal dose of subcutaneous regular insulin every 6 hours plus sliding scale insulin. There is no fixed standard regimen of insulin dosage and sliding scale dosage, as it is highly variable among different sources. As stated, the goal is maintaining the glucose level in the 100–200 range. A commonly encountered sliding scale regimen is as follows:

Blood Glucose	# Units Regular SubQ Insulin
0–200	0; call M.D. if <60
201–250	2
251–300	4
301–350	6
351–400	8
>400	10; call M.D.

A serum chemistry (Chem 7) should be checked daily to make sure the patient is not severely hyper- or hypoglycemic, dehydrated, or with a high anion gap. Abnormalities on a chemistry profile can signal the onset of ketoacidosis, which would require intensive management with the assistance of a specialist in diabetic management.

Cardiac-related abnormalities are perhaps the most feared in orthopaedics given the potential to be fatal. Goldman et al[5] have identified the major risk factors associated with a perioperative cardiac event. The most significant factors are myocardial infarction within 6 months of surgery, congestive heart failure, arrythmias, age >70, emergency procedures, and aortic stenosis.

A recent myocardial infarction (<6 months prior to surgery) should lead to postponement of elective surgery, as should untreated congestive heart failure. Patients with known or suspected coronary artery disease should have continuous cardiac monitoring during and after surgery. Invasive hemodynamic monitoring is under the realm of the anesthesiologist and cardiologist and should be strongly considered in patients with severe coronary artery disease undergoing a major procedure, and patients with a recent myocardial infarction, congestive heart failure, or left ventricular dysfunction.

Intraoperatively, close attention must be paid to ensuring adequate oxygenation and avoiding hypo- or hypertension. Transfusion should be used in any instances of symptomatic anemia, and transfusion indications should perhaps not be as rigid for these patients, as they do not tolerate poor oxygenation well. Red blood cell transfusion will serve to increase oxygen-carrying capacity and oxygen delivery to vital structures. Patients on cardiac medications preoperatively should have them continued in the perioperative period.

Patients on corticosteroids require special consideration, as they are at risk for developing postoperative adrenal insufficiency secondary to suppression of the HPA (hypothalamic-pituitary-adrenal) axis. Patients who have taken an equivalent of greater than 7.5 mg of prednisone/day for more than 1 week in the year preceding surgery are at risk of adrenal suppression. In an elective setting, a Cosyntropin (Cortrosyn) stimulation test can be performed to assess the ability of the adrenals to produce endogenous steroids in response to stress. In an emergency setting, one should consider stress dose steroids.

Stress dosing involves administration of 100 mg intravenous hydrocortisone acetate preoperatively, then 100 mg intravenously every 6–8 hours for 24 hours. In minor surgery, the coverage can be stopped at this point and the steroid discontinued or returned to maintenance dose. In major surgery, the dose should be decreased 50% per day until the maintenance dose is reached. Signs and symptoms of adrenal insufficiency include myalgias, arthralgias, hypotension, ileus, eosinophilia, and hyponatremia. If these develop, then the dose should be increased.

Controversy exists over the amount of stress dose needed and whether it is necessary at all, as high doses of corticosteroids are immune suppressive and can delay wound healing. Friedman et al[6] question the need for stress dosing, even in patients on chronic steroids, as there were no instances of adrenal insufficiency in their series of patients undergoing orthopaedic procedures while being maintained on their preoperative prednisone dosage in the perioperative period.

The use of stress dose steroids should thus be carefully weighed and individualized based on the medical profile of each patient and extent of procedure. Any signs of postoperative adrenal insufficiency should be aggressively treated.

The preoperative evaluation of the orthopaedic patient is thus highly dependent on the medical profile of that patient and the procedure that he is undergoing. The next important area of the perioperative management of these patients is the choice of anesthesia. Regional anesthesia will be discussed in relation to orthopaedic procedures.

REGIONAL ANESTHESIA[2,4,7]

A significant portion of orthopaedic procedures are now performed under regional anesthesia, both in the operating and emergency rooms. Regional anesthesia, as opposed to general anesthesia, has gained popularity in the past decade secondary to the increase in ambulatory surgical procedures. In addition, the ease in which it can provide postoperative pain relief and the ability to decrease the requirements for general anesthetics in combined regional/general cases has led to increased usage by anesthesiologists. Regional anesthesia also avoids the potential hazards of general anesthesia in high-risk patients, and has less side effects of nausea, drowsiness and immediate postoperative pain than does general anesthesia.

Although the majority of regional anesthetics are administered by anesthesiologists for procedures performed in the operating room, the orthopaedic house officer should be familiar with some basic blocks to use in the emergency room for fracture, dislocation, and laceration work, and for common office orthopaedic procedures.

Although regional anesthesia has significant benefits, it is not without danger, as complications can and do occur. These complications include nerve damage from direct infiltration of drug into the nerve as opposed to the perineural tissue, and toxicity reactions from intravenous injection or from exceeding the maximum recommended safe dosage.

The most commonly used agents are lidocaine (Xylocaine) and bupivicaine (Marcaine, Sensorcaine). Lidocaine has a rapid onset (1–3 minutes) and short duration of action (1–2 hours), while bupivicaine has a slower onset (2–10 minutes) and longer duration of action (8–12 hours). Adding epinephrine to the local anesthetic will increase the duration of action.

The maximum recommended dose for local infiltration of lidocaine is 4 mg/kg and for lidocaine with epinephrine is 7 mg/kg. Lidocaine can serve to lower the seizure threshold in high doses. Bupivicaine's maximum recommended dose is 2–2.5 mg/kg without epinephrine and 3 mg/kg with epinephrine. Bupivicaine can also lower the seizure threshold but even more alarming can cause fatal cardiac arrythmias in toxic doses. Ropivicaine is a new agent similar to bupivicaine but with less risk of cardiotoxicity.

Commonly performed regional anesthetics in the upper extremity include interscalene, supraclavicular, axillary, Bier (intravenous regional), hematoma, wrist and digital blocks, with the latter four often performed by orthopaedic surgeons. Spinal and epidural anesthetics are commonly used for lower extremity procedures. Lower extremity peripheral blocks include femoral/sciatic blocks, knee blocks and ankle blocks, with the orthopaedist commonly performing the latter two types. Of essence to any nerve block is meticulous sterile technique to prevent infection.

Bier Block (Intravenous Regional)

Bier block is performed frequently for upper extremity procedures of short duration (preferably less than 60 minutes) that can be done distal to an upper arm tourniquet. It is a useful technique for forearm and wrist fracture reduction, as well as soft-tissue procedures on the forearm and hand.

The technique involves placement of a double tourniquet or two single tourniquets on a patient's upper arm, starting an intravenous cathether distal to the tourniquets and then exsanguinating the extremity and subsequently inflating the upper tourniquet. The local anesthetic is then injected intravenously distal to the tourniquet to initiate the block. Use of bupivicaine is not recommended owing to its potentially fatal cardiotoxicity reaction.

If the patient begins to complain of tourniquet-related pain (pain, numbness), then the distal cuff overlying the anesthetized skin is inflated, and once confirmed to be working, the upper tourniquet is released. The tourniquets can be released at the end of the procedure if the duration of the procedure was long enough (generally 25–30 minutes) to safely release the anesthetic into the bloodstream. If not long enough, then the tourniquet should remain inflated or can be cyclically inflated and deflated to release small amounts until the remainder can be safely released.

Hematoma Block

Hematoma block, or injection of local anesthetic directly into a fracture site, is commonly used to decrease the pain associated with fracture reduction. It is most commonly used for reduction of distal radius fractures but theoretically can be used to aid in reduction of most distal long bone fractures. Although the hematoma block helps with pain relief, intravenous sedation and analgesia are frequently used as adjuncts to help with pain control and relaxation, as hematoma block provides no muscle relaxation, a necessary factor for adequate reduction.

The block is performed by directly palpating the bony deformity to identify the fracture site. The patient will usually provide distinct clues when this site is reached. Once this site is identified, the skin must be thoroughly prepped to create a sterile field, as introduction of a needle through unclean skin can cause bacterial contamination of the fracture site with possible resultant infection.

Upon entering the fracture site, aspirate with the syringe until dark blood is encountered. The local anesthetic can then be introduced into the fracture site. Generally 5–10 ml of a lidocaine/Marcaine mixture is utilized. Care must be taken to avoid intravascular injection. Once the block and sedation have taken effect, the reduction can be performed.

Wrist Block

Wrist block is a technique that is not frequently performed but can be a useful procedure for reducing fractures or performing soft-tissue work in the hand. For complete hand anesthesia, the median and ulnar nerves should be blocked on the volar aspect of the wrist and the superficial radial and dorsal ulnar sensory nerves should be blocked dorsally.

Landmarks for blockade of the ulnar nerve are the flexor carpi ulnaris (FCU) tendon, ulnar artery (palpate pulse), and pisiform bone. The arm is placed in the supine position and the FCU tendon is identified 1 cm proximal to the insertion on the pisiform. The ulnar artery is palpated and a 25-gauge needle inserted between the tendon and artery until paresthesias are induced. The syringe is then aspirated to ensure that the needle is not intravascular, and then 3–4 ml of lidocaine and/or bupivicaine are injected. An additional 1–2 ml may then be injected subcutaneously prior to completely withdrawing the needle.

With the forearm still in the volar position, median nerve block is then performed. The palmaris longus tendon is then identified by having the patient flex his or her wrist against resistance. If present, a 25-gauge needle is inserted just radial to the tendon at the proximal wrist crease to a depth just below the flexor retinaculum, where paresthesias are induced. Aspirate the syringe and then inject 4–5 ml of lidocaine and/or bupivicaine. If resistance is met, slightly withdraw the needle, as resistance may indicate intraneural placement. Inject an additional 1–2 ml in the subcutaneous tissue to block the palmar cutaneous branch. If the palmaris longus is absent (approximately 10% of people), then insert the needle slightly ulnar to the flexor carpi radialis (FCR) tendon.

The sensory nerves on the dorsum of the hand are blocked with the forearm in the prone position. Landmarks are the radial and ulnar styloids and the extensor pollicis longus and brevis tendons (EPL, EPB). The EPL is identified at the radial styloid; a 22- or 25-gauge 3 cm needle is inserted adjacent to the tendon at the styloid level and a subcutaneous wheal is injected in an ulnar direction over to the ulnar styloid (approximately 5–7 ml). The needle is then removed and through the same insertion point is redirected subcutaneously in a radial direction over the EPB tendon (2–3 ml) at the anatomic snuffbox level.

An entire wrist block is not necessary for procedures that can be performed with isolated ulnar, median, or dorsal blocks.

Digital Block

Digital blocks are extremely useful adjuncts for treating fractures, dislocations, lacerations, and nail bed injuries in the fingers. They can also be used to help properly evaluate the extent of open injury *after* a sensory exam has been performed to rule out a digital nerve laceration, as once the block is administered this cannot be assessed. The most important fact to remember is that *epinephrine must not be used in the anesthetic preparation for digital blocks*, as it can lead to vasospasm and potential digital necrosis.

A digital block can be administered through a volar or dorsal approach (dorsal usually less painful) after skin preparation. The 25-gauge needle is introduced dorsally between the metacarpal heads, and the needle is advanced until detected by a finger placed on the palmar aspect of the skin. Local anesthetic (3–5 ml) is then injected as the needle is withdrawn. The same procedure is then performed on the other side of the affected digit, as both sides need to be anesthesized to get an adequate block.

Knee Block

Intraarticular knee blocks are an important technique to know since they are frequently used for performing knee arthroscopy. For an intraarticular injection, the needle can be inserted under the patella medially or laterally. For arthroscopic purposes, the proposed portal sites should be infiltrated in addition to the intraarticular injection.

The knee is flexed 20 to 30 degrees and the superior, inferior, medial, and lateral borders of the patella are palpated and marked. The junction of the medial and inferior borders and lateral and inferior borders are then palpated and marked to identify the inferomedial and inferolateral portal sites, respectively. Approximately 1–2 fingerbreadths above the junction of the superior and medial borders, the superomedial injection site is marked if it is going to be utilized.

The portal sites are then injected subcutaneously with 25-gauge needles with 3–5 ml of local anesthetic This injection should not reach the deep subcutaneous tissue, as fat pad infiltration can make arthroscopic visualization more difficult. If the superomedial portal site is used for an inflow portal, then the needle should be passed deeply onto the anterior femoral cortex and the injection performed while the needle is being withdrawn (5–10 ml are often needed at this site). The intraarticular portion of the injection is then performed with approximately 40 ml of a 1% lidocaine/0.25% bupivicaine mixture.

Ankle Block

Ankle blocks are useful for providing anesthesia to the foot and can be used for foot fracture reduction and various soft-tissue procedures. A total of five nerves must be blocked: sural, deep peroneal, superficial peroneal, saphenous, and tibial.

The sural nerve is anesthetized by palpating the area between the posterior border of the lateral malleolus near its tip and the lateral border of the Achilles tendon. A 22- or 25-gauge needle is then used to make a subcutaneous wheal between these two points with 3–5 ml of local anesthetic.

The deep peroneal nerve is anesthetized by identifying the dorsalis pedis pulse between the EHL and EDL tendons at the level of the ankle joint and then inserting a 22- or 25-gauge needle just medial to the pulse. The needle is inserted perpendicular to bone to a depth where bone is palpated. It is then withdrawn 2–3 mm, and 5–7 ml of solution are injected after aspirating the syringe to make sure the needle is not intravascular.

The superficial peroneal nerve is anesthetized in combination with the deep peroneal nerve by withdrawing the needle from the deep peroneal block and placing it subcutaneously. It is then directed laterally along a line parallel to the line connecting the two malleoli. A subcutaneous wheal is created with 5–7 ml of solution.

The saphenous nerve is anesthetized by subcutaneous infiltration of 3–5 ml of solution at a point 1 cm anterior and 1 cm proximal to the tip of the medial malleolus. It is infiltrated around the greater saphenous vein, and care must be taken to avoid intravascular injection.

The tibial nerve is located immediately posterior to the posterior tibial artery. The structures behind the medial malleolus can be memorized by the mnemonic **T**om, **D**ick **A**nd **H**arry, corresponding to the **T**ibialis posterior tendon, flexor **D**igitorum longus tendon, posterior tibial **A**rtery, tibial **N**erve and flexor **H**allucis longus tendon. The nerve is anesthetized by palpating the posterior tibial pulse and then inserting a 22- or 25-gauge needle just posterior to this and perpendicular to the medial malleolus. Paresthesias are often elicited, and 5–10 ml of solution are then injected. Care must be taken to avoid intraarticular injection.

Digital blocks in the toes are not commonly performed and can be done with the same technique as described for the hand. Once again, *solutions with epinephrine should not be used for any digital blocks (fingers or toes).* Epinephrine solutions can be used for the other blocks described above.

POSTOPERATIVE CARE

Once the operative procedure is completed, postoperative management becomes the key to successful outcome. Three essential components of the postoperative management of orthopaedic patients are pain management, DVT prophylaxis, and judicious use of antibiotics (prophylaxis and treatment). These three parameters should be a central part of all postoperative orders for nonambulatory surgery in addition to the patients preoperative medications and as needed (PRN) medications such as antipyretics (acetaminophen), antiemetics, and laxatives. The initial postoperative patient evaluation is also an essential part of complete and effective postoperative care.

Pain Management[8,9]

Perioperative pain management is an extremely important aspect of both ambulatory and inpatient orthopaedic procedures, as ineffective pain management will lead to a dissatisfied patient and can also lead to medical complications, wound and surgical site healing problems, and difficulty with rehabilitation. In the ambulatory setting, uncontrolled pain with associated nausea and/or vomiting can lead to delays in discharge and possibly require unwanted hospital admissions. Recent advances in perioperative pain management have apparently enhanced pain control and decreased adverse outcomes. These techniques include patient-controlled analgesia (PCA), regional anesthetics (spinal, epidural, and peripheral blocks), nonnarcotic analgesics, and preemptive analgesia.

Postoperative pain, until recently, was predominantly managed with oral and/or injectable opioids on an intermittent fixed-dose basis. This regimen is not always effective, as there can often be a delay in administration of these medications and their onset of action varies between patients, thus there may be gaps in pain control, with the patient experiencing significant pain before the medication is administered or before it takes effect. In fact, this regimen has been shown to provide ineffective pain control in approximately one-half of all postoperative patients. Most opioids also have a high potential for abuse. Opioids can be effective for many procedures and generally are used for variable amounts of time after discharge from the hospital.

Administration of opioids with the premedication just prior to surgery, as well as adjunctive use of NSAIDs can be effective in decreasing postoperative opioid requirements. Newer techniques of perioperative pain management aim to eliminate the analgesic gaps encountered with intermittent fixed-dose opioids.

Patient-controlled analgesia (PCA) devices allow the patient to self-administer frequent small doses of analgesics to eliminate gaps in pain control by maintaining therapeutic analgesic concentrations in the central nervous system. The physician prescribes the medication and sets limits to the demand dose administered, continuous infusion dose, lockout interval, initial bolus dose, and maximum dose per unit time (usually 4-hour maximum). This regimen is generally effective with high levels of patient satisfaction. Once the initial postoperative pain has diminished (1–3 days), the patient can be converted from PCA to oral medications in preparation for discharge.

The use of spinal and epidural anesthetics with catheters placed for postoperative pain management has gained recent popularity in lower extremity surgery. The mechanism is stimulation of spinal opioid receptors, which leads to inhibition of substance P release, effectively decreasing the intensity of incoming painful stimuli. Epidural anesthetics have also been associated with lower rates of DVT in arthroplasty surgery in addition to providing excellent pain control[10]. Side effects are similar to those of oral opioids, but severe ventilatory depression can occur if the dosage is not managed effectively. Narcan (naloxone) can be used to reverse any unwanted effects of spinal opioids. Local anesthetics are routinely coadministered through the catheters and should be discontinued several hours prior to initiating physical therapy or ambulation to allow for recovery of motor and sensory function. Concurrent use of opioids and local anesthetics decreases the dosage requirements for both medications.

Peripheral nerve blocks, as discussed earlier in this chapter, can be used to provide effective postoperative pain relief by initially utilizing long-acting agents and/or continuous infusion through catheters. Negative aspects include inability to perform an accurate neurologic examination, and inability to detect if the postoperative splint is providing too much compression or if the patient is developing a compartment syndrome, as pain cannot be effectively monitored. Major advantages are the ability to use blocks for ambulatory surgery (especially upper extremity) and potential for rapid mobilization to allow for early rehabilitation.

The use of nonnarcotic analgesics such as NSAIDs pre- and/or postoperatively has been shown to effectively decrease narcotic requirements in the postoperative period. Ketorolac (Toradol), the only current NSAID available for intravenous use, has demonstrated a significant opioid-sparing effect even in procedures associated with severe postoperative pain[11] and may potentially be effective as the sole analgesic in minor procedures. NSAIDs act at the site of tissue trauma by providing an antiinflammatory effect but can have systemic effects such as GI upset and ulceration, renal and hepatic toxicity, and antiplatelet effects, and thus must be used carefully. Concurrent use of NSAIDs, opioids, and local incisional anesthetics ("balanced analgesia") effectively decreases the required efficacious dose for all of these medications and may help avoid the unwanted side effects of each. This concept is especially useful in ambulatory surgery.

Preemptive analgesia refers to preincisional administration of NSAIDs, opioids, and incisional or nerve blocks alone or in combination with each other. The rationale is to decrease and/or prevent noxious input to the central nervous system. This input can cause hyperexcitability to the painful stimuli in the affected area. Preemptive analgesia with local anesthetic and opioid combinations has documented efficacy in orthopaedic procedures[12]. Using these combinations also effectively decreases the therapeutic doses necessary for each individual medication.

Significant advances have thus been made in management and control of postoperative pain in recent years. These have been effective for both ambulatory and inpatient procedures previously associated with high pain levels. This allows for more rapid mobilization and earlier rehabilitation, which helps prevent postoperative morbidity. In addition, patient satisfaction is improved, which is perhaps the greatest achievement in improved postoperative pain management.

DVT/PE

Deep venous thrombosis (DVT) represents a significant problem in orthopaedics, as nearly all patients undergoing orthopaedic procedures, especially those involving the lower extremity, are at risk of developing postoperative thrombosis and pulmonary embolism (PE). It is estimated that venous thromboembolism is responsible for the death of up to 200,000 patients in the United States annually[13]. Fortunately, the number of emboli contributing to deaths in orthopaedic patients is much lower; however, the problem must be taken seriously.

Given the high rates of venous thromboembolism, prophylaxis is warranted, especially in elective lower extremity procedures and trauma procedures. The incidence of DVT in patients undergoing hip or knee arthroplasty or hip fracture surgery is 50%–80% if prophylaxis is not utilized. Proximal DVTs, or those most likely to embolize to the lungs, occur in up to 35% of elective THAs, 20% of elective TKAs, and 35% of hip fracture procedures, and fatal PE occurs in up to 4%, 1% and 10%, respectively, in these groups without prophylaxis against thromboembolism[14]. All patients with orthopaedic trauma, especially pelvic fractures, are also at high risk for DVT/PE, with the young multiple trauma patient having a 1%–2% risk of PE if left unprotected.

Risk factors for DVT/PE include advanced age, venous disease, tobacco use, high-dose estrogen therapy, prior or current malignancy, genetic predisposition (Protein C or S deficiency, Antithrombin III deficiency, dysfibrogenemia, lupus anticoagulant), prolonged surgery, immobilization, and prior history of DVT/PE[14]. In addition, a recent consensus conference on antithrombotic therapy, classified orthopaedic patients as being in the "very high risk" category for developing a thromboembolic event and recommended prophylaxis for these procedures[13].

Unfortunately, DVT/PE is difficult to diagnose on clinical means alone. Approximately 70%–80% of all venous thrombi are unsuspected. The classic presentation of a warm swollen leg with tenderness to palpation and a palpable venous cord does not occur in most instances of DVT. Detectable pulmonary embolus classically presents with pleuritic chest pain, dyspnea, tachycardia, hemoptysis, and sometimes impaired mentation; however, up to 75% are asymptomatic. Regrettably, most deaths secondary to PE occur within 30 minutes of the embolic event and thus anticoagulant treatment would be ineffective if started after the acute event.

Diagnosis of DVT, if clinically suspected, is confirmed by radiographic modalities such as venogram, duplex ultrasound, and MRI. Venogram is considered the gold standard for diagnosis; however, it is invasive and can cause allergic reactions and phlebitis. Duplex ultrasound has shown excellent accuracy for detecting proximal leg (thigh) DVTs but is less accurate (88% sensitivity) in diagnosing calf DVT[15]. Although calf DVTs are felt by many to be inconsequential, they still can propogate to the proximal venous system in approximately 15%–20% of cases[16]. MRI is another good option for diagnosing DVT; however, the cost remains high. The most accurate means of diagnosis for any given institution may vary dependent on the proficiency and experience of the radiologist and technologist for each technique, and thus the radiologist should be consulted in a suspected case of DVT to determine which method he or she feels would be most accurate. For suspected cases of pulmonary embolism, ventilation/perfusion (V/Q) scans remain the primary means of confirmation, with pulmonary angiography being an option for "indeterminate" cases on V/Q scanning.

The most effective form of DVT prophylaxis is highly controversial. Various strategies include the use of aspirin, dextran, intermittent pneumatic compression devices (IPC), low-dose unfractionated heparin (LDUH), adjusted dose heparin, low molecular weight heparin, and coumadin. In addition, hypotensive epidural anesthesia has demonstrated efficacy in preventing postoperative DVT in arthroplasty patients[10]. Chapter 12 discusses the dosages and mechanisms of action of each method. The efficacy of each will be briefly presented here.

The efficacy of any method of DVT prophylaxis is studied most frequently in patients undergoing hip and knee arthroplasty. Aspirin, through its antiplatelet action, would be expected to provide an effective measure of prophylaxis; however, pooled data from multiple series has shown no relative risk reduction compared with other regimens in THA and TKA surgery[13]. Low-dose unfractionated heparin shows some risk reduction, but the incidence of DVT in pooled data is still >30%. Dextran was slightly more effective than aspirin; however, it may cause volume overload, which can potentially be harmful in elderly patients with cardiac disease, and also frequently causes headaches and nausea.

Intermittent pneumatic compression (IPC) devices promote blood flow through the deep venous system of the lower limb and also serve to enhance fibrinolytic activity. They do not increase the risk of bleeding and are not associated with significant side effects. Devices generally are calf high or applied just to the feet. They have proven efficacy in reducing calf thrombi[17], but have not demonstrated efficacy in reducing proximal thrombi, with rates approximating 15%–20%. For this reason, they are not often used as a sole means of prophylaxis in arthroplasty surgery but are frequently used in conjunction with other measures. One problem with these devices is a lack of patient compliance with their use, as they tend to be uncomfortable. These devices remain popular for intra- and postoperative use in spinal surgery.

Adjusted-dose heparin given intravenously with dosage based on maintaining the activated partial thromboplastin (APTT) time just above the upper limits of normal (40–50) has proven efficacy in DVT prophylaxis after hip surgery[13]. Problems with this regimen include frequent use of costly lab tests to accurately adjust the APTT and a significant risk of bleeding complications. Unfractionated heparin has also been associated with thrombocytopenia and paradoxical thrombosis. Despite the inconvenience of utilizing adjusted-dose heparin therapy, it is often an important adjunct for patients with a history of thromboembolism or for patients on coumadin therapy preoperatively who require immediate postoperative anticoagulation until their coumadin levels become therapeutic.

Low-dose coumadin therapy, with the goal of treatment being an international normalized ratio (INR) of 2.0 to 3.0, has documented efficacy in prophylaxis after THA but less efficacy after TKA[18–20]. Prior to the introduction of low molecular weight heparins, it was perhaps the most common method of prophylaxis used in North America. Controversy exists over beginning coumadin use preoperatively or immediately postoperatively, as it often takes 2–3 days to achieve therapeutic, nontoxic levels. An advantage of low-dose coumadin is that it can be continued postdischarge once the dosage is adjusted properly. Monitoring is necessary to ensure that levels remain therapeutic and nontoxic and thus adds expense. Controversy also exists as to the appropriate length of postoperative prophylaxis.

Low molecular weight heparin derivatives have proven clinical efficacy in comparison with other accepted means of prophylaxis in well-controlled clinical trials, with potentially fewer side effects than unfractionated heparin[20–25]. Because of concerns over bleeding complications, the first dose is often given 12–24 hours postoperatively. To date enoxaparin (Lovenox) has been utilized in most clinical trials, but other preparations are currently being clinically tested. The most effective dosage of Lovenox is 30 mg subcutaneously every 12 hours. Advantages are that it can be given unmonitored and has proven efficacy, with disadvantages being potential bleeding complications.

Hypotensive epidural anesthesia also has demonstrable efficacy in decreasing postoperative thrombosis in THA patients[10]. It is felt that significant blood loss leads to activation of the clotting cascade and that the decreased blood loss associated with hypotensive epidurals will prevent activation and thus not lead to a "hypercoagulable state."

Placement of an IVC filter (Greenfield filter) represents another option for those patients unable to take pharmacologic therapy, those with demonstrable thrombosis preoperatively who require nonelective surgery, and those with a history of thromboembolic disease. This procedure is not without complications and should be used only under strict indications.

Recommendations for DVT prophylaxis based on the 1995 American College for Chest Physicians consensus conference[13] included the use of low molecular weight heparin, low-dose coumadin, or dose-adjusted unfractionated heparin in total hip arthroplasty. Adjuvant prophylaxis with IPC devices was deemed acceptable, but LDUH, aspirin and Dextran were considered less effective modalities. For total knee arthroplasty, low molecular weight heparin was considered treatment of choice and IPC devices were considered an acceptable alternative.

Controversy continues over length of prophylaxis postoperatively, as patients with no or discontinued therapy remain at risk for developing DVT with propagation for an indeterminate time period[26]. Recent studies show 17% and 39% rates of DVT up to 1 month postoperatively in nonprophylaxed patients[27,28]. This issue becomes increasingly problematic with the advent of short hospital stays (4–5 days) after joint replacement secondary to policies and pressures of third-party payers. The majority of DVTs occur within the first week postoperatively[29] and these patients are being discharged from the hospital during this high-risk period; thus, continuing prophylaxis becomes an important issue. The type of agent and length of necessary postoperative prophylaxis (and treatment of known DVT) are now being actively investigated in clinical trials[27,28,30].

Antibiotics

The use of prophylactic antibiotics is an important adjunct in the prevention of surgical wound and deep periprosthetic infections. In orthopaedics, first-generation cephalosporins are administered in most instances immediately preoperatively in clean cases. In patients with significant penicillin allergies (swelling, anaphylaxis), vancomycin is usually administered.

The timing of prophylactic antibiotics is important. Classen et al[31] found that giving antibiotics within 2 hours of surgical incision led to lower wound infection rates than giving them earlier, intraoperatively or postoperatively. This suggests that antibiotics must have sufficient plasma levels at the time of incision to most effectively decrease the likelihood of wound infection. It has been demonstrated that bone and serum levels of cephalosporins are maximal within 60 minutes of drug administration[32]. The house officer should thus order the antibiotic to be administered "on induction" for any patients receiving prophylactic therapy. For those receiving ongoing therapy, the current antibiotics can be continued on their usual schedule.

The length of prophylactic therapy is also controversial in clean cases. For outpatient procedures, patients usually receive just one preoperative dose of cephalosporin and no postoperative antibiotics with low infection rates in most instances. For inpatient procedures not involving prostheses, spinal instrumentation or open fractures, utilizing antibiotics postoperatively may not be necessary. Garcia et al[33] found a single preoperative dose of cefonocid equally effective as 3 and 5 perioperative doses of cefamandole in prevention of wound infections. Most surgeons, however, prefer 24 hours of postoperative prophylaxis for inpatient cases involving suction drains to provide antimicrobial coverage for the foriegn body (drain). In arthroplasty and spinal instrumentation procedures, 24 hours of postoperative prophylaxis is routinely given. In open fractures, this generally continues until definitive wound management is achieved.

Utilization of antibiotics for treatment of documented infection, as opposed to prophylaxis, is constantly changing based on emergence of new organisms and new resistance patterns of existing organisms. The central tenet in treating infection is the administration of specific antibiotics based on culture and sensitivity results rather than prolonged treatment with multiple broad spectrum agents, which can select out resistant organisms. In cases of abscesses, chronic osteomyelitis, septic arthritis, periprosthetic infection, and aggressive soft-tissue infection, surgical drainage and debridement of infected tissue remain the critical factors in infection eradication, and antibiotics provide a supportive role.

New trends in antibiotic therapy include home administration of antibiotics through central or peripheral catheters to attempt to control costs of inpatient care. Antibiotic levels must be checked in all cases but especially in these instances to ensure that adequate levels are achieved to eradicate the infection. Outpatient treatment of orthopaedic infections is usually performed in conjunction with an infectious disease specialist.

Postoperative Check

All patients should be evaluated by a physician after their procedures to ensure that they are not experiencing any procedure-related or medical problems. This is especially true for those patients being admitted to the hospital, as their procedures are generally more extensive than outpatient procedures, but outpatients must also be thoroughly evaluated prior to discharge.

The postoperative check begins wth a review of the patient's vital signs and drain output (if applicable). It is not unusual for patients to be slightly febrile postoperatively, especially after long procedures under general anesthesia, but excessively high fevers (103–105°F) may signify the presence of malignant hyperthermia, which is a potentially fatal condition. The anesthesiologist is more familiar with treating this uncommon condition, but in the emergent situation the orthopaedist may need to take action. Core cooling and oxygen must be immediately administered and intravenous dantrolene pushed beginning at 1 mg/kg and continuing until symptoms resolve up to a total dose of 10 mg/kg. A high fever in a patient with an open fracture or contaminated wound could signal the onset of aggressive soft-tissue infection such as gas gangrene or necrotizing fasciitis, and the wound must be immediately inspected and the patient returned to the operating room for further debridement if aggressive infection is present.

Tachycardia may signal symptomatic anemia in cases associated with high blood loss. A CBC should be ordered in these cases. Tachycardia is also a normal physiologic response to pain, so the patient's pain level must be assessed. Brady- or tachycardia can also signify a primary cardiac abnormality and an ECG should be ordered if the patient is not in pain or not anemic. Arrythymias deserve cardiac consultation. Tachycardia with tachypnea and hypoxia can signify pulmonary or fat embolism and must be rapidly treated and evaluated.

Tachypnea postoperatively should be evaluated with a chest radiograph and pulseoximeter reading once determined that it is not a response to excess pain. Oxygen should be administered if the patient is uncomfortable or has oxygen saturation below 92%–94%. In a trauma patient with long bone fractures, tachypnea can signify the onset of fat embolism syndrome (see next section). In a patient with an interscalene block, tachypnea may occur secondary to a pneumothorax from aberrant needle placement during the block, and a chest radiograph should be ordered. An ABG should be considered if any patient does not rapidly respond to oxygen administration, especially if he is at high risk for pulmonary embolism.

Hypertension may represent a physiologic response to pain and generally does not become tremendously problematic in the postoperative period. Hypotension is more problematic and can signal hypovolemia, bleeding, or a cardiac event. Hypovolemia can be corrected with fluid resuscitation if ongoing bleeding is not the underlying cause. Drain output should be checked and if excessive, a CBC and coagulation profile should be ordered. If a coagulopathy is present, it should be corrected. If the coagulation profile is normal and ongoing blood loss continues, then wound exploration should be considered. If euvolemic with normal hematocrit and still hypotensive, then an ECG and serum chemistries should be ordered to rule out acute cardiac event or electrolyte abnormality.

A thorough neurovascular examination focused on the operated or injured extremity is the next important step in the postoperative evaluation. In cervical spine surgery, all four extremities must be evaluated, and in thoracolumbar surgery, the lower extremities must be evaluated.

The splint or dressing should first be checked to make sure it is not saturated with blood or serous fluid. Most postoperative forms of immobilization will be noncircumferential splints, as opposed to circular casts, to allow for swelling of the extremity without constricting it. These dressings still can be constrictive if they become blood soaked and will not expand.

Pulses should then be checked if the dressing will allow for access. If just the fingers or toes are accessible, then they should be checked for capillary refill. Certain injuries such as pediatric supracondylar humerus fractures, knee dislocations, and severe open tibia fractures are frequently associated with vascular injuries, and in these cases the dressing can be partially split to allow access to check pulses. In older patients with peripheral vascular disease, a doppler examination may be necessary. One must also remember that a palpable pulse does not rule out a compartment syndrome if that diagnosis is suspected.

Any pulse abnormalities should be considered an emergency. Constrictive dressings should be loosened all the way down to the level of the skin and the extremity palpated to make sure the compartments are soft if the procedure or injury potentially predisposes the patient to compartment syndrome. If the pulses still remain abnormal with loosening of the dressing and the patient is not hypothermic (vasoconstriction) or hypotensive, then consideration should be given for urgent arteriogram or surgical exploration. If hypothermic or hypotensive, then these should be corrected and the pulses reassessed.

A special circumstance is in digital replantation or revascularization where temperature probes are often in place. Decreased temperature in relation to the control probe and the other digits can signal impending or actual vascular compromise, and the microvascular surgeon should be notified immediately.

Extremity sensory examination provides clues to nerve injury or impending compartment syndrome. It is not useful in the setting of regional anesthesia, as sensory function may still be blocked at the initial postoperative evaluation. In the upper extremity, the autonomous zones of the median, radial, and ulnar nerves should be tested and pin prick and two-point discrimination assessed at the fingertips. In the lower extremity, pin prick should be tested in the individual dermatomes and in the sensory zones of the nerves supplying sensation to the foot. Light touch can also be tested in all areas. Paresthesias may present secondary to prolonged tourniquet ischemia, and these should improve over time. Paresthesias associated with impending compartment syndrome will worsen over time if the compartment is not decompressed. If there is doubt over this diagnosis, then compartment pressures should be measured.

The motor examination completes the neurovascular assessment. Radial, median, and ulnar function can be tested in the upper extremity as long as the patient's fingers extend beyond the distal aspect of the splint. Radial function is assessed by extension of the thumb IP joint (EPL), median function assessed by opposition of the fingers to the thumb, and ulnar function assessed by the patient crossing his or her fingers.

Lower extremity motor function is assessed by asking the patient to dorsi- and plantar flex his or her toes (entire foot if not splinted). Dorsiflexion of the great toe assesses EHL function, which is indicative of deep peroneal nerve function. One must assess this carefully, as a flicker of dorsiflexion may actually be rebound motion from plantar flexion and vice versa, rather than representing true motion. Simply asking the patient to wiggle his or her toes is not sufficient in differentiating true function from rebound. Examining all motor groups in the lower extremity is important in spinal surgery.

Patients undergoing total hip arthroplasty should have the position of their operated leg checked to ensure that it is not dislocated. Positions of shortening, adduction, and internal rotation may signify posterior dislocation, while abduction and external rotation may signify anterior dislocation. If in doubt, order a portable A-P pelvis to rule out dislocation.

The final step in the postoperative check is attending to any laboratory studies that may have been ordered in the initial postoperative period. All abnormalities in the postoperative check must be addressed immediately to avoid any untoward consequences.

This examination should be repeated on a daily basis for any inpatients with any changes in status being further investigated.

Fat Embolism Syndrome[34]

Fat embolism syndrome is discussed in this section because it is a potentially fatal, yet preventable, postoperative complication of orthopaedic trauma. It generally occurs in young healthy patients with closed lower extremity long bone fractures. The incidence is approximately 1%–2% of all fracture patients and 2%–4% of all patients with multiple fractures.

The syndrome consists of respiratory insufficiency (tachypnea, hypoxia), confusion, and a petechial rash occurring 24–72 hours after the injury. The rash is caused by embolic fat, is transient, and generally occurs on the face, neck, and conjunctiva. Other signs include fever, tachycardia, retinal changes, jaundice, and anxiety. ABGs demonstrate hypoxia, ECG shows tachycardia with possible ST changes, and chest radiographs may show fluffy pulmonary infiltrates. In addition, the hematocrit level may fall, the prothrombin time may be prolonged, and fat globules may be present in the urine, blood, sputum, and CSF.

Pathogenesis is not fully understood, and the syndrome is secondary to either embolization of fat marrow into the lung or secondary to the effects of oxidation of fat to free fatty acids causing endothelial damage in the lungs and other tissue.

Treatment involves maintaining adequate oxygenation with supplemental oxygen, and in severe cases, may require intubation with positive pressure ventilation. The use of corticosteroids remains controversial without proven efficacy for treatment once the syndrome exists, but with possible prophylactic benefit. Early recognition is crucial because once the syndrome becomes advanced, there is a 10%–15% mortality rate.

Prevention remains the key to avoiding this complication. Proper fracture splinting prior to surgical treatment, utilization of oxygen in the preoperative period, and perhaps, most important, early stabilization of long bone fractures are the key factors necessary to prevent this potentially fatal condition.

References

1. Goldman DR, Brown FH, Guarnieri DM. Perioperative medicine: The medical care of the surgical patient. 2nd ed. New York: McGraw-Hill, 1994.
2. Loach A. Orthopaedic anesthesia. Boston: Little, Brown & Co., 1994.
3. Merli GL, Weitz HH. Medical management of the surgical patient. Philadelphia: WB Saunders, 1992.
4. Wedel DJ. Orthopedic anesthesia. New York: Churchill Livingstone, 1993.
5. Goldman L, Caldera DJ, et al. Cardiac risk factors and complications in non-cardiac surgery. Medicine 1978;57:357–370.
6. Friedman RJ, Schiff CF, Bromberg JS. Use of supplemental steroids in patients having orthopaedic operations. J Bone Joint Surg 1995;77-A:1801–1806.
7. Pinnock CA, Fischer HBJ, Jones RP. Peripheral nerve blockade. New York: Churchill Livingstone, 1996.
8. Joshi JP. Postoperative pain management. Int Anest Clin 1994; 32(3):113–126.
9. Riegler FX. Update on perioperative pain management. Clin Orthop 1994;305:283–292.

10. Lieberman JR, Huo MM, et al. The prevalence of deep venous thrombosis after total hip arthroplasty with hypotensive epidural anesthesia. J Bone Joint Surg 1994;76-A:341–348.

11. Fragen RJ, Stulberg SD, et al. Effect of Ketorolac tromethamine on bleeding and on requirements for analgesia after total knee arthroplasty. J Bone Joint Surg 1995;77-A:998–1002.

12. McQuay H, Carroll D, Moore R. Postoperative orthopaedic pain: the effect of opiate premedication and local anesthetic blocks. Pain 1988;33:291–295.

13. Clagett GP, Anderson FA, et al. Prevention of venous thromboembolism. Chest 1995;108:312S–334S.

14. Paiement GD, Mendelsohn C. The risk of venous thromboembolism in the orthopedic patient: epidemiological and physiological data. Orthopedics 1997;20:7S–9S.

15. Grady-Benson JC, Oishi CS, et al. Postoperative surveillance for deep venous thrombosis with duplex ultrasonography after total knee arthroplasty. J Bone Joint Surg 1994;76-A:1649–1657.

16. Oishi CS, Grady-Benson JC, et al. The clinical course of distal deep venous thrombosis after total hip and total knee arthroplasty, as determined with duplex ultrasonography. J Bone Joint Surg 1994; 76-A:1658–1663.

17. Westrich GH, Sculco TP. Prophylaxis against deep venous thrombosis after total knee arthroplasty. Pneumatic plantar compression and aspirin compared with aspirin alone. J Bone Joint Surg 1996;78-A:826–834.

18. Amstutz HC, Friscia DA, et al. Warfarin prophylaxis to prevent mortality from pulmonary embolism after total hip replacement. J Bone Joint Surg 1989;71-A:321–326.

19. Paiement GD, Wessinger SJ, et al. Routine use of adjusted low dose warfarin to prevent venous thromboembolism after total hip replacement. J Bone Joint Surg 1993;75-A:893–898.

20. RD Heparin Arthroplasty Group. RD Heparin compared with warfarin for prevention of venous thromboembolic disease following total hip or knee arthroplasty. J Bone Joint Surg 1994;76-A:1174–1185.

21. Colwell CW, Spiro TE, et al. Use of Enoxaparin, a low molecular weight heparin, and unfractionated heparin for the prevention of deep venous thrombosis after elective hip replacement. A clinical trial comparing efficacy and safety. J Bone Joint Surg 1994;76-A:3–14.

22. Fauno P, Suomalainen O, et al. Prophylaxis for the prevention of venous thromboembolism after total knee arthroplasty. A comparison between unfractionated and low molecular weight heparin. J Bone Joint Surg 1994;76-A:1814–1818.

23. Fitzgerald, RH; Spiro, TE et al.: A randomized and prospective comparison of enoxaparin (a low molecular weight heparin) and warfarin

in the prevention of thromboembolic disease following total knee arthroplasty. Orthop Trans 1995;19:355.

24. Planes A, Vochelle N, et al. Prevention of postoperative venous thrombosis: a randomized trial comparing unfractionated heparin with low molecular weight heparin in patients undergoing total hip replacement. Thromb Haemost 1988;60:407–410.

25. Turpie AG, Levine MN, et al. A randomized controlled trial of a low molecular weight heparin (enoxaparin) to prevent deep venous thrombosis in patients undergoing elective hip surgery. N Engl J Med 1986;315:925–929.

26. Trowbridge A, Boese CK, et al. Incidence of post-hospitalization proximal deep venous thrombosis after total hip arthroplasty. A pilot study. Clin Orthop 1994;299:203–208.

27. Nilsson PE, Bergquist D, et al. The post-discharge prophylactic management of the orthopedic patient with low molecular weight heparin: enoxaparin. Orthopedics 1997;20:22S–25S.

28. Planes A, Vochelle N. The post-hospital discharge venous thrombosis risk of the orthopedic patient. Orthopedics 1997;20:18S–21S.

29. Sikorski JM, Hampson WG, Staddon GE. The natural history and aetiology of deep venous thrombosis after total hip replacement. J Bone Joint Surg 1981;63-B:171–177.

30. Hyers TM, Hull RD, Weg JG. Anti-thrombotic therapy for venous thromboembolic disease. Chest 1995;108:335S–351S.

31. Classen DC, Evans RS, et al. The timing of prophylactic administration of antibiotics and the risk of surgical wound infection. N Engl J Med 1992;326(5):281–286.

32. Williams DN, Gustilo RB, et al. Bone and serum concentrations of five cephalosporin drugs. Relevance to prophylaxis and treatment in orthopaedic surgery. Clin Orthop 1983;179:253–265.

33. Garcia S, Lozano ML, et al. Prophylaxis against infection. Single dose cefonocid compared with multiple dose cefamandole. J Bone Joint Surg 1991;73-A:1044–1048.

34. Gleis GE, Seligson D. Diagnosis and treatment of complications. In: Browner BD, Jupitor JB, Levine AM, et al., eds. Skeletal Trauma. Philadelphia: WB Saunders, 1992.

Chapter 10

Pediatric Orthopaedics

Pediatric orthopaedics is a subspecialty within the field unlike any other. This broad field covers many issues and topics not touched upon by other areas of orthopaedics. This chapter will attempt to briefly cover the major topics of pediatric orthopaedics in order to give the junior resident a base-line level of knowledge.

BIRTH INJURIES

Obstetric Brachial Plexus Injury[1,2]

Obstetric brachial plexus injury has steadily dropped in frequency over the past half-century and, most recently, a rate of 0.87 per 1000 births was documented in 1981. The clinical presentation is similar to a fractured clavicle or a separation of the proximal humerus that can occur at birth, with the affected extremity usually hanging motionless at the infant's side. These other two entities usually resolve in approximately 7–10 days.

The cause of nerve injury in obstetric palsy is usually traction. Nerve traction is usually associated with fetal malposition, shoulder dystocia, cephalopelvic disproportion, high birth weight, or the use of forceps.

Type 1 is also known as Erb's palsy, affecting the C4, 5, and 6 roots. The shoulder is adducted, internally rotated, and contractures soon develop. The elbow often lacks active flexion. Erb's palsy is four times more common than Types 2 and 3. It also has the best prognosis of the birth palsies.

Type 2 is known as entire brachial plexus or Erb-Duchenne-Klumpke palsy. Roots C5–T1 are normally dysfunctional. This type is easily noted, since both motor and sensory deficits are present and the arm is virtually placid. This type of palsy has the worst prognosis.

In Type 3 (lower plexus or Klumpke palsy), the roots of C8 and T1 are involved, causing limited flexion of the fingers and wrist, poor interosseous function, and a Horner's syndrome.

Four out of five patients are completely recovered by 12 months of age. Overall therapy should be aimed at preventing contractures while awaiting neurologic recovery. If the biceps or the deltoid has not started to function by age 2–3 months, function will usually not return. In this case, an EMG should be performed to confirm a total absence of electrical activity. If electrical activity is nonexistent, microsurgical techniques are employed for internal neurolysis and grafting to the affected roots.

Children sometimes do not present until 1–2 years of age, and contractures may already be present requiring joint releases. L'Episcopo described a procedure transferring the latissimus dorsi and the teres major to the lateral aspect of the humerus, causing them to become shoulder external rotators. Two procedures that have been described to treat weakness or loss of elbow flexion include Clark's pectoral transfer and the Steindler flexorplasty, which involves the proximal attachment of the flexor pronator origin from the elbow to a position on the humerus. Procedures for wrist extension are similar to those used for radial nerve palsies and involve the transfer of the FCR or the FCU to the extensor carpi radialis brevis. The wrist flexors can be strengthened by a brachioradialis transfer.

Congenital Muscular Torticollis[1]

Congenital muscular torticollis is the most common cause of torticollis (rotatory deformity of the neck) in the infant and young child. Other causes include retropharyngeal infections, cervical spine anomalies, ophthalmologic disorders that may cause the child to have to tilt his head in order to see normally, and brain tumors of the posterior fossa.

Some think that torticollis is caused by intrauterine crowding, pointing out that 20% of children with congenital muscular torticollis will have developmental hip dysplasia and/or metatarsus adductus. Most of these children have a history of a breech presentation or difficult delivery. However, congenital muscular torticollis has been reported in children with normal births and even those born by C-section. There tends to be a familial tendency.

The latest theory is that a compartment syndrome occurs as a result of trauma to the soft tissues of the neck at the time of delivery. This results in degeneration and fibrosis of the muscle fibers.

These children often present at 4 weeks of life, when a palpable mass is noted in the neck. This mass disappears over time, leaving only the muscular contracture and resultant neck deformity. A very careful examination of the hips must be performed at diagnosis. Radiographs of the cervical spine should also be obtained at the time of diagnosis in order to rule out a bony anomaly.

If the deformity persists, skull and facial deformities can occur within the first year of life (plagiocephaly). If the deformity is untreated for several years, the level of the eyes and ears can become unequal (a considerable cosmetic deformity).

Treatment initially consists of passive stretching exercises, and some series report up to 90% success. Surgery is recommended when the deformity persists after 1 year of age. Surgical treatment includes a unipolar or bipolar release of the sternocleidomastoid muscle.

ORTHOPAEDIC SYNDROMES

An orthopaedic syndrome should be suspected if a characteristic malformation is encountered. A syndrome should also be suspected if all four extremities are affected, if deformities are symmetric, or if there are associated nonorthopaedic anomalies. The importance of understanding syndromes is that it enables the orthopaedic surgeon to better manage the particular patient and plan surgical intervention more appropriately.

Neurofibromatosis (NF)[1,2]

Neurofibromatosis is the most common single gene disorder in humans, affecting 1 out of 3000 newborns. The gene for NF1 (von Recklinghausen's disease) has been mapped to the long arm of chromosome 17 and accounts for 85% of all cases of neurofibromatosis. Central NF (NF2) is characterized by bilateral acoustic neuromas with minimal peripheral findings.

Neurofibromatosis is an autosomal dominant disorder (AD) with a 100% penetrance, though half the cases are thought to be secondary to sporadic mutation associated with advanced paternal age. NF is a neural crest disorder, so the skin, brain, and spinal cord are affected.

The diagnosis of NF1 requires two or more of the following features. Patients can have at least six café-au-lait spots (discreet, tan spots), measuring 5 mm in diameter in children and 15 mm in adults. Patients can have two neurofibromas (composed of the Schwann cells and fibrous connective tissue); these can be cutaneous or covered by darkly pigmented skin. They can be highly vascular and lead to limb gigantism, facial disfigurement, and invasion of the neuraxis. Patients can have freckles in the inguinal or axillary regions (good diagnostic markers). Additionally, patients can have an optic glioma, two or more Lisch nodules (hamartoma of the iris), distinctive osseous lesions (vertebral scalloping or cortical thinning), or a first-degree relative with NF1.

Musculoskeletal manifestations include scoliosis, a nonunion of a long bone, overgrowth of a part of a bone or a curious bone lesion. Most scoliosis curves in NF are similar to idiopathic scoliosis curves and can be managed similarly. Rarely, these curves take on a dystrophic pattern. Dystrophic curves are short and sharp, resulting in a thoracic kyphoscoliosis typically involving four to six segments. Radiographs frequently demonstrate vertebral scalloping, enlarged foramina, penciling of the transverse process or ribs, severe apical rotations, or the presence of a paraspinal mass. Dystrophic curves are refractory to brace treatment. The goal of surgery in dystrophic curves is spinal stabilization, and fusions are normally performed in situ. MRI and CT scans are helpful in preoperative planning to help identify vertebral or dural abnormalities.

Posterior fusion with instrumentation is indicated for patients with less than 50 degrees of kyphosis. Anterior fusion with strut grafting and posterior fusion with instrumentation is indicated for patients with more severe kyphosis. In younger patients, both anterior and posterior fusion are routinely performed to avoid a "crankshaft" phenomenon. Some surgeons perform routine augmentation of the posterior fusions mass at 6 months postoperatively because of the high pseudarthrosis rate.

Pedicle erosion in the C-spine can result in instabilitiy or kyphosis. Posterior fusion with autogenous bone graft and halo stabilization is indicated for these patients. Pseudarthrosis of the tibia often occurs following an increasing anterolateral bow that is obvious in early infancy. Creating surgical union is a challenge, and amputations are not infrequent. Pseudarthrosis can also occur in the ulna, radius, femur, and clavicle.

Approximately 5% of patients with diagnosed neurofibromatosis will develop a CNS malignancy such as an optic nerve glioma, an acoustic neuroma, or an astrocytoma. There is also risk of malignant degeneration from neurofibroma to a neurofibrosarcoma. Children with neurofibromas have a propensity to develop other malignancies such as Wilms' tumors or rhabdomyosarcoma.

Children with NF are frequently short and have large heads. Fifty percent have some sort of intellectual handicap. Hypertension secondary to renal artery stenosis or pheochromocytoma is frequently documented.

Arthrogryposis[1]

Arthrogryposis represents a group of about 150 syndromes, all of which have obvious joint contractures present at birth. Some types such as arthrogryposis multiplex congenita and Larsen syndrome involve all four extremities. Other types of arthrogryposis are referred to as distal arthrogryposis and involve the hands and feet. Another subset of this condition is referred to as pterygia, which is notable for the skin webs across the knees and elbows.

Arthrogryposis multiplex congenita is notable for tubular limbs lacking skin creases and having diminished muscle mass. The elbows and knees are typically extended and the hips are usually flexed. The joints are pain-free with a firm, elastic block to movement beyond a limited range of movement. The hips may be dislocated unilaterally or bilaterally. Scoliosis develops in approximately one-third of patients. Clubfeet are always present.

The viscera are typically without deformation, though a stiff jaw and a mobile tongue lead to respiratory infections and failure to thrive in some infants. The face is not dysmorphic, and intelligence is normal. Initial feeding difficulties and delayed language development should not be mistaken for retardation.

The cause is unknown, though intrauterine crowding may predispose to this entity. Some suggest an intrauterine viral etiology because the number of anterior horn cells in the spinal cord is decreased and, like polio, sensory function is maintained while motor function is lost.

Evaluation includes neurological studies, enzyme tests, and muscle biopsy to distinguish between a neurologic and myopathic etiology. Biopsy reveals increased fibrosis and fat. Initial treatment consists of passive stretching and dynamic splinting. Perinatal fractures are not infrequent, as joint contractures make the birthing process difficult. Unilateral dislocated hips should be opened and reduced, while bilateral dislocated hips may be left alone, as these patients are not prevented from walking because of their hips. Knee flexion contractures are typically treated with posterior capsulotomy. Supracondylar osteotomies in the femur are recommended toward the end of growth if this can possibly improve ambulation. A severe and resistant clubfoot is characteristic of this condition. Clubfeet do not respond to casting, and posteromedial release often fails, necessitating revision surgery that sometimes includes a talectomy.

Upper extremity surgery is aimed at allowing the patient to feed himself and perform perineal care. Indications for spine surgery are similar to those for other neuromuscular scoliosis.

Other forms of arthrogryposis include Larsen syndrome, which is characterized by multiple congenital dislocations of large joints, a characteristic flat face, scoliosis, and cervical kyphosis. Typically, both knees, both hips, and both elbows are dislocated along with the presence of bilateral club feet. The cause is unknown, with both AD and AR inheritance patterns demonstrated.

Down Syndrome (Trisomy 21)[1,2]

Down syndrome is the most frequent chromosomal abnormality, with a frequency of 1 per 660 live births. Its incidence is associated with advanced maternal age. The general features include a flattened face, mental retardation, congenital heart disease (usually a septal defect), duodenal atresia, and leukemia (1%). Hyperthyroidism, diabetes, and infections are common, and there appears to be some evidence of premature aging.

Short stature and ligamentous laxity are cardinal features. Half have scoliosis, with 99% demonstrating an idiopathic pattern. The incidence of spondylolisthesis is approximately 6%, with L4–L5 and L5–S1 being most commonly involved. The presence of flat acetabulae and flared iliac wings allow for accurate diagnosis in the newborn prior to chromosome analysis. Slipped capital femoral epiphyses occur frequently and appear to have a higher than expected risk for osteonecrosis. The knee tends to be in valgus with a subluxated or dislocated patella. Asymptomatic, flexible planovalgus feet are common.

There are many abnormalities involving the upper cervical spine including instability at the occiput-C1 junction, odontoid dysplasia, lamina defects at C1, spondylolisthesis, and precocious arthritis in the midcervical region. Patients undergoing general anaesthesia should have cervical spine radiographs performed preoperatively. Atlantoaxial instability (C1–C2) in Down syndrome has received a great deal of attention. Currently, all children with Down syndrome who wish to participate in contact sports should have lateral flexion-extension C-cpine radiographs prior to participation. If the atlantodens interval (ADI) exceeds 4.5 mm, the odontoid is dysplastic, or if the patient has neurological signs or symptoms, there should be restrictions on sports that involve possible trauma to the head and neck and the patient should be followed up at regular intervals.

Posterior cervical wiring at C1–2 with autogenous iliac crest bone graft and postoperative halo immobilization is recommended in some symptomatic patients. Surgery should be performed with trepidation, as the Down syndrome patient appears to be at much greater risk of postoperative neurological complication following cervical fusion than the general public. Preoperative cardiac evaluation is essential.

CEREBRAL PALSY[1,2,3]

Introduction

Cerebral palsy is a nonprogressive neuromuscular disorder with an onset before 2 years of age resulting from an injury to an immature brain. It is often referred to as static encephalopathy by pediatricians. Frequent causes include prenatal intrauterine factors, perinatal infections (PORCH infections), prematurity, anoxic injuries, head injuries, intracranial bleeds, and meningitis.

The brain lesion in cerebral palsy is permanent and nonprogressive. Nevertheless, disease progression is not static, because growth and maturation produce a wide variety of changing musculoskeletal problems in the child with CP.

Cerebral palsy has an incidence of 1–7 per 1000 children throughout most of the world. This disease is thought to be most common where prenatal and perinatal care are poor. Cerebral palsy occurs 12 times more in twin pregnancies than singleton pregnancies. Cerebral palsy is classified according to neuropathic type and anatomic region.

Neuropathic Types

Spasticity results from lesions of the pyramidal systems of the brain. This type of CP is characterized by increased muscle tone and hyperreflexia. This type of CP is most common and most ammenable to orthopaedic treatment.

Athetosis refers to dyskinesia caused by an extrapyramidal lesion. Athetosis is characterized by purposeless, slow, writhing movements. This type of CP is less common and is more difficult to treat.

Children with mixed CP have pyramidal and extrapyramidal lesions and involvement demonstrating a combination of spasticity and athetosis with total body involvement. Ataxic cerebral palsy is uncommon, and it is usually the result of cerebellar dysfunction.

Anatomic Patterns

Quadriplegia or total involvement describes children with all four extremeties affected. These children typically have lower IQs and higher mortality rates, and they are usually unable to walk. Children with diplegia often have both lower extremities involved much more than their upper extremities; most diplegics eventually walk. Their IQs are often normal. In hemiplegia, one side of the body is often involved, with the upper extremity more affected than the lower. These children often develop early "handedness." These children are usually able to walk regardless of treatment. A focal vascular or asymmetric infectious lesion is the most likely cause for hemiplegia. Seizure disorders are most commonly seen with this type of involvement, usually beginning before age 2.

Orthopaedic Assessment and Management

A thorough history must include birth and developmental details (e.g., independent sitting by 6 months or walking by 12 months), while physical examination is focused on locomotor profile. The orthopaedic surgeon should also check for persistence of primitive reflexes in his or her physical examination (please see the section on pediatric physical examination).

The orthopaedic physical examination should focus on muscle strength grading and selective control, muscle tone evaluation (spastic, athetoid, or mixed), and joint and muscle contracture at each of the major joints. One should also assess linear, angular, and torsional deformation of the spine and long bones and fixed hand or foot deformities. It is also important to appraise balance, equilibrium, and standing, walking, or sitting (in wheelchair) postures.

Surgery to improve gait and ambulation is entertained for the child usually over 3 years old with spastic CP and voluntary motor control. Initial treatment includes soft-tissue procedures in effort to prevent bony abnormality. Later, bony procedures may be required in effort to improve gait mechanics.

Only 20% of the children with spastic quadriplegia eventually walk. Subsequently, the goals for this population include a straight spine and a level pelvis in order to sit comfortably in a wheelchair. One should attempt to keep the hips located and painless. Ideally, the hips should flex at least 90 degrees for comfortable sitting and extend to at least 30 degrees of flexion for helping with pivot transfers. The hips should have enough abduction to allow room for perineal care. Mobile knees that flex adequately for sitting and plantigrade feet for wearing shoes and positioning on footplates of the wheelchair are also important. Surgical intervention is often indicated to maintain the aforementioned parameters if physical therapy and a stretching regimen have failed.

Additional modalities include selective posterior rhizotomy performed by neurosurgeons to reduce spasticity in the lower extremities by balancing muscular tone at the level of the anterior horn cells of the spinal cord. Botulinum A toxin is occasionally injected intramuscularly (especially in the gastrocnemius) to temporarily decrease dynamic spasticity in effort to improve ambulation. Physical therapy, manipulation and casting, and orthotics also have a role in the management of the cerebral palsy patient.

Neuromuscular Scoliosis

Neuromuscular scoliosis occurs in approximately 25% of CP patients. This type of scoliosis is different from idiopathic scoliosis. It develops earlier and it is more likely to be progressive. Unlike adolescent idiopathic scoliosis, it frequently progresses beyond skeletal maturity. It is also less responsive to orthotic control and is more likely to require surgical intervention.

Observation alone is required for curves less than 25–30 degrees that have not demonstrated progression. Curves greater than this require at least an attempt at orthotic treatment. Most quadriplegic patients do not obtain any meaningful curve control from bracing. At best, an orthosis may slow curve progression and allow time for beneficial growth in an immature spine prior to definitive surgical stabilizaion.

Once the curve exceeds 40 degrees in magnitude, it is likely to continue and surgery is indicated. Posterior segmental spinal fusion is done using two rods with cross links connected to the spine by multiple hooks and/or sublaminar wires. Fusion is facilitated by autogenous iliac crest or rib graft or sometimes allograft.

Fusions usually extend from the upper thoracic region to L5 or, more commonly, the pelvis. Fusions should include the pelvis if pelvic obliquity exceeds 10 degrees from the intercrestal iliac line compared with the inferior endplate of L4 or the superior endplate of L5, when measured on a sitting A-P radiograph. Anterior spine surgery is usually not required unless the curve will not be correctable to <50–60 degrees from only a posterior approach. This judgment is made from the preop bending films. Anterior internal fixation is rarely required when posterior fixation is utilized. Usually, anterior and posterior operations are performed in the same surgical setting rather than staging the procedures. Pulmonary function tests, nutritional parameters (prealbumin, transferrin), and total lymphocyte count should be checked prior to surgery for neuromuscular scoliosis.

Hip Problems

Patients with CP experience hip problems because of muscle imbalance (primarily contractures of adductor and flexor muscles), acetabular dysplasia, pelvic obliquity, excessive femoral anteversion, increased femoral neck valgus, lack of weight bearing, and maldirected resultant force vectors across the hip joint. Concern for hip instability is particularly warranted in children with less than 30 degrees of abduction and hip flexion contractures greater than 20–25 degrees. Hip dislocation should be prevented in all but the most severely involved children. A positive Galeazzi's test is another sign of hip subluxation or dislocation. If in doubt, an A-P pelvis can help distinguish between hip pathology and worsening contractures about the hip in children with CP. Hips that are subluxated rarely cause discomfort, but if they progress to dislocation, up to 50% of cerebral palsy patients will have increased pain. Additionally, hip dislocation allows the formation of increased contractures, making perineal care more difficult and worsening sitting balance.

Hips at risk often progress to subluxation or dislocation unless treated. Adductor tenotomy and often psoas tenotomy is a relatively simple first step after bracing and stretching have failed. Postoperatively, many surgeons utilize abduction casts or splints several weeks to months in order to avoid recurring contractures. Anterior branch and complete obturator neurectomy are rarely indicated.

Hip subluxation is defined as the uncovering of more than one-third of the femoral head and a break in Shenton's line, with the femoral head maintaining at least some contact with the acetabulum. Preoperative planning should often include plain radiographs and, occasionally, an arthrogram and/or a CT scan to better understand the pathoanatomy. Prior to 9 years of age, a patient with unilateral subluxation is often best treated by bilateral surgery, since the contralateral hip is often abnormal and will likely become increasingly so when unilateral surgery is performed. Patients often need a femoral varus derotation osteotomy. However, if the neck shaft angle is not abnormal, a proximal femoral derotation osteotomy will suffice. Varization should be performed to restore normal anatomy with a neck shaft angle of 120–125 degrees. Greater amounts of varization are acceptable in nonambulatory children. These procedures are frequently performed with adductor tenotomy and iliopsoas tendon release. If acetabular dysplasia is present (acetabular index greater than 25 degrees), it should be corrected. Frequently, the acetabular deficiency is superior and posterior requiring a shelf augmentation, a Dega procedure, or a pericapsular procedure.

Hip dislocations are treated by relocation procedures, accepting the dislocation, by proximal femoral resection, hip arthrodesis (rare), or total hip arthroplasty. If the dislocation occurred within the past year, most surgeons suggest performing an anterior open reduction combined with adductor and psoas tendon releases, proximal femoral shortening, varization, and derotation osteotomy. Acetabular dysplasia, if present, should be addressed at the same time. If the hip has been dislocated for longer than 1 year and is painless, no treatment is required. If the hip is painful, a proximal femoral resection with muscle interposition is probably indicated, though painful recurrence is frequent owing to continued muscle spasticity.

Knee Flexion Deformity

Knee flexion deformity is typically associated with hip flexion contractures and a crouched gait. It may also be the result of calcaneous deformity causing exaggerated dorsiflexion at the ankle. It is important that all pathology be addressed at the time of surgery to appropriately manage a crouched gait. This is a situation in which gait analysis can be very helpful. Knee flexion deformity is typically caused by spastic hamstring muscles that lead to muscle shortening and a fixed capsular contracture of the knee. The medial hamstrings are often the major offenders.

Hamstrings require lengthening when straight leg raising cannot exceed 70 degrees above the horizontal or when the popliteal angle demonstrates a >45-degree lack of full extension (popliteal angle <135 degrees) when the patient is supine and the hip is flexed to 90 degrees. Nonambulators are treated with tenotomy of the gracilis and the semitendinosis and division of the fascia overlying the semimembranosis and, if needed, the biceps femoris. Ambulators are treated with lengthening and repair of the aforementioned muscles. Postoperatively, these patients are managed in long leg casts or knee immobilizers for 6 weeks. Ambulators can ambulate as tolerated with braces on if no bony procedures have been performed.

There is sometimes cospasticity of the rectus femorus muscles. This situation requires concomitant transfer of the distal rectus femoris tendon to the sartorius, gracilis, semitendonosis, or iliotibial band. This will prevent a stiff knee gait in which adequate knee flexion in the swing phase is not achieved, thus interfering with foot clearance.

Foot and Ankle Equinovalgus

Foot and ankle equinovalgus is typically seen in patients with spastic diplegia. This is caused by triceps surae overactivity, weakness of the tibialis posterior muscle, and relative overpull of the peroneal musculature. This deformity is typically in the subtalar joint but can be present in the ankle joint and weight-bearing A-P radiographs of the ankle should be studied as part of the preoperative planning.

If the subtalar valgus is mild and supple, an AFO or a UCBL orthosis can often control the deformity. Moderate deformity can often be improved by peroneus brevis lengthening. More severe deformity not responsive to an orthosis is typically treated by subtalar arthrodesis (Grice procedure). Other methods of correcting a supple valgus hindfoot deformity are by a medial displacement oblique osteotomy of the calcaneous or by calcaneal neck lengthening osteotomy. These procedures have the advantage of preserving subtalar motion and not disturbing the growth potential of the hindfoot. Fixed hindfoot valgus is ignored in the nonambulator whose feet are shoeable. Triple arthrodesis is reserved for the 12–13 year nonambulator with shoeing problems or the ambulator with painful feet.

Hindfoot Equinus

Hindfoot equinus is a less involved but frequently seen entity that typically results in "toe-walking" owing to overactivity of the triceps surae musculature. Mild cases can be treated by stretching and bracing (AFO). Serial casting is sometimes used to stretch a tightened heelcord in order to get into a braceable position (at least neutral). Surgical z-lengthening is used for refractory cases. Intramuscular botulinum toxin injections into both heads of the gastrocnemius are now being used with and without serial casting to treat dynamic deformity.

MYELOMENINGOCELE[1]

Introduction

Neural tube defects are grouped together under the generic terms myelodyplasia, spinal dysraphism, and spina bifida. These are not to be confused with spina bifida occulta, which is a radiographic finding referring to the lack of fusion of the spinous process of the lower lumbosacral spine without neurologic implication. Neural tube defects are subdivided into four subtypes: meningocele, myelomeningocele, lipomeningocele, and rachischisis.

A meningocele is a cyst involving only the meninges, without any neural elements. This condition requires surgical closure by a neurosurgeon, but rarely requires further treatment.

A myelomeningocele refers to abnormal neural elements in a meningeal sac. The sac can be any size, form, or location along the spine. CNS abnormalities including Arnold-Chiari malformations and hydrocephalus are common. A lipomeningocele is a meningeal sac containing a lipoma that is closely involved with sacral nerves. These lesions are often epithelialized at birth, and these children may not have hydrocephaly or any CNS abnormality. Neurological function may be nearly normal at birth but it can decline with growth. Rachischisis is a complete absence of skin and sac with exposure of muscle and the presence of a dysplastic spinal cord. Occasionally even bone is exposed.

Etiology

Approximately 6000 infants are born each year with neural tube defects. The inheritance is multifactorial. The overall incidence of neural tube defects is 0.15% among Caucasians and 0.04% among African-Americans. There is evidence that the mothers of these children have an inherent disorder of folate metabolism. These abnormalities appear to occur between the third and fourth weeks of gestation. It is unclear whether the defect is caused by a lack of closure of the spine or whether the defect is caused by the rupture of the previously closed neural tube.

Classification in myelodysplasia is usually demonstrated by the cord or root level at which the patient has bilateral antigravity musculature. The three major associated sequelae include hydrocephaly and associated hydrosyringomyelia, Arnold-Chiari deformity, and tethered court syndrome.

Most children with hydocephalus require a ventriculoperitoneal (VP) shunt. In young children, shunt failure is accompanied by nausea, vomiting, and headache. In older children, symptoms include increased irritability, decreased motor function, decreased attention span, increased scoliosis, and increased paralysis. Unresolved hydrocephaly eventually causes the formation of a hydrosyringomyelia, which results in neurological changes (even in the upper extremities) and progressive scoliosis.

The Arnold-Chiari deformity is caused by the associated hydrocephaly. Most of these children have a Type 2 Arnold-Chiari deformity, which is characterized by displacement of the medulla oblongata caudally through the foramen magnum, requiring cervical roots to take an upward course in order to reach their appropriate foramina. In the infant, this can cause periodic apnea, stridor, nystagmus, weak or absent cry, and upper extremity spasm and weakness.

Following sac closure at birth, there is a tendency for the spinal cord to become adherent to the repair site. As the child grows, this attachment produces a tethering that disallows the spinal cord to migrate cephalad during growth. Although many children have a tethering of the spinal cord, very few actually develop symptoms of the condition and require surgical release. Pain in the low back, buttocks, and posterior thighs appears to be the prominent symptom in tethered cord syndrome. Occasionally, an increase in scoliosis (especially increased lordosis) or changes in bladder function can be seen. The diagnosis of tethered cord syndrome is made on clinical evaluation. Surgical release rarely provides complete return of lost function.

Latex Hypersensitivity

Latex hypersensitivity is a severe immediate type allergic reaction to latex that occurs in up to $\frac{1}{3}$ of children with myelomeningocle. All patients should be asked about a history of swelling or itching of the skin after contact with any rubber products (balloons or dental examinations). All patients, regardless of history, should have surgery performed in a latex-free environment.

Treatment of Specific Deformities

Spine deformities are usually progressive and cause severe disability in the myelomeningocele patient. The most obvious deformity is the incomplete posterior arch in the lumbosacral spine. Other malformations such as hemivertebrae, diastematomyelia, and unsegmented bars may be present anywhere along the spine and may affect treatment.

Neuromuscular Scoliosis

The neuromuscular scoliosis in children with myelomeningocele appears at 2–3 years of age, often becoming severe by age 7. Factors affecting surgical outcomes include the high infection rate secondary to chronic urinary tract infections, poor nutritional factors, and the poor skin quality in the area of the meningocele repair that gives minimal coverage to the instrumentation.

Neuromuscular scoliosis occurs in almost 100% of the patients with a thoracic level. This rate tends to decrease as one considers more caudal levels. For example, an L4 myelomeningocele is only associated with scoliosis 60% of the time, with only 40% requiring surgical treatment. A C-shaped scoliosis is usually caused by muscle weakness, asymmetric levels of paralysis, and/or spastic hemiplegia. Hydromyelia or hydrosyringomyelia often results in an S-shaped curve in the thoracic or the thoracolumbar region. A tethered cord typically causes an increasing lordotic deformity in the lumbar region. Congenital malformations are frequently seen alone or with any of the above deformities.

Treatment of Neuromuscular Scoliosis

A sitting radiograph of the spine evaluation should be performed annually beginning at age 1. Radiographic progression is often the reason for performing an MRI. An MRI of the head and cervical spine evaluates the hydrocephalus, Arnold-Chiari malformation, and VP shunt if present. The remainder of the spine should also be scanned and evaluated for the appearance of syrinx or hydromyelia or other spinal pathology (lipomas, dermoid cysts).

If the spine is balanced and the curve is <30 degrees, observation is probably indicated. However, if the curve is greater than 30 degrees or the center of gravity falls outside of the pelvic base of support, progression of the deformity is almost assured. In children less than 7 years old, a trial of bracing is indicated if the curve is supple and can be corrected easily. One must look out for pressure sores in areas of insensate skin.

In treating the patient with suspected tethered cord, the tethered cord should be released either before (usually preferable) or during the scoliosis surgery. The fusion should run from neutral vertebra to neutral vertebra (see section on idiopathic scoliosis) and the end vertebra should be located within the stable zone. The treatment of the myelomeningocele spine is complicated by the open vertebral arch, which makes distal attachment of instrumentation less secure unless it is completely bypassed. The levels of fusion depend on the age of the child, the location of the curve, the level of paralysis, and the ambulatory status. Traditionally , the lumbosacral joint was included in the fusion mass because of the difficulty getting a firm attachment to the lower lumbar vertebrae. Newer methods of fixation allow the clinician to stop the fusion in the lumbar spine, if necessary. Inclusion of the lumbosacral joint increases the risk of a pseudoarthrosis and instrument failure. On the other hand, successful fusion of the sacrum may deprive an ambulatory patient of the ability to walk. In wheelchair-bound patients, fusion of the lumbosacral segment may transmit much of the angular and rotational movements of the trunk directly to the interface between the patient's skin and the wheelchair, causing increased frequency of skin breakdown. If the surgeon decides not to include the pelvis, he or she runs the risk of continued progression at the LS junction.

A child <8 years old with a progressive curve that is uncontrollable in a brace should be treated with segmental rod instrumentation without spinal fusion. Also, if the child has not reached adolescence (pubic hair, Risser 1) and surgical intervention is required, the anterior and posterior spine should be fused to prevent curve progression and possible crankshaft phenomenon.

Segmental instrumentation is used for these patients, since it allows better control over the spine and postoperative immobilization is not required. As with prior systems, distal fixation in the lumbar region is difficult and extension to the pelvis is frequent. In general, anterior and posterior fusion are required in the region of the lumbar spine. With greater deformity, anterior instrumentation seems to be beneficial, but this is controversial.

Hip Problems

The function of the hip joint depends largely on the neurological level of the myelodysplasia. Most children are born with reduced hips unless they present in a breech position.

The thoracic-level paraplegic child does not have sensation or muscle control over the lower extremities. In general, hip dislocation is rare in the thoracic level paraplegic because of the lack of muscle function around the hips. Increased muscle tone should be treated by muscle release, and progressive scoliosis causing pelvic obliquity should be treated, as well. Surgery on the hip joint is generally avoided since this can lead to stiffness, which can be quite detrimental. A dislocated hip, if present, does not interfere with the overall function of the child, and in fact, does not prevent the child from even ambulating with an appropriate orthosis. Despite this, most thoracic-level children give up walking by the time they are 8 or 9 years old and use a wheelchair simply because the energy expenditure of independent ambulation is too great. PT and stretching are important for maintaining a functional range of motion.

Upper lumbar paraplegia (L1–L2) results in patients having sensation in the anterior hip and thigh. A higher rate of hip dislocations occurs because the iliopsoas and adductors produce hip flexion and adduction contractions. These patients are treated by maintaining an adequate range of motion by PT and, if needed, surgical release of the iliopsoas and adductor tendons. If an adequate range of motion can be obtained, the dislocated hip does not necessarily cause disability for either walking with an orthosis or sitting.

The lower lumbar paraplegic (L3–L5) has sensation below the knee. Muscle function includes hip flexion, adduction, knee extension and weak knee flexion. Hip dislocation is most common at the L3/L4 level, and the natural history of the hip in these patients is progressive dysplasia and finally dislocation, since the hip flexors and adductors overpower the hip extensors and abductors.

Various tenotomies and muscular transfers have been shown to improve hip stability. Osteotomies and capsular plications around the hip run the risk of creating stiffness, and treatment strategies involve identifying the exact level of the paraplegia and whether the hip subluxation/dislocation is unilateral or bilateral. Hip dysplasia in paraplegics with an L2 level and above almost never warrants these aggressive measures, while those L5 and below nearly always do. Most would not treat bilateral dysplasia in L3 paraplegics, while most would treat unilateral dysplasia in an L4 paraplegic. The true "gray zone" is the unilateral dysplasia in an L3 and a bilateral in an L4. These children will often require correction of coxa valga with a varus derotational osteotomy, as well as correction of acetabular dysplasia with a Pemberton or Shelf acetabuloplasty. The stiffness is rarely a problem if all procedures are done at the same time but may be quite troublesome if the patient requires repeated procedures.

Knee Problems

Knee problems generally involve worsening muscle and capsular contracture, possibly leading to bony deformity. Treatment involves stretching and sometimes surgical release of the hamstrings, quadriceps, or the iliotibial band (Ober-Yount procedure).

Foot Problems

Foot problems are frequent owing to muscle imbalance and insensitivity. The primary objectives are to obtain plantigrade, braceable feet. Patients must be taught to look for pressure sores that can lead to nonhealing ulcers and, finally, amputation.

Ankle valgus is frequent and often progressive. It can be followed using A-P radiographs of the ankle and treated with a medial malleolar screw, a hemiepiphysiodesis, or a distal tibial osteotomy. A rigid talipes equinovarus (clubfoot) owing to muscle imbalance is not infrequently refractory to serial casting. Postero-medial releases are performed, but recurrence rates are high. Excessive tibial torsion is often encountered because of muscle imbalance. A supramalleolar osteotomy can improve cosmesis and, sometimes, ambulation.

CONGENITAL UPPER EXTREMITY DEFORMITIES

Radial Club Hand[1,4]

Radial club hand is a defect of the upper extremity with an incidence of approximately 1 in 30,000 births. This defect is caused by damage to the apical ectoderm on the anterior aspect of a developing limb when the embryo is 3–4 weeks old. Many cases were linked to maternal intake of thalidomide (a sedative) during pregnancy during the early 1960s. No obvious genetic tie has been established.

This syndrome is associated with VACTERLS anomalies—scoliosis, heart defects (patent ductus arteriosis, VSD, tetralogy of Fallot), tracheoesophogeal fistulae, imperforate anus, renal agenesis, and hydronephrosis. Most cases are bilateral, and the spectrum ranges from complete absence of the radius to hypoplasia of the radius that is barely notable. The thumb is usually absent, but occasionally, it is underdeveloped and lies more distal than usual. Additionally, the radial side of the carpus is nearly always deficient, and likewise, there are deficiencies and abnormalities of the muscle, tendons, and nerves of that extremity. The median nerve typically divides midway down the forearm into two branches, the radial most of which serves as the radial nerve for the hand. The ulnar digits are more functional and have a greater range of motion. In the preoperative assessment, it is important to note the range of motion of the elbow. A centralization procedure is generally contraindicated if there is not at least 90 degrees of elbow flexion, because the procedure may make it difficult for the child to bring his hand to his mouth.

Centralization is the most commonly performed procedure for radial club hand due largely to its cosmetic benefit. In this procedure, a slot is removed from the center of the carpus (usually the lunate and part of the capitate). The ulna is subsequently inserted into the slot and held in position by a K-wire that passes from the third metacarpal into the distal ulnar epiphysis. Children without thumbs may gain a true functional benefit if index finger pollicization is performed.

Congenital Radial Head Dislocation[1,5]

Congenital radial head dislocation is an abnormality of unknown incidence. It is most frequently discovered when the child is approximately 5 years old and sustains some elbow trauma and a radiograph demonstrates a radial head dislocation. Radiographs demonstrate hypoplasia or absence of the capitellum in 80% of the patients. A dome-shaped radial head is often seen, as well.

Congenital radial head dislocation does not appear to exist as an isolated unilateral anomaly. Patients will either have a similar anomaly on the contralateral side or they will have some other congenital abnormality.

Sixty-five percent of these dislocations will be posterior. Supination is the most restricted range of motion. Most of these elbows do not require treatment. Some patients will request radial head excision for appearance. Excision does not improve elbow range of motion. If at all possible, radial head excisions should be postponed until skeletal maturity.

Congenital Radioulnar Synostosis[1,6]

Congenital radioulnar synostosis is a rare entity owing to failure of longitudinal segmentation in the forearm, resulting in a persistent fibrous or osseous (more common) bridge between the proximal ulna and radius. The child is usually brought to the orthopaedic surgeon in early childhood when the parents discover that the child does not pronate and supinate the forearm normally. The condition occurs unilaterally and bilaterally. Physical examination should focus on the rotational position of the forearm and how functional that position is. Most patients are quite functional since the forearms tend to be in moderate pronation, allowing writing and handling of objects. If the condition is bilateral, patients may benefit if one of the extremities is supinated to allow perineal care. Efforts to surgically take down the synostosis have generally been unsuccessful. Proximal osteotomies to reposition the forearm are complicated by high rates of neurovascular compromise and compartment syndrome. Most patients are treated nonoperatively.

Syndactyly[1,2]

Syndactyly is a very common congenital hand anomaly describing the union of two phalanges. It is more common in white males and tends to involve the ring and long fingers. These anomalies are described as being simple (skin only) or complex. Complex syndactyly involves shared bony, neurovascular, or tendinous structures (anything more than skin). Involvement can be complete (the entire length of the digit) or incomplete. Digits should be separated in early childhood and nearly always necessitate a skin graft. Separation prior to 1 year of age is sometimes warranted if one of the digits is tethering the growth of the other. This often occurs in the ring-small finger syndactyly.

Polysyndactyly[1,2]

Polysyndactyly describes a condition in which digits are duplicated. This is the most common congenital hand deformity, and it is seen most commonly in blacks. These extra digits tend to be on the ulnar side of the hand and are usually treated with amputation. These digits can be composed of soft tissue only, bony tissue, and, rarely, a fully formed digit including a metacarpal.

PEDIATRIC SPINE

Idiopathic Scoliosis[7]

Idiopathic scoliosis refers to the lateral deviation and rotation of the spine without an obvious identifiable source. Idiopathic scoliosis is classified into adolescent, juvenile, and infantile types. Most of our focus will be on adolescent idiopathic scolisis. Infantile idiopathic scoliosis presents at 2 months to 3 years. Juvenile idiopathic scoliosis is discovered in 3–10-year-olds. Adolescent idiopathic scoliosis refers to curvature and rotation of the spine in children older than 10.

There seems to be a hereditary component to the adolescent type with AD transmission of variable penetrance and expression.

This very common problem is frequently diagnosed at school screening programs. Girls are diagnosed with adolescent idiopathic scoliosis seven times more frequently than boys.

Important historical details at presentation include the age of the patient, the age of menarche, the current height of the child and the height of the child's parents, any recent growth spurts, and of course, any recent trauma to the trunk or lower extremities. Existing neurological disorders, bowel or bladder dysfunction, spasticity, and lower extremity dysfunction must also be ruled out. Physical examination should include inspection of the shoulders for symmetry, inspection of the spine for trunk shift, rib hump, or skin stigmata (e.g., café-au-lait spots or dimpling). One should also rule out leg length inequalities and abduction or adduction contractures about the hips. A careful neurological examination testing sensation, strength, and deep tendon reflexes is an important part of the workup. A-P and lateral radiographs of the TLS spine should be performed if there appears to be significant curvature. The Cobb angle can be measured to quantify the curvature of the spine in the A-P plane. The A-P radiograph can also be used to assess skeletal maturity based on the ossification of the iliac crest apophysis (Risser sign). A lateral radiograph should demonstrate thoracic hypokyphosis and can also rule out spondylolisthesis. Of course, congenital anomalies should be ruled out on these radiographs, as well. An MRI should be obtained if there appears to be an absence of thoracic hypokyphosis or rotational deformity, a left-sided thoracic curve, or rapid curve progression. An MRI is also indicated for early onset scoliosis (age less than 10 years old) or for neurological signs or symptoms.

Treatment is aimed at controlling curve progression. Options include observation, bracing, and surgery. Exercise and electrical stimulation have not been shown to be beneficial. Curve control is desirable for cosmesis and to prevent curve progression beyond 70–90 degrees, which will result in measurable pulmonary dysfunction. The risk of curve progression is more likely with curves greater than 20 degrees, presenting age less than 12 years old, and Risser stage of 0 or 1 at presentation.

Idiopathic curves <30 degrees can be observed until they demonstrate 5 degrees or more of curve progression. When curves progress more than 5 degrees or exceed 30 degrees, bracing strategies are employed. Well-molded TLSO braces are standard and should be changed every 1 to 2 years in order to provide appropriate correction. Some still prefer a Milwaukee brace for upper thoracic curves. After brace fitting, the child should have a radiograph inside the brace to see how much correction is actually attained. Braces should be worn 16 to 23 hours per day, depending on the physician's preference. The goal of bracing is to control and reduce curve progression. The brace will not correct the curve. Once a child is fitted in a brace, radiographs may be performed with the child in the brace at 6-month intervals. Documented progression within the brace should prompt radiographs outside the brace.

Once curves progress beyond 50 degrees, bracing offers little benefit. If a curve has progressed to 50 degrees in an immature child, surgical treatment is usually recommended because of the high risk of continued progression. An individual who has reached skeletal maturity and has a curve around 50 degrees should be warned that his or her curve will continue to progress at a slow rate as he or she ages. Most curves of 50 degrees at maturity will progress an additional 15–30 degrees over a lifetime. Thoracic curves progress more than lumbar ones after maturity. Most patients with curves of this magnitude opt for fusion rather than risking further curvature and the cosmetic and possible pulmonary ramifications. Curves around 30 degrees at skeletal maturity have a much smaller chance of progression. Bracing is typically discontinued at skeletal maturity.

Most surgeons today are utilizing CD (Cotrel-Dobousset) and TSRH (Texas Scottish Rite Hospital) type implants to allow segmental fixation and some rotational correction while maintaining sagital plane contours. Sublaminar wiring offers excellent fixation but has a slightly greater risk of neurological injury. It is reserved for neuromuscular scoliosis by most surgeons.

Choosing fusion levels is one of the most challenging aspects of scoliosis surgery. There is a measurable increase in the rate of low back pain if the fusion extends down to L4. These rates seem to increase if the fusion extends to L5. It is rarely necessary to fuse to the pelvis for idiopathic scoliosis. Harrington recommended fusing from one level above and two levels below the vertebrae that fall within the Harrington stable zone. King and Moe identified five patterns of curves and made treatment suggestions on each of the five curves (Figs. 10.1, 10.2).

Anterior release should often be used with posterior fusion

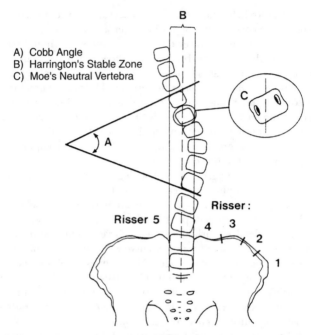

A) Cobb Angle
B) Harrington's Stable Zone
C) Moe's Neutral Vertebra

Figure 10.1. Measurements for idiopathic scoliosis. Note the Cobb angle (A), Harrington's stable zone (B), Moe's neutral vertebra (c), and Risser staging. (Reprinted with permission from Miller MD. Review of orthopaedics. Philadelphia: WB Saunders, 1992:141.)

in stiff curves that have progressed to the point that they are not correctable to better than 50 degrees using only a posterior approach. Anterior fusion with or without instrumentation may be used to save fusion levels in the thoracolumbar or lumbar spine, or it may be used in younger patients in order to prevent a "crankshaft phenomenon."

The most disastrous complication of posterior spinal fusion for idiopathic scoliosis is an iatrogenic neurologic injury. Attempting excessive correction and the use of sublaminar wires are risk factors. Many surgeons utilize a wake-up test and a clonus test intraoperatively to help rule out damage to the spinal cord. Some surgeons use somatosensory evoked potentials for posterior fusion to lessen the risk of nerve damage. Other surgical complica-

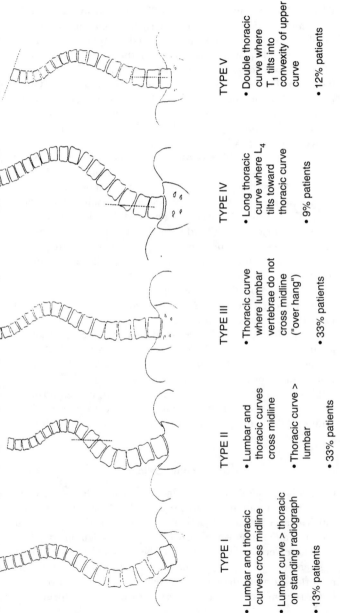

Figure 10.2. Five King types of scoliotic curves. (Adapted from King HA, Moe JH, Bradford DS, et al. The selection of fusion levels in thoracic idiopathic scoliosis. J Bone Joint Surg 1983;65A:1302–1313.)

TYPE I

- Lumbar and thoracic curves cross midline

- Lumbar curve > thoracic on standing radiograph

- 13% patients

TYPE II

- Lumbar and thoracic curves cross midline

- Thoracic curve > lumbar

- 33% patients

TYPE III

- Thoracic curve where lumbar vertebrae do not cross midline ("over hang")

- 33% patients

TYPE IV

- Long thoracic curve where L_4 tilts toward thoracic curve

- 9% patients

TYPE V

- Double thoracic curve where T_1 tilts into convexity of upper curve

- 12% patients

tions include pseudarthrosis (1%–2%), wound infection (1%–2%), implant failure because of early hook cut-out or late rod breakage, and rarely, transfusion-related complications. Failure to re-create adequate lumbar lordosis in these patients can create "flatback syndrome," which causes early fatigue and/or pain owing to the loss of the spine's normal sagittal curve. Other late complications include the "crankshaft phenomenon," which occurs because of continued anterior growth with a posterior fusion. This is why both anterior and posterior fusions are suggested in children who are less than 10–12 years old.

Infantile idiopathic scoliosis is more common in Europe and in boys with curves often having a left thoracic or thoracolumbar pattern. Most of these curves resolve spontaneously, and 85% are nonprogressive. These children should be evaluated for plagiocephaly (skull flattening), congenital dislocation of the hip, congenital heart disease, and mental deficiency. Bracing begins at 35 degrees or with demonstrable progression. Progression in the brace is often an indication for an MRI followed by convex hemiepiphysiodesis and posterolateral fusion.

Juvenile idiopathic scoliosis appears between 3 and 10 years of age. For curves less than 25 degrees, children may be observed until they demonstrate progression. If a child presents with a curve greater than 25 degrees or demonstrates progression of greater than 5 degrees, bracing should be instituted. Bracing should be continued until growth has ceased. If the curve is progressing during brace treatment, fusion should be delayed until the onset of the adolescent growth spurt, if at all possible, to prevent a "crankshaft phenomenon" and to prevent short stature. If this is not possible, both anterior and posterior fusions should be performed.

Congenital Scoliosis[1]

Congenital scoliosis is caused by abnormal vertebral development. Since the anomalies are present at birth, curvature is noted much earlier in life. These curves tend to be rigid and often require early fusion when early progression is demonstrated.

These vertebral anomalies can be classified into failure of segmentation, failure of formation, and mixed problems. It is important to note than a hemivertebra is not an extra vertebra but a remaining portion of a vertebra that did not form completely. Upon initial inspection, these vertebrae must be classified (Fig. 10.3). Careful documentation of the deformity and the magnitude of the curve should be performed initially and at 4–6-month intervals. Seventy-five percent of these curves are progressive. Thoracic curves have the poorest prognosis, with the worst anomaly being a unilateral unsegmented bar accompanied by a contralateral hemivertebra. Other anomalies with a poor prognosis are (in order, beginning with the poorest) a unilateral unsegmented bar, a double convexed hemivertebra, a single free convexed hemivertebra, and a block vertebral anomaly.

Children diagnosed with a unilateral unsegmented bar with contralateral hemivertebra or a unilateral unsegmented bar should undergo an immediate anterior and posterior spinal fusion because these curves have a tendency to progress so rapidly.

Hemivertebra may be single or multiple and balanced or unbalanced. The relation of the hemivertebra to adjacent vertebra is critical because it gives one an idea of the growth potential of the convexity of the curve. Fully segmented hemivertebrae have the greatest potential for steady progression. Partially segmented curves have a less rapid progression. Incarcerated hemivertebrae (nonsegmented hemivertebrae) that are "tucked in" the remainder of the spine may often be observed as they tend to progress slowly.

Upon initial diagnosis, these patients should have a renal ultrasound (20% of these people will have urinary tract anomalies), a cardiac evaluation (10%–15% will have congenital heart defects), and an MRI to uncover any spinal dysraphism.

Orthotic treatment is usually not helpful in these cases, since these curves are rigid and tend to progress. Sometimes bracing can help correct a compensatory curve, since they are usually more flexible. Braces frequently are used postoperatively following casting in children with congenital scoliosis.

When surgery is indicated, same-day anterior and posterior procedures are typically necessary until girls are >10 and boys are >12 years old (to decrease the risk of "crankshaft"). Hemivertebra excision is sometimes indicated at the lumbosacral junction for a hemivertebra causing decompensation of the spine at that level. Hemivertebra excision is combined with correction and fusion around the anomaly. Sometimes an anterior hemiepiphysiodesis and posterolateral fusion are indicated in children <5

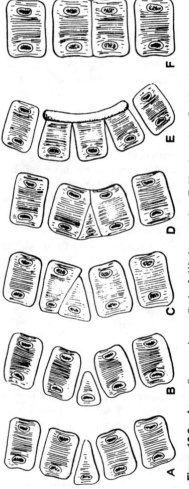

Figure 10.3. Anomalies causing scoliosis. **A.** Wedge vertebra. **B.** Hemivertebra. **C.** A hemivertebra nonsegmented on its cranial surface. **D.** A hemivertebra nonsegmented on both sides. **E.** A unilateral unsegmented bar. **F.** A nonsegmented vertebra (bloc vertebra). (Reprinted with permission from Winter RB. Congenital deformities of the spine. New York: Thieme-Stratton, 1983;12.)

years old who have steady curve progression owing to a fully segmented hemivertebra.

Neuromuscular Scoliosis[1]

Neuromuscular scoliosis frequently affects patients with cerebral palsy, myelodysplasia, spinal muscular atrophy, muscular dystrophies, and various other illnesses. These curves have a variety of clinical presentations and have a very different radiographic appearance when compared with adolescent idiopathic scoliosis. Curves less than 30 degrees can often be managed in a TLSO brace. Curves between 30 and 50 degrees must be watched carefully, as bracing will often fail. Curves greater than 50 degrees are nearly uncontrollable by bracing and subsequently need operative intervention. These operations are associated with higher complication rates compared with stabilization of idiopathic curves.

Scheuermann's Disease[1,2]

Scheuermann's disease is a rigid juvenile kyphosis characterized by vertebral body wedging owing to a growth disturbance of the endplate. The diagnosis is made on the lateral radiograph when more than 5 degrees of wedging exists at three or more adjacent vertebrae. Disc material often herniates through the adjacent endplate (Schmorl's nodes) and can be appreciated on the lateral radiograph. This disease comes in a typical form and an atypical form. The typical form is thoracic kyphosis. Atypical refers to kyphosis of the thoracolumbar junction or the lumbar spine. This form is far less understood.

Pain is the typical presenting complaint rather than deformity. The back pain is usually aggravated with physical activity and improves with rest. The natural history of typical Scheuermann's is relatively well described during adolescence. Little is known about the progression of kyphosis during adulthood after growth is complete.

Radiographic assessment is performed by measuring the Cobb angle on the lateral radiograph. Normal kyphosis is between 20 and 40 degrees. Patients with Scheuermann's tend to have a rigid kyphosis. Flexibility is determined by taking a lateral radiograph of the patient lying over a bolster that is positioned at the apex of the curve. MRIs are required only if there are neurological findings.

Initially, patients are treated with observation and physical therapy. The goals of therapy are to increase the flexibility of the spine, correct excessive lumbar lordosis, stretch the tight hamstring muscles, and strengthen the extensor muscles of the spine. In order for bracing to be an effective modality, studies have demonstrated that the curve must be at least 40% correctable with the brace. A Milwaukee brace is usually prescribed, and compliance is certainly a problem. Bracing is used for pain relief or immature patients with high curves (>50–55 degrees). There is data to suggest that bracing should continue until early adulthood to prevent progression. Patients with curves that are greater than 75 degrees are usually offered surgery. Anterior release followed by posterior fusion is performed unless the curve can be corrected to <50 degrees with only a posterior procedure. Following fusion, a brace or a body cast is worn in order to take stress off the rods while the fusion is healing.

Spondylolysis[1], Spondylolisthesis

Spondylolysis refers to a defect in the pars interarticularis of the vertebrae. Spondylolisthesis, on the other hand, refers to the slippage of one vertebra with respect to the next more caudal vertebra. Spondylolysthesis can occur because of spondylolysis. In children, spondylolysis occurs most frequently at L5, with resultant spondylolysthesis of L5 on S1.

There is a well-known classification developed by Wiltse describing spondylolisthesis. Type 1 is a congenital anomaly of the L5–S1 facet allowing forward slippage of L5 on S1. Type 2 is isthmic spondylolisthesis and is the most frequent type seen in children. In this type, a lesion in the pars interarticularis allows forward slipping on the vertebral body on the next most caudal vertebra. Type 2A refers to a lytic fracture of the pars (stress fracture). Type 2B refers to an elongated but intact pars interarticularis. Type 2C refers to an acute fracture of the pars interarticularis. Type 3 is a degenerative spondylolisthesis (seen in adults), Type 4 refers to a traumatic spondylolisthesis, and Type 5 is a pathologic spondylolisthesis. Some also refer to a Type 6, which refers to postsurgical spondylolisthesis because of excessive resection of neural arches and facets.

Spondylolysis and spondylolisthesis have never been reported at birth and have never been seen in an individual who does not stand or sit upright. The incidence rises from 0 at birth to 4% at 6 years of age to 6% at 14 years of age. The incidence is higher in boys and higher in Caucasians. Alaskan Eskimos have been seen to have rates as high as 25%–50%. Progression occurs after diagnosis in about 5% of the population. When it occurs, it appears to be linked with disc degeneration.

There appears to be some hereditary tie to spondylolysis and spondylolisthesis, but trauma is considered to be a major factor. Many have theorized that spondylolysis is a stress fracture of the pars owing to repetitive microtrauma. This is supported by a higher incidence of spondylolysis in female gymnasts, college football linemen, and weight lifters.

A dull ache in either the low back or buttocks is the most frequent presenting complaint. Patients tend to be 10–15 years old in the middle of an adolescent growth spurt. Radicular symptoms are rare but, when present, are typically in the L5 distribution. Physical examination is notable for flattening of the buttocks, increased lumbar lordosis, and a waddling gait. Patients often have restricted forward bending and a limited straight leg raise because of hamstring tightness.

Radiographic evaluation includes A-P, lateral, and oblique views of the spine in the painful area. A lateral view can allow one to visualize the slip in spondylolisthesis. An oblique view helps one visualize the pars defect (disruption in the neck of the "Scotty dog") in spondylolysis. In the "Scotty dog," the nose is the transverse process, the dog's eye is the pedicle, the ear is the superior articulating facet, the neck is the pars interarticularis, its back is the lamina, and its front paw is the descending articular process. Slip percentage is calculated by visualizing the lateral radiograph and comparing the amount of slip by dividing the forward displacement over the sagittal diameter of the inferior vertebral body (usually S1). One should also measure the slip angle, which measures the kyphosis at the area of the slip. One does this by drawing a tangential line to the posterior aspect of the sacrum and by drawing a perpendicular line to it. One then draws a line parallel to the superior endplate of L5 and measures the angle between the two lines. One should also take note of anatomic changes such as the trapezoidal shape of L5 and the rounded dome shape of S1 when present. Preoperative flexion and extension views can give one an idea of how much flexibility there is at the defect. Bone scan is often utilized in deciding whether spondylolysis is chronic or acute and can affect treatment. CT or MRI imaging is used when there is a neurologic defect that needs further delineation.

Spondylolysis is typically low degree and can usually be treated with observation if the child is without pain. If the child has discomfort, a reduction in activity is the first treatment modality. Bracing is indicated if a child has pain and a bone scan reveals recent fracture of the pars. Healing usually takes 3–4 months, and resumption of all activity is allowed afterward. Arthrodesis is rarely required for spondylolysis. Rarely, a one level L5 to S1 posterolateral fusion is performed for cases not improved with nonoperative treatment. When the pars defect is at L4 or higher, nonoperative treatment is encouraged. If this management fails, many suggest wire fixation from the spinous process to the transverse process with bone grafting of the pars defect.

Nonoperative treatment for spondylolisthesis is indicated for slips less than 50%. The child should be checked annually with radiographs to rule out slip progression until skeletal maturity. If the patient is symptomatic, activity should be restricted. TLSO bracing is performed when pain does not resolve with activity modification. Surgical stabilization is performed for children who have slips greater than 50% and smaller slips that do not respond to conservative therapy. Usually, an L5 to S1 fusion without instrumentation will suffice unless L5 is displaced so anteriorly that the fusion must also incorporate L4. L4 is included so the fusion mass is more vertical, subsequently reducing the shear stress on the fusion mass. Nerve root decompression is only needed if there is obvious weakness and sensory deficit. Typically, pain resolves with fusion. When decompression is required, the Gill procedure with removal of the "loose" lamina of L5 is performed. Reduction of the spondylolisthesis is rarely performed, since fusion in situ yields excellent results even in high-grade slips. Some reduction maneuvers may increase the risk of nerve root injury by 20%–30%. With slips greater than 75%, some believe that some reduction is necessary in order to achieve a fusion mass without excessive shear stress. With greater than 100% spondylolisthesis (spondyloptosis), an L5 vertebrectomy is sometimes indicated. Instrumentation is rarely necessary, but sometimes it can be used in mature adolescents if the pedicles are large enough to accommodate transpedicular fixation. Instead of instrumentation, patients are usually immobilized postoperatively in a body cast with a leg extension for 4 months, followed by TLSO bracing until the fusion is solid. When scoliosis is associated with spondylolisthesis, the two entities can be treated separately as long as the scoliosis is noted to be the standard adolescent idiopathic type.

Low Back Pain

Low back pain in children is a rare entity that should be taken seriously. Acute back pain can be associated with conditions requiring aggressive care such as cystitis, osteomyelitis, and tumors. Workup should begin with A-P, lateral, and oblique views of the spine to rule out a pars defect (spondylolysis). Then a CBC, ESR, and a bone scan should be performed to rule out evidence of discitis, vertebral osteomyelitis, fracture, and tumor. Osteoid osteoma "lights up" on bone scan and is not an infrequent cause of persistent LBP in children with and without scoliosis. If these tests are negative, the child can usually be treated with NSAIDs and activity modification.

LOWER EXTREMITY ABNORMALITIES

In-toeing[1]

In-toeing is a frequent cause for visits to the orthopaedic surgeon. Femoral anteversion is the most common cause of in-toeing followed by tibial torsion and metatarsus adductus. However, as the child learns to walk, the femoral anteversion usually corrects to normal adult values by age 6 or 7 (about 15 degrees), and most children eventually walk with the toes pointing relatively straight ahead. Bracing has not been shown to improve this condition. Surgery is rarely required for excessive femoral anteversion. Open (plate fixation) and closed (intramedullary nail) femoral osteotomies are sometimes performed for cosmesis during the teen years.

Internal tibial torsion is a common cause of toeing-in. Tibial torsion measures the relationship of the knee axis to the ankle axis and can be determined by flexing the knee 10–15 degrees, aligning the patella to be directed anteriorly, and then comparing the angle between the midpoints of the lateral and medial malleoli with that of the thigh. Normally, the intermalleolar axis is externally rotated about 25 degrees relative to the knee and the femur. Less than this would indicate some degree of internal tibial torsion and the foot would tend to point in or toe-in. This problem is likely caused by fetal positioning and usually disappears by age 4–5. The opposite problem, toeing-out because of external tibial torsion occurs less frequently. Bracing is not helpful. Supramalleolar osteotomies with smooth pin fixation performed at around 8 years of age can improve cosmesis.

The third cause of in-toeing is metatarsus adductus. This entity is discussed later in the chapter under foot disorders.

Genu Varum[8]

The challenge for the general orthopaedist is to distinguish between physiologic genu varum and pathologic conditions that may result in functional and cosmetic problems if left untreated. Parents will frequently notice genu varum when the child first begins to ambulate. Genu varum is physiologic until the age of 18–24 months, and no treatment is necessary. Overcorrection to excessive genu valgum is often seen between ages 3 and 4. Correction to physiologic valgus is usually complete by 5–6 years of age. Early walking (prior to 12 months) is often seen in black children and may be a factor in increased physiologic bowing. Internal tibial torsion is often associated with physiologic genu varum.

Examinations should include height and weight percentiles in an effort to rule out a dwarfing condition. The amount of femoral anteversion, tibial torsion, and lateral knee laxity should be routinely assessed. When there appears to be a localized deformity in either the distal femur or the proximal tibia, or if the child is short, full-length standing A-P radiographs should be obtained with the patellae pointed directly forward.

In physiologic bowing, both the distal femur and proximal tibia will both demonstrate some varus bowing without an acute angular component and both physes will appear normal without medial physeal changes. Treatment of physiologic genu varum is periodic observation and examination, as well as reassurance for anxious parents.

Tibia vara, or Blount's disease, is characterized by an abrupt varus deformity of the proximal tibia. There are both infantile (onset before 5 years old) and late onset or adolescent (onset after 6 years of age) types. Infantile idiopathic tibia vara is seen more frequently in black females and obese children who begin to walk earlier than normal. Involvement is bilateral in 80% of the patients. Late onset tibia vara is usually unilateral and has a greater prevalence in black male and obese children.

Acute angulation of the proximal tibia will often be noted on physical evaluation, and a lateral thrust indicating laxity of the lateral ligamentous complex is often seen during gait observation. Radiographs frequently demonstrate medial fragmentation of the proximal tibia metaphysis. In later stages, medial physeal depression and varus angulation of the metaphysis develop. In the end stages of Blount's disease, an osseous bridge between the epiphysis and metaphysis can develop. These radiographic changes are often less obvious in late onset tibia vara. A metaphyseal-diaphyseal angle greater than 16 degrees is strongly correlated with the later development of tibia vara. If the angle is less than 9 degrees, the risk of Blount's is actually quite small, and observation may continue to be the treatment. The rotation of the lower extremity can have a 1–4-degree effect on the radiographic measurement of this angle.

Langenskiold outlined six stages of tibia vara that are helpful for classification as well as prognostication. Many will use a KAFO brace during Stages 1 and 2 if the child is less than 3 years old, while others do not think that bracing alters the natural history. If the tibia vara progresses despite bracing, most authors suggest a proximal tibial valgus osteotomy prior to the child's 4th birthday, since this seems to decrease the likelihood of recurrence. In children >4 years old, most will still opt for an osteotomy but will often add other procedures in an effort to improve outcomes. Physeal bar resection, if present, is often attempted, though this is unreliable. Others perform a lateral proximal tibial hemiepiphysiodesis or lateral proximal tibial stapling to reduce the likelihood of recurrence.

Other causes for tibia vara include vitamin D resistant rickets, renal osteodystrophy, metaphyseal chondrodysplasia, achondroplasia, osteogenesis imperfecta, and fibrocartilaginous dysplasia. The metabolic abnormalities in vitamin D resistant rickets and in renal osteodystrophy must be medically controlled prior to engaging in surgical treatment.

Genu Valgum[9]

Like genu varum, the challenge with genu valgum is to distinguish between physiologic and pathologic forms. One must remember that genu valgum is greatest between ages 3 and 4 and that the normal amount of valgus should be achieved by approximately age 6. Physiologic genu valgum can be accentuated by fat thighs, ligamentous laxity, and flat feet. Additionally, excessive femoral anteversion and compensatory external tibial torsion can also create the appearance of exaggerated genu valgum.

Pathologic causes include idiopathic, posttraumatic, metabolic, neuromuscular, infectious, and generalized disorders. Idiopathic causes include lateral femoral hypoplasia that can be diagnosed when lateral femoral condyle height is less than 70% of that of the medial femoral condyle. Trauma is the most common cause of pathologic genu valgum. Salter-Harris fractures Types 3, 4, and 5 of the proximal tibia pose a great risk for angular deformity. Meanwhile, any injury including Salter-Harris 1 and 2 injuries to the distal femur can be associated with physeal damage owing to the convoluted anatomy of that growth plate. Prior to diagnosing a child with a medial or lateral ligamentous injury about the knee, one should probably perform stress films in order to rule out a physeal injury, since the physis is often weaker than the ligament. A Cozen's fracture of the proximal tibia can result in tibia valga caused by hyperemia and the resultant overgrowth of the proximal medial tibia. The metabolic effects of rickets and renalosteodystrophy are quite similar on the physes. Despite this similarity, vitamin D–resistant and vitamin D–deficient rickets are typically associated with a varus deformity of the knee, while renal osteodystrophy is typically associated with a valgus deformity. Metabolic conditions have to be maximized prior to operative interventions. Genu valgum is often seen in children with neuromuscular disorders such as cerebral palsy, and this is often exacerbated by pes valgus and/or excessive external tibial torsion, which causes the foot to be rotated externally relative to the knee. This alignment leads to a significant valgus moment at the knee during ambulation. In paralytic conditions such as myelodysplasia or polio, genu valgum is thought to be caused by contracture of the iliotibial band.

Prior family history and developmental milestones must be documented. Physical examination should pay close attention to anatomic tibiofemoral angle, rotational deformities, and the laxity of the medial collateral ligament. If children >7 years old with genu valgum have greater than 15–20 degrees of tibiofemoral angulation and are below the 25th percentile in height, a single weight-bearing A-P radiograph of the lower extremities is indicated. The appearance of the physis and the mechanical and anatomic axes of the femur and tibia should be evaluated in order to identify the cause and location of the valgus deformity.

Children who are <10 years old and have a tibiofemoral angle of greater than 15–20 degrees and/or an intermalleolar distance of more than 8 cm, should be examined and radiographed every year. If these findings persist after 10 years of age, spontaneous correction is unlikely to occur and most authors recommend surgical intervention. Options include partial epiphysiodesis, hemiepiphyseal stapling, or an osteotomy using stable internal fixation or external fixation. Osteotomies are relatively large procedures with significant neurovascular complications. These include compartment syndromes, ischemia owing to stretch or compression of the anterior tibial artery and neuropraxia because of traction on the peroneal nerve.

Osteochondritis Dissecans[1,2]

Osteochondritis dissecans typically occurs in the lateral aspect of the medial femoral condyle (and also in the capitellum) when the underlying bone becomes avascular and the cartilage subsequently becomes involved. The involved cartilaginous fragment becomes loose and displaces. Trauma appears to play a role. A-P and lateral radiographs of the knee, as well as a tunnel view of the knee flexed 20–30 degrees, often demonstrate the lesion. An MRI shows the extent of avascularity in the underlying bone and may show evidence of cartilage damage. Additionally, MRI can rule out other causes of knee pain. This is important, since many OCD lesions are asymptomatic. If an OCD lesion is discovered incidentally and the patient is asymptomatic, no treatment is necessary. If the knee is painful, sports and activities should be limited. Nonsteroidals, quadricep strengthening exercises, and sometimes a knee immobilizer should be employed until symptoms improve. If pain persists despite conservative therapy, arthroscopy should be performed. At arthroscopy, if the articular cartilage appears to be dull and damaged, this region should be debrided and the subchondral bone drilled using a K-wire to induce the proliferation of fibrocartilage by bringing new blood flow to it. If the chondral fragment can be flipped up, the bony base can be roughened with a curet and the fragment can be pinned in position with a biodegradable screw. If a loose body has occurred leaving bare bone, the bone is drilled using a K-wire and the loose body is removed. Occasionally, the loose body can be replaced if it has become loose acutely. Again, fixation is typically a biodegradable screw or pin. The prognosis of OCD lesions in children is excellent, in teenage children the prognosis is intermediate, and in adults the prognosis tends to be poor. In particular, OCD lesions present on the weight-bearing portion of the articular cartilage tend to be difficult to repair.

Osgood-Schlatter Disease[2]

Osgood-Schlatter disease is an apophysitis of the tibial tubercle caused by overuse that occurs in young teenagers. Pain and swelling about the tubercle are the chief complaints. Examination reveals tenderness of the tubercle, but activity is rarely limited. Radiographs sometimes show irregularity and fragmentation of the tubercle. Treatment involves nonsteroidals and limitation of activity. This process is self-limited and causes no long-term damage. Surgical intervention is very rare.

Congenital Pseudarthrosis of the Tibia[1]

Congenital pseudarthrosis of the tibia occurs in 1 in 190,000 people. In this condition, the tibia bows anterolaterally in early childhood, usually progressing to pathologic fracture. Bilateral cases are rare. Anterolateral bowing is typically discovered in the first or second year of life. It may be distinguished from genu varum because the bowing is in the distal part of the tibia and because it occurs unilaterally. Fracture tends to occur by age 2–3 years. In fact, cases fracturing after age 5 are called late onset and typically run a different course. This condition is associated with neurofibromatosis 55% of the time. There is no evidence that cases associated with neurofibromatosis have a lower rate of successful treatment. Radiographically, there is typically antero-lateral bowing at the junction of the middle and distal thirds of the tibia. A fibular pseudarthrosis tends to be present.

This entity is treated initially by clamshell bracing in an effort to prevent fracture. It is not clear whether this actually works. Once a fracture has occurred, electrical stimulation offers a 55%–85% chance of union and is not invasive. Unfortunately, this treatment does not allow correction of the angular deformity and requires long-term casting. Intramedullary rod fixation with a bone graft offers a 90%–100% chance of union but tends to cause ankle stiffness and does not provide the opportunity to correct shortening though it can correct angular deformity. Free vascularized bone graft offers a 90%–95% chance of union and adds bone stock, as well as length. This is unfortunately a very expensive procedure requiring specialized skill. Use of an external fixator to create compression then distraction causes union 90%–100% of the time, but there is a high risk of refracture with this method. Unfortunately, once union occurs, the chance for refracture is high no matter the treatment selected. Patients need to be protected until they reach skeletal maturity and possibly for their entire life. Scanograms should be performed intermittently to identify any subsequent leg length deformities in the tibia and the ipsilateral femur. Parents should be warned initially that multiple fractures and multiple operations are often required. Once a patient has had three operations, many pediatric orthopaedists believe that an amputation is indicated. In this case, a Boyd or a Syme is performed distal to the pseudarthrosis. An amputation through the pseudarthrosis can risk formation of a painful spike at the end of the stump. Prior to Boyd or Syme amputation, the pseudarthrotic tibia can be rodded and bone grafted to correct angulation. After amputation, a prosthesis helps provide support of the pseudarthrosis while giving the patient a functional lower extremity. This modality should not be considered a failure, since the biology of this disease entity seems to be quite variable. Amputation occurs in at least 5% of the cases.

Developmental Dysplasia of the Hip (DDH)[1,2,10]

Developmental dysplasia of the hip, previously referred to as congenital dysplasia of the hip, can be classified into typical and teratologic types. Teratologic dislocations are typically prenatal dislocations that are not reducible at birth. This type of dislocation is usually seen in the presence of other congenital abnormalities. Typical cases of DDH can be divided into subluxatable, dislocatable (positive Barlow's), and dislocated but reducible hips (positive Ortalani's).

All infants should be screened in the neonatal ward. Most cases of DDH are picked up in the first few days of life. Some high-risk infants should be considered for ultrasound examination. Risk factors for DDH include first-born child, female sex (85%), breech presentation (30%–50%), oligohydramnios, and a positive family history (>20%). Associated conditions include metatarsus adductus (10%), calcaneovalgus feet, and torticollis (20%).

During the first 3 months of life, the Ortalani test (a reduction maneuver) and the Barlow test (a subluxating or dislocating maneuver) are frequently used. The child must obviously be quite relaxed in order to perform these tests. Inexperienced examiners will often confuse the high-pitched click made by a soft-tissue band with the low-pitched clunk typical of a hip subluxating causing unnecessary anxiety. When the child reaches 3 months, the side with a dislocated hip will have developed an adduction contracture, and asymmetric abduction will be noted. This is frequently a very subtle sign. Additionally, a Galeazzi test can be performed in which the child is supine and his femora are made perpendicular to the examination table and the height of their distal ends are compared. The side of the dislocated hip will not be as high as the reduced hip, causing a positive Galeazzi test. When the child begins walking, an abduction limp, toe walking, or increased lordosis can be signs of a dysplastic or dislocated hip.

Radiographic examination is difficult to perform on the infant since most of the bones have not ossified. An A-P pelvis can be obtained and Hilgenreiner's, Perkin's, and Shenton's lines should be evaluated (Fig. 10.4). A break in Shenton's line is often a subtle clue to a dislocated hip. The acetabular index (angle) can be measured, and serial radiographs over time can identify whether the hip is improving or worsening. An angle of <25 degrees is normal when the infant is >3 months old. In hip dysplasia, <30 degrees is probably acceptable when the child is 1 year old, though the physician should continue to follow the hip radiographically to make sure that an osteotomy is not indicated. Ultrasound is very user-dependent but is used as a screening tool in Europe. In the United States, screening with ultrasound is not thought to be cost effective. Here, we use it to assess high-risk infants only and to assess treatment with a Pavlik harness. Other practioners prefer to use a Chassler-Lapine radiograph to demonstrate the position of the femoral head after placement in a Pavlik harness.

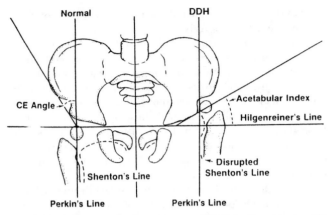

Figure 10.4. Radiographic evaluation of DDH. (Adapted from Morrissy RT, Weinstein SL. Lovell and Winter's pediatric orthopaedics. 4th ed. Philadelphia: Lippincott-Raven, 1996:915.)

During the first 6 months of life, a dislocated hip can be reduced and treated initially with a Pavlik harness. Proper application of the harness is critical. The hip should be flexed to approximately 110 degrees and abduction should be performed to the point at which it is well within the "safe zone." The "safe zone" marks the point between adduction, where dislocation occurs, ranging to maximal abduction, where the risk of avascular necrosis is great. Ultrasound is often used to confirm hip reduction in the Pavlik harness. If the hip fails to remain reduced after 2–3 weeks in the Pavlik harness, this method of treatment should be abandoned. If the hip remains reduced in the Pavlik, the child should remain in the harness for a period equaling twice the child's age at diagnosis plus 6 weeks. Using this rule, a newborn diagnosed with a dislocated hip should only require 6 weeks of treatment.

If the child fails treatment with a Pavlik harness or is 6–18 months of age when a dislocated hip is diagnosed, the child should undergo examination under anesthesia, arthrogram, closed reduction, and spica casting in a stable position. This treatment should be followed by an MRI or CT scan to confirm that the hip is located. Many surgeons will use Bryant's traction prior to closed reduction to reduce the tension on the soft tissues and reduce the risk of AVN.

If this treatment is unsuccessful or if the child is greater than 18 months of age, open reduction should be performed following preliminary traction. Most would incorporate a femoral shortening osteotomy, as well, to decrease the risk of AVN, and depending on the situation, a pelvic osteotomy may also be included. Open reduction is typically performed through the anterior Smith-Peterson approach between the sartorius and the tensor fascia lata. Many prefer to perform an open reduction as early as 12 months of age in order to get a perfect reduction and to make sure that the acetabulum is clear of soft tissue.

Of children diagnosed with a DDH at birth (hip is subluxatable, dislocatable, or dislocated), 90% of these children will normalize without any treatment within the first 6 weeks of life. In a patient who is less than 6 months old with a positive Barlow's test, the Pavlik harness is successful more than 90% of the time. If the patient has a positive Ortalani test and is less than 6 months of age, treatment with a Pavlik is successful 80% of the time. Patients who go on to closed reduction also have high success rates. It is generally thought that if the hip is reduced prior to the child's first birthday, the risk of long-term disability is small.

Legg-Calvé-Perthes Disease (Coxa Plana)[1,11]

Legg-Calvé-Perthes disease is a self-limited deformity of the femoral head that occurs in boys at a 3 to 1 ratio compared with girls. The pathogenesis is thought to involve bone necrosis owing to recurrent injury to the circumflex arteries. Other theories involve femoral head ischemia secondary to tamponade of the retinacular vessels. More recently, clotting factors and possibly endocrine abnormalities have been implicated as possible factors. Though children with Perthes disease are euthyroid, they have been noted to have higher levels of free thyroxine and free triiodothyronine.

The usual age at presentation is 4–8 years old. Children frequently present with a painless limp that has been present for weeks or months. Pain, when present, is often referred to the knee by the femoral nerve or the medial thigh by the obturator nerve. On physical examination, limited internal rotation and abduction of the hip compared with the contralateral hip are the most consistent findings. The gait may have a gluteus medius lurch, and a Trendelenburg test is often positive. An apparent leg length discrepancy is sometimes because of an adduction contracture. However, significant shortening can occur if severe coxa plana (head flattening) has developed later in the disease. Ten percent to twenty percent of cases are bilateral, and the hips are frequently at different stages. Both hips should be radiographed at the initial presentation.

Initial evaluation involves A-P and frog-leg lateral radiographs of both hips. The radiographic differential diagnosis includes multiple epiphyseal dysplasia, spondyloepiphyseal dysplasia, hypothyroidism, Gaucher's disease, trichorhinophalangeal syndrome, and steroid use. Most of these are bilateral conditions. One must also consider Meyer's dysplasia, which is a growth anomaly of both femoral head epiphyses. In this syndrome, both femoral heads appear to be radiographically identical, unlike bilateral cases of Perthes disease in which the hips are typically at different stages.

Waldenstrom classified radiographic findings based on the evolutionary phase of the disease. During the initial phase, the physis becomes irregular and the femoral head becomes more radiodense and smaller while the cartilage space of the hip is wider. The increased density of the head occurs because the surrounding bone has a normal blood supply and thus appears osteopenic compared with the avascular segment. The cartilage space appears wider because it is receiving a normal blood supply and continues to grow relative to the femoral head. Following subchondral fracture, the fragmentation stage begins. Fragmentation is caused by the reabsorption and creeping substitution of necrotic bone by vascular connective tissue. The third stage is reossification, which is characterized by new bone formation. Finally, Waldenstrom's fourth stage is the healed stage in which the head and neck demonstrate varying amounts of residual deformity.

The Catterall classification is the most widely used in Perthes disease. In Group 1, there is only anterior and central involvement with no metaphyseal involvement. In Group 2, there is about 50% involvement anterolaterally with the medial and lateral pillar portions of the femoral head intact. In Group 3, about 75% of the head is involved including the lateral column with a diffuse metaphyseal reaction. In Group 4, the entire head is involved. Catterall suggested that Groups 1 and 2 have favorable outcomes without treatment, while Groups 3 and 4 have a poorer prognosis and require treatment.

Other classifications include the Salter-Thompson classification based on the extent of subchondral fracture. In Group A, less than half the femoral head is involved, while in Group B more than half the femoral head is involved. More recently, a new classification has been proposed by Herring, and this is favored by many pediatric orthopaedic surgeons. This classification compares the height of the lateral epiphyseal pillar during early fragmentation stage with that of the normal contralateral epiphysis. In Group A, the lateral pillar retains its original height and shows minimal radiographic changes. In Group B, the lateral pillar may show density changes and some height loss but retains at least 50% of its original height. In Group C, the lateral pillar is characterized by radiolucencies and collapse to less than 50% of the contralateral height

The main objective in the treatment of Perthes disease is to minimize the development of residual hip deformity in an effort to reduce the likelihood of early hip arthritis. Catterall described "head at risk signs" that included Gage's sign (a radiolucent "V" on the lateral side of the epiphysis), calcification lateral to the epiphysis, lateral subluxation of the femoral head, a horizontal physis, and a metaphyseal cyst. These signs were previously thought to be important prognostically, but two recent reports have shown that the only "head at risk" sign that was important was lateral subluxation. It appears that the two most important prognostic indicators are prolonged limitation of hip motion and the age of onset of the disease. Oddly enough, the earlier that patients get Perthes disease, the better their outcome. Patients who develop Perthes after age 8 are more likely to develop severe osteoarthritis because the femoral head and acetabulum have less remodeling potential as the child ages. Stulburg demonstrated that the only patients who have osteoarthritis in early adulthood were patients in whom the femoral head appears flattened and the acetabulum appears unaffected at the end of the healing phase.

In Stulburg's review, he staged Perthes disease according to eventual deformity in order to estimate the risk for osteoarthritis. Stage 1 demonstrated essentially no deformity in the healing phase. Stage 2 demonstrated coxa magna, indicating that the femoral head was 10% larger than the contralateral head. Stage

3 demonstrated an oval-shaped head that was often larger than the contralateral side. Stage 4 demonstrated a flat head. In Stages 2, 3, and 4, the femoral neck was often shortened and there was often increased acetabular slope, but the acetabulam was always congruent with the femoral head. In Stage 5, the femoral head was deformed, but the acetabulum and femoral neck were normal. Therefore, in Stage 5, patients are left with an incongruous joint. Stages 1 and 2 demonstrated no increased risk for osteoarthritis. Stages 3 and 4 demonstrated mild to moderate arthritis in their 50s and 60s. Stage 5 demonstrated severe arthritis before age 50.

Treatment of patients with Perthes disease is aimed mostly at those with onset between 6 and 9 years old. It is thought that patients who have Perthes prior to age 6 will have adequate time to remodel and will subsequently have little deformity. Patients who develop Perthes after age 9, on the other hand, will likely have a bad outcome regardless of what treatment is performed because of little remodeling time prior to skeletal maturity. Unfortunately, treatment of Perthes disease has little scientific basis, and the literature offers little evidence to suggest the superiority of one treatment over another.

The cornerstones of treatment include maintenance of range of motion and containment (prevention of subluxation). Restoration of motion is obtained with nonsteroidals and occasionally bed rest and traction. Resistant cases may be treated with serial Petrie abduction casts in an effort to stretch out the soft tissues and increase motion (especially abduction). Motion must be regained prior to beginning any form of containment treatment. Also, prior to beginning containment treatment, it is important to ensure that the hips can be contained congruently and that there is no hinge abduction because of femoral head flattening. A Von Rosen view of the pelvis may demonstrate this, but, if this is equivocal, arthrography is often useful in showing which position is best for containment. Children who are 6 or 7 and have persistent or recurrent synovitis, lateral subluxation, involvement of the lateral pillar, or involvement of nearly 50% of the femoral head are typically treated with closed containment strategies. This typically involves the Scottish-Rite orthosis, which consists of two thigh cuffs connected by an abduction bar. This has replaced the Petrie casts that were used in the past. This treatment strategy is continued until there is evidence of reossification of the lateral epiphysis.

Children who are 8 or 9 years old and have persistent or recurrent synovitis, lateral subluxation, involvement of the lateral pillar, involvement of nearly 50% of the femoral head, or have failed closed containment strategies are candidates for open containment. These strategies include proximal derotation osteotomies of the femur and various pelvic osteotomies designed to improve acetabular coverage of the femoral head. An arthrogram is often done prior to performing the femoral osteotomy in order to find the best position for the osteotomy. Varus corrections should be limited to 20 degrees because a short leg and an abductor lurch can be more pronounced with varus angulation greater than that. Many studies have demonstrated that operative treatment provides an improved outcome compared with the natural history of Perthes disease, but, in reality, good studies with rigorous controls are lacking in today's literature.

Slipped Capital Femoral Epiphysis (SCFE)[1]

Slipped capital femoral epiphysis refers to a deformity occurring in adolescence in which the proximal femoral metaphysis externally rotates and displaces anteriorly from the capital femoral epiphysis, which stays reduced in the acetabulum. This is the most common hip disorder in the adolescence age group with an incidence of 2 cases per 100,000 people. Boys are more affected than girls. The average age of onset is 12.1 years for boys and 14 years for girls. Most of these children tend to be overweight and skeletally immature, though about one-third have a normal morphotype. The incidence of bilateral involvement is 20%–40%. Black children have a higher incidence than whites. Increased mechanical shear forces on the physis associated with obesity have been thought to cause SCFE, but endocrine reasons such as hypothyroidism, growth hormone deficiency, and hypogonadism have also been implicated.

Children present with an antalgic gait and complain of severe hip pain. Up to half of patients complain *only* of knee pain, so the practitioner must be alert and suspicious. SCFE has traditionally been categorized into four groups depending upon the length of symptoms. Preslips have no symptoms of pain but have a notably widened physeal plate. Acute slips have had symptoms for less than 3 weeks and are unstable. They often have displacement easily visualized on radiograph. Chronic slips have had symptoms of pain for greater than 3 weeks and often have evidence of displacement radiographically. These hips are stable. Acute or chronic slips occur when patients report a prodrome of knee or hip pain that has been present for a long time but has recently been exacerbated and worsened. These hips are unstable.

SCFE is graded radiographically by the amount (a percentage) of slip that has occurred between the epiphysis and the metaphysis best seen on the frog-leg lateral. Generally speaking, treatment should be fixation of the epiphysis to the metaphysis with one cannulated screw (6.5 or 7.3 mm). Screw placement is preceded by percutaneous guide pin placement into the anterolateral femoral cortex on the distal aspect of the femoral neck and into the center of the capital femoral epiphysis perpendicular to the physis in both the A-P and lateral planes. Some surgeons prefer to use two pins if the slip is acute. Most pediatric orthopaedic surgeons currently use only one pin, arguing that the minimal mechanical advantage gained by two pins is not worth the increased risk of complications. The two primary complications are avascular necrosis (AVN) and chondrolysis. AVN is largely caused by the initial displacement prior to patient presentation. Despite this, the risk of AVN clearly goes up when hips are reduced from their displaced position. One study demonstrated a 40% incidence in reduced hips. Chondrolysis occurs when the screw is protruding into the joint. If a pin enters a joint during the procedure and is promptly removed, no harm has been done. The problem arises when the pin is inadvertantly left in the joint and it is not appreciated during the procedure. The "approach-withdrawal" technique should be used with the image intensifier once the pin or pins are in place to ensure that no pins remain in the joint. Even moderate amounts of chondrolysis leads to hip degeneration. Blacks and individuals who are casted to treat SCFE appear to be more prone to chondrolysis. Most surgeons use one screw for both acute and chronic situations and avoid performing any reductions in order to reduce the risk of AVN and chondrolysis.

Subtrochanteric osteotomies are performed if residual deformity is causing a decreased range of motion at 2 years after the SCFE has been treated. The natural history of SCFE is progressive joint degeneration, with one study demonstrating more than 40% joint narrowing at 35 years follow-up. Patients who go on to develop degenerative joint disease typically have a pistol grip deformity of the proximal femur.

Transient Synovitis of the Hip[1]

Transient synovitis of the hip is the most common cause of childhood hip pain. Children can be affected as early as 9 months of age through their teen years, but most cases occur between 3–8 years of age. This is a diagnosis of exclusion that should only be considered after others have been ruled out. Other possibilities include pyogenic arthritis, osteomyelitis of the femoral neck or pelvis, tuberculous arthritis, JRA, acute rheumatic fever, Perthes disease, tumor, trauma, and SCFE. As in these other conditions, children typically present with a limp and an antalgic gait if they are willing to bear weight at all. The extremity is often held in a flexed and externally rotated postion in effort to decrease intracapsular pressure. Etiologies include active or recent infection, trauma, or allergic hypersensitivity. Lab values are nonspecific, with the WBC count averaging 10,000–14,000 and ESR around 20 mm/hour. The child's temperature is typically less than 38°C. Radiographs are usually normal.

Treatment involves bed rest and nonsteroidals. Skin traction is no longer recommended, except for recurrent cases. Aspirin should be avoided in a child with an active viral infection because of the association with aspirin and Reye's syndrome. Routine aspiration of the hip is not therapeutic but may assist in ruling out other more serious etiologies of hip pain. If rest and NSAIDs are not helpful, the parents should be instructed to bring the child back for re-evaluation.

Proximal Focal Femoral Deficiency (PFFD)[1,2]

Proximal focal femoral deficiency is a term applied to a condition in which the femur is short and there is an absence of continuity between the femoral neck and shaft. This congenital defect was at one time associated with the use of thalidomide, but most cases today are idiopathic without evidence of a hereditary cause. In this deformity, the thigh is of varying lengths and the hip is often flexed, abducted, and externally rotated. The hip abductors and extensors are present but are frequently dysfunctional. The knee frequently lies near the groin and is often quite unstable. In 45% of the cases, there is associated ipsilateral fibular hemimelia (see below). The foot often has an equinovalgus deformity and there are often deficient lateral rays of the foot.

The Aitken classification is the most commonly used because it has some clinical relevance (Fig. 10.5). Children with Types A and B typically have a better prognosis because they have a hip joint that can sometimes be functional. Type A can be distinguished from Type B because there is no osseous connection between the head and shaft in Type B. Types C and D are typified by an absent femoral head and a severely dysplastic and even absent acetabulum. The prognosis for these patients is much poorer owing to the absence of a relatively normal hip joint.

TYPE		FEMORAL HEAD	ACETABULUM	FEMORAL SEGMENT	RELATIONSHIP AMONG COMPONENTS OF FEMUR AND ACETABULUM AT SKELETAL MATURITY
A	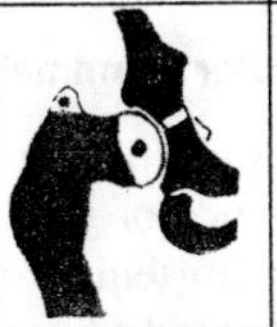	Present	Normal	Short	Bony connection between components of femur Femoral head in acetabulum Subtrochanteric varus angulation, often with pseudarthrosis
B	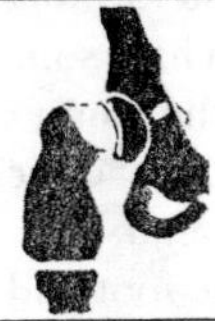	Present	Adequate or moderately dysplastic	Short, usually proximal bony tuft	No osseous connection between head and shaft Femoral head in acetabulum
C	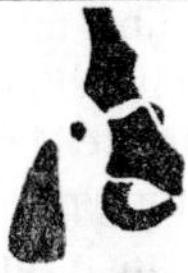	Absent or represented by ossicle	Severely dysplastic	Short, usually proximally tapered	May be osseous connection between shaft and proximal ossicle No articular relation between femur and acetabulum
D	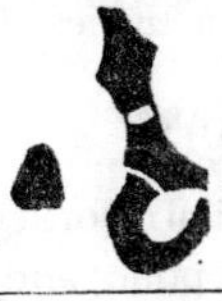	Absent	Absent Obturator foramen enlarged Pelvis squared in bilateral cases	Short, deformed	(none)

Figure 10.5. Aitken classification of proximal femoral focal deficiency. The four types of deficiency. (Reprinted with permission from Tachdjian MO. Pediatric orthopedics. 2nd ed. Philadelphia: WB Saunders, 1990:556.)

Types A and B are often treated with limb lengthening of the affected extremity, depending on knee stability and the condition of the leg. Types C and D are often treated with a knee fusion and a Boyd or Syme amputation. Growth arrests to the affected side will allow the extremity to be shortened enough to allow room for a high-functioning prosthetic knee.

Congenital Hypoplasia of the Femur

Congenital hypoplasia of the femur is a related condition in which there is up to 10% shortening of the femur compared with the contralateral femur. These children do not have the varus angulation seen in children with PFFD, but they do have significant anterolateral femoral bow, as well as a valgus deformity of the knee. Absence of the cruciate ligaments is frequent in this condition. Many of these patients also have ipsilateral fibular hemimelia.

Longitudinal Deficiency of the Fibula (Fibular Hemimelia)[1]

Longitudinal deficiency of the fibula includes a wide spectrum of abnormalities ranging from complete absence of the fibula with missing lateral rays of the foot to mild shortening of the fibula without any foot abnormality. The ipsilateral tibia is also shortened accordingly. These children will often have some femoral shortening and lateral condylar dysplasia of the femur causing valgus at the knee. These children also have ACL deficiencies with absence of the tibial spine and often have a tarsal coalition.

Treatment depends on the condition of the foot and ankle, as well as on the amount of shortening in the tibia and fibula. Mild cases may need a shoe lift or require limb lengthening. Severe foot and ankle involvement is often best treated by a Syme or Boyd type amputation and early prostethic fitting prior to age 1. If this is done, these children can become extremely functional and can participate at high levels of sporting activities.

Leg Length Discrepancies (LLD)[1,12]

Leg length discrepancies are caused by congenital disorders, such as PFFD and DDH; paralytic disorders, such as polio; and myelodysplasia; infections; tumors; and trauma. Leg length discrepancies must be addressed in order to prevent the following problems: 1) increased energy expenditure during ambulation;

2) cosmetically altered gait; 3) use of a shoe lift; 4) equinus contracture of the ankle; 5) scoliosis and low back problems; and 6) late degenerative arthritis of the hip. Leg length discrepancies should be measured on physical examination using blocks on the shortened extremity and radiographically using scanograms or orthoroentograms. Using radiographic measurements, the patient's growth can be plotted on the Green-Anderson graph or Moseley straight-line graph. These radiographs should be performed and the results plotted annually so the practitioner can see a trend. Skeletal age should be determined at every visit by obtaining a left hand and wrist radiograph, which can be compared with normal standards in an atlas. One should plan surgery based only on the anticipated discrepancy at maturity, not the present discrepancy. This data can be obtained using either the Green-Anderson data or the Moseley straight-line graph.

Growth discrepancies <2 cm at maturity can easily be treated with a shoe lift or ignored. Leg length discrepancies of 2–5 cm are typically well-treated with an epiphysiodesis. The appropriate time and location of the epiphysiodesis is determined using the straight-line graph or using the Green-Anderson data. On average, the distal femur contributes $\frac{3}{8}$ inch (0.9 cm) of growth annually, the proximal tibia contributes $\frac{2}{8}$ inch (0.6 cm) of growth annually, and the distal tibia contributes $\frac{1}{8}$ inch (0.3 cm) of growth annually until the male is 16 or the female is 14 years of age. This is easy to remember since it is $\frac{3}{8}$, $\frac{2}{8}$, and and $\frac{1}{8}$ as one moves down the extremity. It is important to attempt to make the knees level at maturity if at all possible. This can affect the level and location of the epiphysiodesis.

Lengthening techniques are used for discrepancies >6 cm. Most lengthenings utilize the Ilizarov principles, which include a metaphyseal corticotomy in which the medullary canal and blood supply are preserved followed by gradual lengthening of 1 mm per day. This lengthening requires the placement of a ring external fixator (Ilizarov apparatus).

Children with a leg length discrepancy that cannot be treated by epiphysiodesis or lengthening can sometimes be treated by femoral shortening. These are often performed in the subtrochanteric region to avoid relative lengthenings of the quadricep muscles and subsequent temporary weakness of the knee. Shortenings can also be performed in the midshaft using a closed nailing technique to avoid excessive scarring.

CERVICAL SPINE DEFORMITY

The cervical spine deformities that will be discussed include Klippel-Feil syndrome and os odontoideum. Torticollis was discussed earlier in the section on birth injuries.

Klippel-Feil Syndrome[1,2]

Klippel-Feil syndrome is typified by congenital fusions of the cervical vertebrae. Half of the patients present with the classic triad of low posterior hairline, short neck, and limited neck motion. Anomalies associated with Klippel-Feil syndrome are congenital scoliosis, Sprengel's deformity, renal anomalies, deafness, synkinesis (mirror movements), pulmonary dysfunction, and congenital heart disease. Renal ultrasound and pediatric evaluation should be part of the normal workup.

A-P and lateral C-spine films, as well as flexion/extension views, are needed to assess hypermobility and possible instability. An MRI should be obtained if there is concern for neurological dysfunction. Children with Klippel-Feil syndrome who develop mechanical symptoms should be treated with activity restriction, cervical traction, soft collars and analgesics. When neurologic symptoms arise because of instability, surgical fusion, often from C1 to 2 with a Gallie fusion, should be undertaken.

Os Odontoideum[1,2]

Os odontoideum is an entity in which the tip of the odontoid process is separated by a wide transverse gap from the remainder of C2. The frequency of this entity is unknown but is thought to be caused by damage to the base of the odontoid or damage to the epiphyseal plate during the first few years of life interrupting blood supply. Children often present with neck pain, and there is often some concern of an acute dens fracture, but this is not the case. Typically, the os odontoideum is an oval or round ossicle with a smooth sclerotic border.

FOOT PROBLEMS IN CHILDREN

Clubfoot (Congenital Talipes Equinovarus)[1]

Clubfoot is a complex foot deformity that consists of hindfoot equinus, forefoot, and heel varus, and an adducted forefoot. The overall incidence is approximately 1 per 1000 children. Boys are affected twice as often as girls, and half of all cases are bilateral. Despite strong evidence for genetic causes of clubfoot, many support extrinsic causes. Many think that intrauterine crowding is the primary reason for clubfoot, but this is not supported by an increased occurrence of the deformity in high birth-weight babies or multiparity. There are also data gained from the examination of stillbirths that point to a possible germ plasm defect during embryological development. Others think that the obvious relationship with arthrogryposis, myelomeningocele, and other inherited disorders indicates that neuromuscular causes are responsible for clubfoot deformities. Practitioners should be aware that clubfeet that are associated with constriction band syndrome, diastrophic dwarfism, arthrogryposis, and myelomeningocele are different, often more severe entities than idiopathic clubfeet and should be treated more cautiously.

Examination of the patient with a clubfoot should include thorough examination of the spine, looking for signs of deformity, examination of the neck to rule out torticollis, inspection of the hips to rule out DDH, and evaluation of the lower extremities to rule out pathologic torsional deformities. Parents should be told that a clubfoot will always be smaller and stiffer than the contralateral foot. Additionally, the ipsilateral calf will be smaller. There is a wide spectrum of severity, ranging from postural clubfeet that are easily treated with serial casting to resistant clubfeet that, despite casting, usually require operative intervention. In these children, the hindfoot will obviously be in equinus and varus, and the calcaneus itself will be in severe equinus, causing an easily palpable fat pad that is empty. The tibionavicular interval will be extremely small and often will be absent in severe clubfeet. The normally palpable sinus tarsi will be absent. The forefoot will be supinated and adducted.

When clubfeet have been resistant to efforts at serial casting every 1–2 weeks, radiographs should be obtained. These should include A-P and lateral views, as well as stress dorsiflexion and plantar-flexion lateral views. The most obvious radiographic finding is "parallelism" on the A-P views and the stressed lateral views. This means the relationship between the calcaneus and the talus remains constant despite full plantar or dorsiflexion. Additionally, Kite's angle, which refers to the talocalcaneal angle on the A-P view, will be less than 20 degrees and near 0 degrees. This angle is normally 20–40 degrees. The forefoot is often obviously adducted on the A-P view. In the normal foot, the long axis of the talus should be in line with the axis of the first metatarsal or pass just medial to it. The calcaneocuboid axis normally passes between the fourth and fifth metatarsals. In a clubfoot, these radiographic landmarks are clearly disrupted. Additionally, metatarsal "stacking" is notable on the lateral view, indicating forefoot supination.

The untreated severe congenital clubfoot develops progressive deformity as the patient matures. In the severe situation, the patient ultimately develops a large callous on the dorsolateral aspect of the foot that he uses for weight bearing. Progressive arthritic changes develop requiring extensive shoe modifications. Despite these modifications, these patients ultimately develop severe pain during ambulation and are forced to live with severely compromised feet.

The goal of treatment of the congenital talipes equinovarus is to get a functional, pain-free, plantigrade foot with adequate mobility and without sign of excessive wear (callous). Depending on one's definition of a clubfoot, serial casting has varying levels of success. Most pediatric orthopaedists think that a true clubfoot cannot be treated by casting alone. Many will utilize preoperative casting in order to help stretch the skin and the neurovascular structures in anticipation of surgical posteromedial release (PMR). This procedure releases all the posteromedial structures as necessary to get the foot in a plantigrade position. It is preferably performed around 6–9 months of age. PMR includes division of the calcaneal and navicular heads of the adductor hallucis, Z-lengthening of the PTT, FDL, and FHL, as well as the Achilles tendon. Also released are the tibiotalar and talonavicular ligaments, as well as the spring ligament. The calcaneocuboid capsule is opened by some surgeons. Additionally, many will open the posterior aspects of the ankle and the subtalar joints, as well as release the calcaneofibular ligament and the posterior talofibular ligament, and release portions of the superficial and deep deltoid. Other structures that can be released for severe clubfeet include the plantar fascia and the interosseous talocalcaneal ligament. Many surgeons use pins to keep the foot in position following surgery.

Patients who are older and have recurrent clubfeet, or were simply late in presentation, are often treated with revision PMR with a medial opening and/or lateral column shortening osteotomy. When children are 10 to 12 years old or older, triple arthrodesis may be the only option. Children who have surgery for clubfoot reconstruction require reoperation 25% of the time. This number probably rises if surgery is delayed.

Metatarsus Adductus[1,2]

Metatarsus adductus refers to adduction of the forefoot with varying degrees of forefoot supination. There is no associated hindfoot equinus or varus, and, in fact, the heel is often in slight valgus. The incidence is 1 per 1000 live births, and the male-to-female ratio shows minimal male predominance. This defect is thought to be the result of tight intrauterine packing and is associated with hip dysplasia and torticollis. Bleck observed that the line bisecting the heel should pass through the second and third toes in the normal foot. Metatarsus adductus was judged to be normal, mild, moderate, or severe depending on the location of this line as it exited the foot distally. Most children with metatarsus adductus demonstrate some progression until age 1–2 years, when the deformity begins to regress, resulting in a completely normal foot or a mild flatfoot deformity. Treatment is given to children with some rigidity. Modalities include simple stretching and observation, plaster casts, and corrective shoes. Surgical management of metatarsus adductus is rarely undertaken and involves high complication rates. The usual indications are for a child older than 3–4 years old with residual metatarsus adductus. Multiple complications including painful scars, and AVN of the second or third cuneiforms and late degenerative arthritis can occur. Rarely, multiple metatarsal osteotomies are performed for this problem.

Congenital Calcaneovalgus Foot[1]

Congenital calcaneovalgus foot is the most frequent deformity seen at birth, occurring in 30%–50% of all live births. In this condition, the foot is acutely dorsiflexed and the dorsum of the foot is actually in contact with the anterior shin. It is thought to be caused by intrauterine positioning. This deformity is usually supple, and the foot can be put into some plantar flexion and supination. This condition nearly always resolves without any treatment at all. This benign condition must be differentiated from congenital vertical talus, which is a fixed deformity with a rounded sole and in which the hindfoot is actually in equinus.

Flexible Flatfoot[1]

Children with a flexible flatfoot have little or no longitudinal arch when standing. The arch is re-created when the child assumes a sitting position or when he is instructed to go up on his toes. In the child who is greater than 2–3 years old, the absence of these two features may indicate that the child has a stiff flatfoot, which is often a pathologic entity. Children <3 years old frequently have a minimal longitudinal arch and because of excessive ligamentous laxity, may have flatfeet that are quite severe in appearance. For the most part, flexible flatfeet tend to be completely asymptomatic for children and have not been documented to cause disablity in adulthood.

Most patients will be able to report another family member with similar feet. Mostly people with flat feet have a bilateral deformity. It is crucial that the foot is clearly supple with normal subtalar and midtarsal motion. It is also important to make sure that the heelcord is not tight, since this can lead to progressive midfoot breakdown and lead to arthritis in the adult.

There is no evidence that use of supports or corrective shoes will lead to permanent formation of a longitudinal arch. If a patient gets symptomatic relief from an orthotic, one should encourage the patient to purchase an off-the-shelf product if at all possible to keep down costs. The most common treatment is a $\frac{1}{8}$-inch sole wedge and a Thomas heel.

Surgical management is never indicated for a child. In the adolescent nearing skeletal maturity, surgery may be indicated only when the flatfoot is severe and painful. Possible procedures include sliding calcaneal osteotomies or calcaneal lengthening procedures.

Congenital Vertical Talus (CVT)[1]

Congenital vertical talus, often known as rocker-bottom foot, is caused by an irreducible dorsal dislocation of the navicular on a fixed talocalcaneal complex in which the talus is medially rotated and plantar flexed and the calcaneous is everted and in equinus. This rare entity is frequently associated with other congenital anomalies. Up to 10% of children with myelodysplasia have CVT. This condition is also associated with DDH, arthrogryposis, and trisomy 13, 14, 15, and 18. In isolated cases of CVT, there appears to be a genetic connection in which transmission is by an autosomal dominant trait with incomplete penetrance.

Clinically, the plantar aspect of the foot is rocker-bottom in appearance. The heel is in fixed equinovalgus and the head of the talus is palpable medially on the sole. The patient often bears weight on the talar head, causing a painful callous. Additionally, the forefoot is abducted and slightly dorsiflexed at the midtarsal joint. This condition is usually easy to distinquish from the more common calcaneovalgus foot or the flexible flatfoot. Radiographically, the head of the talus is medial and plantar, with the most posterior portion of the talus actually in contact with the distal tibia. The navicular, which ossifies at age 3, is usually not visible at the time of diagnosis, but it rests on the dorsal surface of the talus. Diagnosis is confirmed by obtaining a lateral stress plantarflexion view demonstrating that the relation of the talus to the navicular bone is fixed and the talocalcaneal angle is unchanged.

Serial casting with manipulation is tried initially but is rarely helpful. Early aggressive surgery with soft-tissue release, tendon lengthening, reduction, and pinning of the talonavicular and subtalar joints prior to age 12 months offers the best chance for a normal foot. If children are between 1 and 2 years of age, many will often include a subtalar fusion, as well. Subtalar fusion can be performed as late as 6–8 years of age with some benefit. Once children are older than this, correction can only be performed by triple arthrodesis usually requiring excision of a large portion of the talus. Talectomy and excision of the navicular are no longer accepted as surgical options.

Congenital Oblique Talus[1,2]

Congenital oblique talus is a talonavicular subluxation similar to CVT, but is less severe, since the navicular can be reduced on the talus with plantar flexion of the forefoot. This condition should be treated nonoperatively with observation and sometimes a UCBL insert.

Cavus Foot[1]

Cavus foot is a complex deformity consisting of elevation of the longitudinal arch. The condition is referred to as cavovarus when the first metatarsal is in hyperflexion. When the calcaneous is in excessive calcaneus position (opposite of equinus) because of weakness of the calf musculature, the condition is referred to as calcaneocavus foot.

These deformities are usually owing to neuromuscular diseases causing muscle imbalance, producing deformity. Charcot-Marie-Tooth (CMT), Friedreich's ataxia, CP, polio, tethered cord, and myelodysplasia are frequent causes of this abnormality. Management guidelines can be found in those sections.

Tarsal Coalition[1,2]

Tarsal coalition is a fibrous, cartilaginous, or bony connection of two or more tarsal bones leading to a rigid flatfoot. This autosomal dominant disorder is frequently referred to as peroneal spastic flatfoot, but, in reality, peroneal spasiticity is rarely noted, though these muscles are typically contracted and pain is elicited during attempted inversion of the hindfoot. The most frequently involved joint is the calcaneonavicular joint followed closely by the talocalcaneal joint (usually the middle facet).

Patients present with a vague insidious aching pain that worsens with activity and improves with rest. Many think that the onset of pain correlates with the age at which the bar ossifies. Symptoms usually begin at age 3–5 in talonavicular coalitions, 8–12 in calcaneonavicular coalitions, and 12–16 in talocalcaneal coalitions. Pes planus and ankle valgus are often clinically apparent.

Radiographic evaluation includes A-P, lateral, and oblique views. The calcaneonavicular coalition is typically visualized on the 45-degree oblique view. The "anteater nose," a prolongation of the anterior aspect of the superior calcaneous, is frequently seen in the lateral view in those with a calcaneonavicular coalition. Talocalcaneal coalition is best seen on the Harris heel view, which demonstrates obliteration of the middle facet, which is typically dorsal to the medial aspect of the posterior facet. Other secondary radiographic changes include talar beaking, broadening or rounding of the lateral process of the talus, and narrowing of the subtalar joint. Sometimes a ball and socket ankle develops, perhaps to compensate for lost subtalar motion. CT scans are used for diagnosing coalitions, ruling out multiple coalitions, and for documenting the area involved by a particular coalition. Since we are not sure how many patients with a single symptomatic coalition have multiple coalitions, many suggest that all patients have CT scans.

Initial treatment should be conservative, since many adults have asymptomatic tarsal coalitions. First-line therapy should involve activity modification, NSAIDs, and orthotics. Secondary treatments may involve joint injection with a steroid preparation and 3–6 weeks of immobilization in a short leg walking cast. Injection of the peroneal muscles, nerve blocks, and manipulation under anesthesia are no longer advised.

The main indication for surgery is persistent pain despite nonoperative modalities. For calcaneonavicular bars, resection of the bar and interposition of the extensor digitorum brevis is the treatment of choice and has been successful in several trials. Talocalcaneal coalitions are more difficult to treat. Bar resection is indicated when less than 50% of the articular surface is involved and there are no degenerative changes or malalignment. If these conditions are not met, subtalar arthrodesis is probably indicated. If the bar is to be resected, many use fat for interposition. A calcaneal osteotomy is sometimes utilized to bring the heel out of valgus. In patients who have diffuse degenerative changes, triple arthrodesis may be performed, though this is not indicated until late adolescence or adulthood.

Accessory Navicular[1]

Accessory navicular is the most common accessory bone in the foot. This a normal variant seen in up to 12% of the population. It is often associated with flatfoot and can cause arch pain with overuse. On physical examination, these patients have a prominence on the medial aspect of the foot and have tenderness at the talonavicular joint near the insertion of the PTT. The pain is exacerbated by foot inversion against resistance. The accessory navicular is typically best seen on the external oblique radiographic view of the foot. Symptoms tend to improve by activity and/or shoe modification. Temporary immobilization may decrease discomfort. Surgical management is indicated for resistant cases and involves resection of the navicular with repair of the posterior tibialis tendon where the ossicle is excised.

Kohler's Disease[1,2]

Kohler's disease is thought to be secondary to osteonecrosis and occurs in children around 4–5 years of age. They present with midtarsal pain that is present with weight bearing and relieved by rest. Radiographically, the tarsal navicular is seen to densify, fragment, eventually narrow, and then later actually reconstitute. It is a self-limiting phenomenon that should be treated with a walking cast for 3–6 weeks.

Freiberg Infraction[1,2]

Freiberg infraction is a rare clinical condition found in adolescents complaining of pain over the second metatarsal head. The etiology is unknown, though some suggest it is owing to a short second metatarsal. Radiographically, the physis demonstrates irregularity and collapse. If the physis is closed, the metatarsal head is often enlarged, flattened, and irregular. Treatment is nearly always nonoperative and initially includes various orthotic devices including metatarsal bars. Occasionally, a walking cast may be effective in reducing symptoms.

Sever's Disease[1,2]

Sever's disease is calcaneal apophysitis that frequently occurs in children who are overweight and physically active. These children present with heel pain and tenderness over the posterior portion of the calcaneous. A lateral radiograph of the foot will often demonstrate irregularity of the calcaneal apophysis.

The differential diagnosis of heel pain in children includes unicameral bone cysts, aneurysmal bone cysts, and osteoid osteoma. Tarsal coalition, osteomyelitis, or septic arthritis should be ruled out. Rarely, a fracture or tendonitis can be the source of discomfort. Rheumatologic conditions like JRA or Reiter's syndrome should also be ruled out. Treatment should begin with nonsteroidals and heelcord stretches. Restriction of activities and heel cups and pads are secondary modalities.

Idiopathic Toe Walking[1]

Children who present with toe walking must be evaluated for CP, muscular dystrophy, spinal dysraphism, and myopathies. Children who are found to have none of these disorders are thought to be idiopathic toe walkers. Clinical examination is aimed at ruling out any neurological disorder and then evaluation of the tightness of the heelcord. If the child's foot can be dorsiflexed beyond neutral with the knee extended, the child should be placed in an AFO to attempt to break his ambulatory pattern. If the heelcord is tight, serial casts should be placed until his heelcord is loose enough to allow him to get into an AFO. Hoke tendo-Achilles lengthening is indicated for appropriate candidates who continue to toe walk after age 6–7 years.

Polydactyly[1]

Polydactyly is a common foot deformity in which one or more toes are duplicated. This tends to run in families, and duplication is more often on the lateral aspect of the foot. Patients present shortly after birth or when they have difficulty wearing shoes. In complicated cases, operative intervention should be postponed as long as possible to allow as much ossification as possible for better resection and subsequent reconstruction. Operative planning involves avoiding scars that will cause painful shoe wear and planning reconstruction of tendons or collateral ligaments.

INFECTIONS

Osteomyelitis[1]

Osteomyelitis occurs frequently during childhood because of blood sludging in the metaphysis where small arterial loops empty into venous sinuses, resulting in turbulence and poor flow. Hematogenous seeding of the bone just distal to the physis occurs in these venous pools, creating bone abscesses because of poor phagocytosis in this region. Osteomyelitis has a predilection for the fastest growing regions (e.g., distal femur and proximal tibia). An abscess will often collect just beneath the periosteum, causing pressure necrosis on the cortical bone. This bone may die and subsequently form a sequestrum.

Like in septic arthritis, the chief presenting complaint is often refusal to bear weight, limping, or disuse of an extremity. Fever and other systemic signs may be present but often are not. Occasionally, the child will present with a tender, warm, swollen region over a bony metaphysis. In history taking, one should try to understand how long the child has been ill and whether any antibiotics have been taken. Chickenpox is a common childhood illness that causes a temporary suppression of immunity often leading to infections by *Staphylococcus aureus* and group A streptococcus.

During the physical examination, the parent can be instructed in range-of-motion assessment if the child is not cooperating. The parent can also be told how to palpate the extremity to assess tenderness.

In a series from the Mayo clinic, only 25% of infants and children with osteomyelitis had a WBC count above normal for their age. ESR elevation is more notable in osteomyelitis than in septic arthritis. This nonspecific indicator will be elevated within 2–3 days of infection onset. A more precise indicator is C-reactive protein (CRP). This will tend to elevate within 1–2 days of the onset of infection and will reduce to normal levels much sooner compared with ESR. Blood cultures will demonstrate the organism between 30% and 50% of the time for both osteomyelitis and septic arthritis. Bone aspirates yield positive cultures 50%–70% of the time. A STAT Gram stain is important to guide early antibiotic coverage. In neonates, group B strep is the most common organism. *S. aureus* is the most common organism overall. *Haemophilus influenzae* is also common in children 6 months to 4 years of age. Emperic therapy is typically cefotaxime (Claforan) in the neonates and cefazolin in older children.

Plain radiographs often demonstrate deep soft-tissue swelling and loss of normal tissue planes. Bone resorption and periosteal reaction are rarely noted. Technetium bone scan is occasionally used to identify the area of pathology in an uncooperative young child who refuses to ambulate and examination does not identify a specific site. The sensitivity and specificity are approximately both 90%. Keep in mind that a "cold scan" can indicate acute devascularization of bone caused by a tense subperiosteal abscess. Aspiration of the bone prior to the bone scan does not alter the results of the scan. An MRI can be useful to help delineate the extent of the infection.

The differential diagnosis for osteomyelitis includes trauma, neoplasm, and bone infarction. The most common malignancy in childhood is leukemia, and many of these children will present with bone pain and systemic manifestations. Anemia and low platelets should arouse suspicion of leukemia. Other less common neoplasms include metastatic neuroblastoma, eosinophilic granuloma, and Ewing's sarcoma. Bone infarctions are frequently seen with Gaucher's disease.

Septic Arthritis[1,2]

Septic arthritis occurs at twice the rate of osteomyelitis in childhood, with its peak incidence in the early years of the first decade.

Similar to osteomyelitis, physical examination is often vague and diagnosis is sometimes difficult. Septic arthritis can be caused by hematogenous spread or by local spread from metaphyseal osteomyelitis. This is especially true in joints in which the metaphysis is intraarticular (hip, elbow, shoulder). Infection in the joint causes rapid cartilage destruction, and septic arthritis is subsequently a surgical emergency. As with osteomyelitis, pain is the leading symptom, with the child refusing to bear weight or refusing to use an extremity. Again, parents can be helpful in performing the physical examination. An infected joint will have an effusion and, if the joint is not covered by large amounts of soft tissue, this can often be palpated. An infected joint usually has a limited range of motion and should be painful through anything but a small range of motion. In the hip, internal rotation, which tightens the hip capsule, is especially painful and limited.

WBC may only be elevated in about a quarter of patients and is not a reliable test. ESR should be elevated above 20 in more than 90% of the cases but is often not elevated until the infection is 2–3 days old. The ESR should not be diminished by previous antibiotic therapy. ESR is unreliable in the neonate in the presence of a significant anemia or in children with sickle cell disease. CRP begins to rise within 6 hours of infection and reaches a peak within 2 days. CRP also begins to drop much sooner than ESR when the infection is being properly treated.

Blood cultures should always be performed, since they are positive 30%–50% of the time. Aspiration of the joint should always be attempted, as it can offer an opportunity for organism identification, as well as cell count. Joint fluid should be sent for Gram stain, culture and sensitivity, cell count and differential (Table 10.1). Positive yields from joint aspirate range from 36%–80% in the literature. When children are less than 12 months of age, the most common organisms are *S. aureus* and group B strep, and empiric antibiotics should include first-generation cephalosporins. When the child is 6 months to 5 years of age, the most common organisms are *S. aureus* and *H. influenzae,* and a second- or third-generation cephalosporin is indicated. During ages 5–12 years old, the most common organism is *S. aureus,* and a first-generation cephalosporin is indicated. From ages 12–18 years old, the most common organisms are *S. aureus* and *N. gonorrhoeae,* and oxacillin and a first-generation cephalosporin should be utilized empirically. Of course, these antibiotic choices should be altered when one has Gram stain and culture

Table 10.1
Synovial Fluid Analysis

Disease	Leukocytes[a]	Polymorphs[a] (%)
Normal	<200	<25
Traumatic	<5000 with many erythrocytes	<25
Toxic synovitis	5000–15,000	<25
Acute rheumatic fever	10,000–15,000	50
Juvenile rheumatoid arthritis	15,000–80,000	75
Septic arthritis	>80,000	>75

[a] The leukocyte count and percentage of polymorphs can vary in most diseases depending on the severity and duration of the process. Overlap greater than shown in these averages is possible.

Morrissy RT. Septic arthritis. In: Gustilo RB, Genninger RP, Tsukayama DJ, eds. Orthopaedic infection: diagnosis and treatment. Philadelphia: WB Saunders, 1989.

information. One should also recall that lumbar punctures should be considered in a septic joint infected by *H. influenzae,* because there is about a 30% risk of meningitis. If an LP is not performed, antibiotic therapy must be able to cross the blood-brain barrier.

Radiographically, joint space widening is often seen in septic arthritis of the hip. This may be caused by the position of external rotation and abduction assumed by the irritable hip to reduce intracapsular pressure. Again, a bone scan is very helpful in identifying the reason that the child is unwilling to ambulate. As with osteomyelitis, specificity and sensitivity are both around 90%. Unfortunately, a bone scan often does not separate bone from joint sepsis. Additionally, it does not differentiate infectious from noninfectious arthritis. This is particularly problematic in the hip, where the differential diagnosis includes transient synovitis and septic arthritis. Again, aspiration of the joint prior to bone scan does not alter the scan.

The differential diagnosis for septic arthritis includes JRA, toxic synovitis, rheumatic fever, and Henoch-Schönlein purpura. In JRA, the child has a more gradual onset of pain and is usually able to remain ambulatory. The synovial fluid leukocyte count is usually less than 100,000 per milliliter, unlike sepsis, where there is usually more than 100,000. In toxic synovitis, there is usually a longer history with both improvement and worsening. In septic arthritis, the pain is usually worse and the motion more restricted than in toxic synovitis. With rheumatic fever, there should be a history of an untreated pharyngitis, febrile illness, or rash owing to group A streptococcus about 2 weeks before the joint swelling began. Henoch-Schönlein purpura is a vasculitis of unknown origin and typically manifests itself with a purpuric rash, abdominal pain, arthritis, and nephritis.

NEUROMUSCULAR DISORDERS

Muscular Dystrophies

Muscular dystrophies are a group of noninflammatory, inherited disorders with progressive degeneration and weakness of skeletal muscle without obvious neurological cause.

Duchenne Muscular Dystrophy[1]

Duchenne muscular dystrophy is the most common type of muscular dystrophy. Transmission is by an X-linked recessive trait, and the disease is characterized by occurrence in males except for rare cases associated with Turner's syndrome. There is a high mutation rate, so positive family history is present in only 65% of cases. This occurs in 1 in 3500 male births.

Duchenne muscular dystrophy (DMD) is often diagnosed when the child is between 3 and 6 years old and is noted to have continued difficulty with independent ambulation. There is progressive weakness in the proximal muscle groups that is most notable in the lower extremities. The gluteus maximus and other hip extensors are the first muscles affected. Patients compensate for this by carrying the weight of their head and shoulders behind the pelvis, creating an exaggerated lumbar lordosis. These children develop mild hip abduction contractures that make standing somewhat precarious. The lumbar lordosis creates excessive anterior tilt of the pelvis. Also one notices pseudohypertrophy of the calves caused by the accumulation of fat around the musculature. The tibialis posterior is one of the last muscles affected, so patients typically develop an inversion or varus deformity of the foot owing to overpowered peroneals. Weakness of the shoulder girdle occurs 3–5 years later and precludes use of crutches for ambulation. Early in the disease, patients will demonstrate a Gower's sign when placed prone or sitting on the floor and instructed to get up. A positive sign is noted when the patient needs to use his hands to push off his legs in order to stand up. These patients are free of sensory deficits. Upper extremity and patellar tendon reflexes are lost early in the disease. Ankle reflexes remain positive until the later stages of the disease.

Serum CPK is markedly elevated in the early stages of DMD. EMG demonstrates reduced amplitude, short duration, and polyphasic motor action potentials. Muscle biopsy shows degeneration with varying amounts of fibrosis and the proliferation of connective and adipose tissue.

Treatment of the patient with DMD includes physical therapy directed toward prolonging muscle use and joint flexibility. AFOs and KAFOs are used as the patient ages and independent ambulation becomes difficult around age 10. Wheelchairs are used after age 10, when the patient begins losing the ability to walk. When ambulation ceases, 90% of patients with DMD develop a progressive kyphoscoliosis that requires posterior fusion from the thoracic spine to the pelvis once the curve is greater than 20 degrees. This will help prevent a kyphoscoliosis that is out of control and can help prolong the patient's life. Other surgeries include release of contractures in order to improve ambulation and improve performance with ADLs. Most of these children develop progressive pulmonary and cardiac difficulties and die before age 20.

Spinal Muscular Atrophy (SMA)[1,2]

Spinal muscular atrophy is characterized by degeneration of the anterior horn cells of the spinal cord, resulting in muscle weakness and atrophy. The loss of anterior horn cells is a one-time event without progression. The progressive muscle weakness that occurs in this disease is a reflection of normal growth exceeding reserve. This disorder occurs in about 1 in 20,000 births, and is divided into three subtypes ranging in severity from severe to mild.

Type 1 (acute Werdnig-Hoffman disease) is clinically apparent before 6 months of age. These children have severe involvement with marked weakness and hypotonia and tend to die prior to their second birthday.

Type 2 (chronic Werdnig-Hoffmann disease) is notable for clinical onset between 6 and 24 months of age. These children are never able to walk but do tend to live into their fourth and fifth decades.

Type 3 (Kugelberg-Welander disease) spinal muscular atrophy has clinical onset after 2 years of age and usually before 10 years of age. Walking is possible until early adolescence, though these children are not able to run. The mobility of these children usually decreases as they age. Like DMD, they will often have pseudohypertrophy of the calves and a positive Gower sign. Unlike children with DMD, they have normal intelligence and function well in society.

These children develop contractures that are difficult to treat and tend to recur after the child becomes wheelchair bound. Children with Types 2 and 3 will also often develop progressive hip subluxation leading to dislocation if they are not followed closely. Soft-tissue releases and sometimes proximal femoral osteotomies are often required. Spinal deformity develops in 100% of the children with Type 2 and a large percentage with Type 3 SMA. The thoracolumbar paralytic C-shaped and single thoracic patterns curve to the right and are the most frequent pattern. One-third of children have an associated kyphoscoliosis. Children with Type 2 SMA have curves that are much more progressive than those with Type 3. Braces are used to delay curve progression when the curve is between 20 and 40 degrees. When the curve is >40 degrees, posterior spinal fusion with segmental spinal instrumentation from the thoracic spine to the pelvis is performed.

Friedreich's Ataxia[1]

Friedreich's ataxia is typified by slow, progressive spinocerebellar degeneration occurring in 1 in 50,000 live births. Friedreich's ataxia typically presents with a triad including ataxia, areflexia of the knees and ankles, and a positive Babinski sign. Onset is typically between 7 and 15 years of age and always before 25 years of age. Other secondary symptoms include dysarthria, scoliosis, pyramidal weakness in the lower extremities, absent upper extremity reflexes, and loss of position and vibratory sense in the lower extremities. Patients also develop clinical evidence of diabetes mellitus and a progressive hypertrophic cardiomyopathy. Ataxia is the primary cause for the loss of ambulation, which usually occurs in the second or third decade. Muscle weakness is a secondary cause (esp. gluteus maximus). Death usually occurs in the fourth or fifth decade owing to progressive hypertrophic cardiomyopathy, pneumonia, or aspiration.

Besides neurologic sequelae, the central orthopaedic problems are cavovarus feet, scoliosis, and painful muscular spasms. Orthotic management with AFOs is usually ineffective for the cavovarus. Surgery includes Achilles lengthening and PTT tenotomy, lengthening, or anterior transfer to the dorsum of the foot. Rigid foot deformities often require triple arthrodesis in addition to soft-tissue procedures. Scoliosis tends to progress to greater than 60 degrees when disease onset is before 10 years of age and tends to remain less than 40 degrees if disease onset is after 10. The cause of the scoliosis in Friedreich's ataxia appears to be the ataxia that causes a disturbance in equilibrium and postural reflexes. Muscle weakness is a secondary factor at best. A TLSO may be useful for curves from 25–40 degrees. Curves greater than 60 degrees require posterior segmental fusion from the thorax to the lower lumbar region. Anterior surgery is rarely required except for large or rigid curves.

Charcot-Marie-Tooth Disease (CMT)[1,2]

Charcot-Marie-Tooth disease is the prototype for a group of inherited neuropathic disorders referred to as hereditary motor sensory neuropathies (HMSN). These neuropathies are broken into seven groups (the first three involve children). HMSN Type 1 refers to an AD disorder that is referred to as peroneal atrophy, Charcot-Marie-Tooth disease, or Roussy-Lévy syndrome. This is a demyelinating disorder typified by a peroneal muscle weakness, absent DTRs, and slow NCVs. HMSN Type 2 is the neuronal form of CMT that is characterized by persistently normal reflexes, sensory and motor nerve conduction times that are only mildly abnormal, and variable inheritance patterns. These two types are clinically similar, though HMSN Type 2 is less severe and tends to have a later onset. Type 3 is an AR disorder referred to as Dejerine-Sottas disease. This typically begins in infancy and is characterized by alterations in nerve conductions and sensory disturbances that delay ambulation and cause deformity at an earlier age.

Orthopaedic manifestations include cavovarus feet, hammer toes, peroneal weakness, and the appearance of "stork legs." Around 5%–10% of children with HMSN develop hip dysplasia usually between ages 5 and 15 years. Scoliosis occurs in approximately 10% of children with HMSN and is managed similarly to idiopathic adolescent scoliosis except that there is an increased incidence of kyphosis.

Most patients are referred to orthopaedic surgeons because of foot deformities. Plantar and medial releases are often indicated in children younger than 10 years old who have a flexible cavovarus deformity. Adolescents with flexible deformity frequently require these releases and tendon transfers including anterior tibialis transfer to the third cuneiform or a split posterior tibialis transfer. Flexor to extensor tendon transfers are sometimes required for claw toes.

If there is any evidence of any foot stiffness, a *Coleman block test* can distinguish a fixed deformity from a supple one. Children who have a mild but fixed deformity may be candidates for the soft-tissue procedures previously mentioned, as well as a calcaneal osteotomy to correct the varus deformity of the hind foot. Stiffer feet may require a midtarsal osteotomy in which the proximal osteotomy cut is through the navicular and cuboid bones and the distal cut is through the cuboid and the three cuneiforms, removing a dorsal and slightly lateral wedge of bone. This is frequently augmented with soft-tissue releases and a calcaneal osteotomy. Adolescents who have reached skeletal maturity and have stiff, severe deformities are candidates for triple arthrodesis. Interphalangeal joint fusions are often performed for claw toes at this point. An extensor hallucis longus transfer to the neck of the first metatarsal (Jones procedure) will help to dorsiflex the first MT.

Additionally, these people also have diminution of distal light touch, position, and vibratory sensation of the hands and feet. Two-thirds also have intrinsic muscle weakness in the hands.

Poliomyelitis[1]

Poliomyelitis is the result of an acute viral infection of anterior horn cells of the spinal cord and certain brainstem motor nuclei. Disease transmission is by the oropharyngeal route initially causing a gastroenteritis. A small percentage of people then have hematogenous spread to the central nervous system. After an incubation period of 6–20 days, the anterior horn cells of the spinal cord are attacked, causing extensive scarring in the region

and loss of motor function to upper and lower extremity musculature. Lower extremities are affected twice as often as upper extremities.

Poliomyelitis is divided into three stages—acute stage, convalescent stage, and chronic stage. In the United States, physicians
rarely see the acute or convalescent stage. The chronic stage is
sometimes seen when a child has been adopted to an American
home from a nonindustrialized nation.

The chronic stage of poliomyelitis begins after 2 years and
this involves the long-term management of deformity resulting
from muscle imbalance. This involves release of soft-tissue contractures, tendon transfers, and bony procedures like osteotomies
and arthrodesis.

Osteogenesis Imperfecta (OI)[1]

Osteogenesis imperfecta is an inheritable disorder of type 1 collagen, resulting in bone and ligament abnormalities. Clinical features include bone fragility, short stature, scoliosis, defective den-
tition, middle ear deafness, laxity of ligaments, blue sclera, and
blue tympanic membranes. Distingishing OI from child abuse is
often difficult. One should keep in mind that fractures from
child abuse most often occur before age 3. Children with OI
tend to present early in life, as well, but they will often have a
positive family history, dental or eye changes, and diffuse radiographic changes.

The disease is thought of by many as a continuum of severity
with different inheritance patterns. In the Sillence classification,
Type 1 (AD inheritance) has bone fragility and blue sclerae with
onset of fractures around preschool age. Type 2 (AR inheritance)
is lethal in the perinatal period, with children often being born
with multiple fractures and dark blue sclerae. Type 3 (AR) presents with fractures at birth that heal readily but with progressive
deformity. Sclerae and hearing are normal. Type 4 is of AD
inheritance presenting with bone fragility, normal sclerae, and
good hearing.

Orthopaedic management of patients with Type 1 OI involves
standard fracture care. Children with type 2 typically die prior
to requiring orthopaedic help. Types 3 and 4 are the groups that
pose the greatest challenge for the orthopaedic surgeon. Dietary
treatments have not proved effective. Many advocate bracing in

order to prevent fractures. A parapodium is often used to get the child accustomed to an upright posture. Prior to age 5 a closed fracture treatment strategy is elected. After 5, intramedullary rodding of the long bones of the lower extremities has been accepted for managing recurrent fractures and resultant deformity in order to maintain function. The two rods that are most frequently used are Rush rods, which require exchanges as the child grows, and the Bailey-Dubow rods, which elongate as the child grows. Sofield osteotomies are performed for fracture treatment, as well as prevention of progressive bone deformity.

Scoliosis occurs in 50% of the patients and is difficult to treat because bracing is ineffective and curves tend to progress out of control. Current therapy favors posterior fusion using segmental fixation once the curve has progressed beyond 40 degrees.

Radiographs demonstrate thin cortices. Histologically, widened Haversian canals and osteocyte lacunae are visualized. Fracture healing is normal initially, but, unfortunately, defective bone with insufficient collagen is used to repair the fracture, causing recurrent problems.

SKELETAL DYSPLASIAS[13]

Skeletal dysplasias or osteochondrodysplasias are a group of disorders caused by deformities in the development of the skeletal system. These disturbances affect the skeletal spine, pelvis and extremities, resulting in alteration in size and shape. There are more than 160 types of skeletal dysplasias, each distinguishable by clinical, genetic, and radiographic characteristics. The incidence of these disorders, including lethal types, is 1 in 3000 to 5000 births.

Dysplasia refers to deformities caused by an intrinsic bone anomaly. Dystrophy refers to abnormalities created by metabolic or nutritional aberrations. Proportional dwarfism refers to situations in which the extremities and spine are appropriately sized. Disproportionate dwarfism, on the other hand, is divided into short trunk and short limb varieties.

A geneticist should be consulted to help obtain an exact diagnosis, since this may affect treatment strategies. Diagnosing a skeletal dysplasia requires careful history and physical examination. One should measure the patient's adult height because, though all bone dysplasias result in decreased height, the amount

of dwarfism can hint at the final diagnosis. For example, a disproportionate adult with a height of 42″ is likely to have diastrophic
dwarfism, while an adult height of 48″ indicates achondroplasia,
and a height of 52″ may indicate hypochondroplasia.

As mentioned previously, it is important to indicate whether
the patient is a proportionate or disproportionate dwarf. The
most useful ratios include the ratio of the arm span to height
and the ratio of the upper and lower segments of the body. The
physician should determine whether the patient is rhizomelic
(characterized by short proximal segments—humeri or femora),
mesomelic (characterized by short middle segments—forearms
or tibiae) or acromelic (short hands or feet). The normal radius
to humerus ratio is 75% and the normal tibia to femur ratio
is 82%.

It is important to identify dysmorphic features, such as a
depressed nasal bridge, excessive bony prominences, or short
and broad thumbs. Other deformities that should alert one to
the possibility of a skeletal dysplasia include excessive lordosis,
kyphosis, varus or valgus angulation of the extremities, and limited joint motion.

Radiographic evaluation typically should include a lateral
skull view and an A-P pelvis, a lateral lumbar spine, A-P of the hand
and wrist, and A-P and lateral of the knee. These radiographs will
help identify if the defect is mainly epiphyseal, metaphyseal or
diaphyseal. One can also identify whether the spine is involved.

A thorough family history is important, since many of these
dysplasias are autosomal dominant or recessive traits. Laboratory
evaluation is rarely helpful, but it can help to identify treatable
metabolic or endocrine disorders such as rickets or hypothyroidism. Most research in this area is aimed at chromosomal mapping,
which will be utilized to design therapies in the future.

Commonly seen dysplasias include achondroplasia, hypochondroplasia, pseudochondroplasia, dyschondrosteosis, multiple epiphyseal dysplasia (MED), spondyloepiphyseal dysplasia
congenita (SED congenita), spondyloepiphyseal dysplasia tarda
(SED tarda), and diastrophic dysplasia[1].

References

1. Morrissy RT, Weinstein SL, eds. Lovell and Winter's pediatric orthopaedics. 4th ed. Philadelphia: Lippincott-Raven, 1996.

2. Miller MT, ed. Review of orthopaedics. 2nd ed. Philadelphia: WB Saunders, 1996.

3. Skoff H, Woodbury DF. Management of upper extremity in cerebral palsy. J Bone Joint Surg 1985;67-A(3):500–502.

4. Green DP, ed. Operative hand surgery. 3rd ed. 2 vols. New York: Churchill-Livingstone, 1993.

5. Mardaem-Bey T, Ger E. Congenital radial head dislocation. J Hand Surg 1979;316–320.

6. Cleary JE, Omer GE. Congenital radioulnar synostosis: natural history and functional assessment. J Bone Joint Surg 1985;67-A(4):539–545.

7. Green NE. Adolescent idiopathic scoliosis. Spine: state of the art reviews. Philadelphia: Hanley & Belfus, 1990;4(1).

8. Brooks WC, Gross RH. Genu varum in children: diagnosis and treatment. J Am Acad Orthop Surg 1995;3:326–335.

9. White GR, Mencio GA. Genu valgum in children: diagnostic and therapeutic alternatives. J Am Acad Orthop Surg 1995;3:275–283.

10. Barlow TG. Early diagnosis and treatment of congenital dislocation of the hip. J Bone Joint Surg Br 1962;44:292.

11. Skaggs DL, Tolo VT. Legg-Calvé-Perthes disease. J Am Acad Orthop Surg 1996;4:9–16.

12. Moseley CF. A straight-line graph for leg length discrepancies. J Bone Joint Surg 1997;59-A(2):174–179.

13. Beals RK, Horton W. Skeletal dysplasias: an approach to diagnosis. J Am Acad Orthop Surg 1995;3:174–181.

Chapter 11

Arthroplasty

Joint replacements are among the most common procedures performed in orthopaedics. It is essential for the house officer to understand the care of patients undergoing these procedures, as they are often elderly patients with multiple medical problems. The purpose of this chapter is to review the basics of arthroplasty and potential pitfalls and complications associated with the procedures and their postoperative care. This chapter is just an overview and by no means should be considered a comprehensive text on this broad topic.

Total joint arthroplasty refers to replacement of both articulating surfaces of the joint. The most common joints replaced are the hip and knee, with approximately 250,000 of each procedure performed annually in the United States. The shoulder and elbow are the other large joints that have documented success with arthroplasty procedures, but in numbers much lower than the hip or knee. Ankle replacements are rarely performed anymore because of high failure rates and since arthrodesis is such a successful procedure[1,2].

Primary arthroplasty refers to the initial joint replacement and is associated with high success rates and high levels of patient satisfaction[3-7]. Revision or "re-do" procedures are often technically challenging procedures with higher complication and lower success rates than the primary procedures. With increasing life expectancies and expanding indications for primary procedures, the number of revision procedures will increase in the future.

Hemiarthroplasty refers to the replacement of one articular surface of the joint. This is commonly performed in the hip, usually for the treatment of displaced femoral neck fractures in elderly patients, and in the shoulder for complex proximal humerus (usually three- or four-part comminuted fractures) fractures. Some surgeons also prefer hemiarthroplasty for primary shoulder replacements given the complications associated with the glenoid component in total shoulder arthroplasty. In both instances, the proximal femur and the proximal humerus, respectively, are the sides of the joint that are replaced. Hip hemiarthroplasty can be unipolar, with the articulation occurring between the large head component and the native acetabulum, or bipolar, in which there is an additional articulation between outer and inner head bearings. Theoretically, the additional articulation in the bipolar component should reduce acetabular articular cartilage wear. Hemiarthroplasty is not performed in the knee, but unicompartmental replacement of either the lateral or medial compartment is occasionally performed for isolated unicompartmental changes[8].

The remainder of this chapter will concentrate on the individual arthroplasties with their associated controversies, pitfalls, and complications.

TOTAL HIP ARTHROPLASTY

Total hip arthroplasty (THA) is commonly used for degeneration of the hip joint secondary to osteoarthritis (OA), rheumatoid arthritis(RA), avascular necrosis (AVN), post-traumatic changes, and other afflictions of the hip joint. Since the introduction of low friction arthroplasty by Sir John Charnley in the 1960s, this procedure has evolved to be one of the most successful in orthopaedics, with respect to longevity and patient satisfaction[5,7].

Early THAs consisted of a cemented stainless steel femoral component with a cemented polyethylene acetabular component. With the evolution of hip implants, changes have occurred in the materials and their methods of implantation. Currently, most prostheses are made of titanium or cobalt-chrome alloys. Polyethylene remains the most common material for the friction bearing surface; however, with concerns over osteolysis related to the inflammatory response associated with polyethylene debris[9,10], ceramics and metal on metal bearing surfaces are now being reintroduced into clinical studies[11].

Cementless designs of both femoral and acetabular components became popular in the 1980s as a potential means for improved implant longevity secondary to biological ingrowth of the bone to the porous coating of the prosthesis[12,13]. These were formulated in response to aseptic loosening of the cemented components presumed secondary to cement debris. Long-term studies of cementless component survival are currently not available, but early and intermediate results have been encouraging in certain patient populations.

Currently, with modern femoral cementing techniques using a medullary plug, cement gun, canal pressurization and lavage, cement centrifugation and stem centralizers, it is felt that the longevity of cemented components will improve further[14]. Metal-backed porous ingrowth acetabular components are now more commonly used than cemented polyethylene components, as the cemented acetabular components had significant loosening and revision rates at long-term follow-up[7]. A metal-backed acetabular component with a cemented femoral stem (Hybrid THA) has recently gained popularity and was the recommended implantation scheme of choice for THA in a recent NIH Consensus conference[15]. Significant controversy still exists for cemented versus cementless femoral components with strong arguments for and against each option[12,13,16].

With respect to the postoperative care of patients undergoing hip arthroplasty, the house officer must be diligent in recognizing and treating the underlying medical problems that can be exacerbated in the perioperative period. *Medical consultation is often necessary in caring for these patients.* Complications of THA in the postoperative period, in addition to medical problems, include infection, DVT/PE, dislocation, bleeding/anemia, nerve palsy, and femur fracture.

Deep-seated **infection** following THA is uncommon with a rate of less than 1%, using modern surgical techniques[17,18]. Early postop infection (Stage I) occurs within the first 4 months of surgery and generally presents as an acute infection does with pain, fever, elevated white blood cell (WBC) count, and wound drainage. Early infection usually results from an infected hematoma, and these can present difficulty in distinguishing between superficial and deep infection. Prolonged drainage from the surgical incision should raise suspicion for infection in both the early and late postoperative periods even after the drainage has ceased. Treatment of Stage I infections involves operative drainage of the hematoma with culture specific intravenous antibiotics for 4 to 6 weeks. The time course for intravenous antibiotics remains controversial. The goal of treatment of Stage I infection is eradication of infection with salvage of the prosthetic components if possible.

Late infections (Stages II and III) can be more difficult to diagnose and often require radionuclide scanning, joint aspiration, and occasionally open tissue biopsy for diagnosis. Treatment involves resection arthroplasty (removal of prosthetic components) with culture specific intravenous antibiotics and eventual prosthetic reimplantation, if possible. The time span for reimplantation varies based on numerous factors including patient condition, the infectious organism (Gram negatives more difficult to eradicate), and proof of eradication of infection.

Deep Venous Thrombosis (DVT) is a common postoperative problem in THA patients, with a 50% to 80% incidence of documented DVT for those not on prophylactic therapy. It is a feared complication, given the possibility for propagation to a potentially fatal pulmonary embolus. This topic is discussed in detail in Chapter 9.

Dislocation after THA can occur for many reasons including factors related to surgical technique, implant design, and patient profile[19]. Most dislocations are **posterior,** and on examination, the affected leg will be *shortened adducted and internally rotated.* In **anterior dislocations** the leg will be *shortened, slightly abducted and externally rotated.* Dislocations are usually extremely painful and easily diagnosed, but on occasion, especially with continuous postoperative regional anesthetics, they can be painless and overlooked.

Leg lengths should be checked on a daily basis while the patient is in the hospital, and any alteration from the initial postop appearance should prompt analysis with an A-P pelvis radiograph. If dislocated, analgesia and muscle relaxation are necessary to allow for a gentle reduction. Excess force can lead to component migration or femur fracture. On rare occasions with soft tissue interposition, open reduction may be necessary.

Patients at higher risk for dislocation are elderly, THA done for fracture, revision surgery, posterior approach, and those patients who are noncompliant with medical instructions. Treatment after reduction involves formulating an orthosis to counteract the forces that caused the dislocation. For example, an orthosis for a posterior dislocation would prevent the hip from excessive flexion, adduction, and internal rotation. These are designed as abduction orthoses with hinges at the hip joint to limit flexion to approximately 0–60 or 70 degrees. Orthoses for anterior dislocations limit extension and external rotation. For patients with recurrent dislocations and malaligned prostheses, revision surgery may be necessary.

Postoperative **anemia** may occur frequently after hip surgery, especially in revision cases, which tend to be associated with higher volumes of blood loss than primary cases. Strict attention must be paid to hemoglobin and hematocrit levels in the perioperative period, especially since arthroplasty patients tend to be older and often have concurrent medical problems. In addition, these patients require rapid optimization of their medical condition secondary to the trend of shorter hospital stays dictated by third party payers.

A universal hemoglobin or hematocrit level should not be used as a cutoff point to give a transfusion, as each patient has a unique medical profile that should dictate management. Nonautologous transfusions should be based on symptomatic anemia (tachycardia, weakness, dizziness, low urine output) and not given blindly, especially with the concerns over transmission of viral diseases such as hepatitis or HIV. THA patients often donate autologous blood prior to surgery, which is often transfused with less strict guidelines since the concern for disease transmission from banked blood is not present.

Erythropoietic drugs and engineered blood products are currently being formulated and tested to eventually replace the need for banked blood transfusion[20]. The use of hypotensive epidural anesthesia may also decrease the need for postoperative transfusion, as it is associated with less intraoperative blood loss[21].

Nerve palsy is uncommon after primary THA (<1%) but can occur in up to 5% of revision procedures[22]. The sciatic nerve is especially at risk with posterior approaches and with leg lengthening. In revision surgery through a posterior approach, the sciatic nerve is often encased in scar and should be identified early in the case to allow for recognition and protection throughout the remainder of the procedure. When leg lengthening is performed, the surgeon should check intraoperatively to ensure that undue tension is not placed on the nerve. The femoral nerve is at risk with anterior and anterolateral approaches to the hip secondary to retractor placement and anterior capsular release.

Postoperatively, both quadriceps contraction (ask the supine patient to press his or her knee into the bed) and sciatic nerve function (check foot and toe dorsi- and plantar flexion) must be checked daily to assess femoral nerve function. Most nerve palsies are neurapraxias with eventual recovery of function. Those with permanent palsies have significant disability. In cases of sciatic nerve palsy, an ankle-foot orthosis (AFO) should be ordered to prevent heelcord contracture from the associated foot drop.

Vascular injury is rare and is generally recognized intraoperatively, where it can be immediately addressed. In a posterior approach, especially during revision acetabular reconstruction, the **superior gluteal artery** may be at risk during dissection or hardware placement in the sciatic notch region. The **femoral vessels** are at risk with anterior approaches and with anterior capsular release from any approach. Of greatest concern is **intrapelvic vessel** disruption, which can go unnoticed in the operative field but can cause massive bleeding with hypotension and even death. This situation can occur with drilling and screw placement for acetabular prostheses. Regions to avoid are **anterosuperior (iliac vein)** and **anteroinferior (obturator artery)**. The safest regions for screw placement are superior into the ilium and posterosuperior toward the dense cortical bone in the sciatic notch. Care must be taken not to be overzealous in this region either, as the superior gluteal vessels can be injured with an erratic drill or screw.

Femur fracture after THA generally occurs intraoperatively, where it can be recognized and treated immediately, but can also occur postoperatively after trauma or a forceful reduction of a dislocated hip. Any increase in thigh pain or abnormal appearance to the leg should be evaluated with radiographs of the pelvis and femur. If a fracture has occurred, the neurovascular status must be carefully assessed and the patient should be placed in longitudinal traction (i.e., Buck's) for comfort. Treatment will depend on the location and extent of the fracture[23].

Postoperatively, THA patients generally begin rehabilitation on postoperative day one or two. The initial weight-bearing regimen depends on the method of fixation of the prostheses and choice of the individual surgeon. Those involving cementless components will range from NWB to WBAT depending on the surgeon's preference. Those with cemented or hybrid components may range from TDWB to WBAT, but generally most surgeons will allow more weight bearing on cemented rather than cementless components. Those patients with revision surgery using bulk allografts will be NWB for several weeks to months until the graft incorporates. THA patients have needs for special equipment upon discharge including elevated commodes, walkers and sometimes elevated shower seats or hospital beds. Debilitated patients generally will have more equipment needs.

In conclusion, the postoperative management of the THA patient can be among the most challenging in orthopaedics. Things to assess on a daily basis besides the patient's medical condition include *leg lengths, quadricep function, foot and toe dorsi- and plantar flexion and distal pulses.* Deviations from previous examinations should alert the house officer to perform further evaluation of the specific problem.

TOTAL KNEE ARTHROPLASTY

Total Knee Arthroplasty (TKA) is commonly used for degenerative conditions of the knee secondary to OA, RA, post-traumatic DJD, and other less common conditions causing knee joint degeneration. Total Knee Arthroplasty procedures have high patient satisfaction and longevity rates similar to those documented for THA[3,6].

TKA refers to replacement of the medial, lateral, and patellofemoral compartments of the knee. Other reconstructive options in the knee include unicompartmental replacement[8], osteotomy, and arthrodesis, each with specific indications that will not be covered in this text. Controversy in TKA exists over resurfacing the patella (cutting undersurface and replacing with prosthesis), utilizing cemented or cementless components, posterior cruciate ligament sparing versus sacrificing, all-polyethylene tibial components versus metal tibial trays with polyethylene inserts, and simultaneous versus staged bilateral knee replacements. Strong arguments exist for both sides of each controversy and are beyond the scope of this text.

The care of patients undergoing this procedure can be challenging as, once again, the patient population is generally elderly with associated medical conditions. Potential perioperative complications are similar to those of THA and include *infection, DVT/ PE, bleeding/anemia, neurovascular injury, and periprosthetic fracture*[24].

Infection after TKA perioperatively occurs from wound healing problems or from infected hematomas[25,26]. Suspicion should be high if the wound has prolonged drainage (greater than 5 days postop), skin breakdown occurs (full thickness necrosis more ominous than partial), or if the patient has prolonged pain and stiffness with no apparent cause. If a patient has prolonged drainage, or develops a perioperative hematoma causing significant pain and limited range of motion, then serious consideration should be given to stopping therapy and operatively draining the knee. If the knee is infected, then treatment should be initiated with operative debridement and culture specific antibiotics. Controversy exists over arthroscopic versus open irrigation and debridement, the length of antibiotic therapy, and retaining versus removing the prosthesis. In cases of full thickness wound necrosis, plastic surgery consultation should be obtained with strong consideration for flap coverage of the defect, especially if the prosthesis is exposed[27].

Late TKA infections (greater than 4 months postoperatively) should be treated similarly to those of late THA infections with resection arthroplasty, antibiotic impregnated cement spacers, intravenous antibiotics and reimplantation once there is documented eradication of infection. Controversy exists over primary (one stage) versus delayed (two stage) reimplantation and also on the time course for the second stage of two-stage reimplantation. **DVT/PE** risk after TKA is similar to that of THA with respect to the percentage of postop DVTs; however, in TKA the majority of these are distal to the knee, unlike in THA, for which the majority are proximal (thigh). It is felt that the risk of PE is low with distal DVTs, but the chance of a distal DVT propagating proximally into the thigh is approximately 15%–20%, thus distal DVTs should not be discounted. Controversy exists over the type and duration of DVT prophylaxis and is discussed in detail in Chapter 9.

Blood loss after primary TKA is generally less than that of THA. The procedure is generally performed under tourniquet control, and the knee can easily be placed in a compression bandage perioperatively to minimize the potential dead space for blood loss and hematoma to occur. Revision TKA may be associated with higher blood loss, since the procedures tend to be lengthy and often cannot be performed in their entirety under tourniquet control. Preoperative autologous tranfusions are often used and should be strongly considered in the revision setting. Transfusion of nonautologous blood should be performed only for symptomatic anemia to minimize the risks of transfusion-related illness.

Vascular compromise is rare with this procedure but can be a devastating complication[28]. Injury to the popliteal artery can be recognized intraoperatively once the tourniquet is released and represents a vascular emergency requiring intervention of a vascular surgeon for repair or grafting. For those who close the wound prior to releasing the tourniquet, arterial damage would be manifested by absent distal pulses and copious drain output. Pulses must be checked on a daily basis, as any alteration from the norm for that patient may represent occult arterial damage. In addition, if a lateral retinacular release is performed, the superior lateral geniculate artery may cause problematic postoperative bleeding if not avoided or coagulated during the procedure.

Peroneal nerve palsy is another potential complication of this procedure (incidence <1%), and patients especially at risk are those with preoperative valgus deformities and flexion contractures[29]. Dorsiflexion of the foot and great toe (Tibialis anterior and EHL, respectively) and foot eversion (peroneus brevis/longus), as well as sensation in the first dorsal web space should be checked in the recovery room and on a daily basis to assess peroneal nerve function. If a patient develops immediate postoperative paresthesias, then initial treatment involves *removal of immobilizers and tight dressings and flexion of the knee to 20–30 degrees.* With the advent of continuous regional anesthetics, it is difficult to diagnose an impending nerve palsy in an expedient manner, as the patients will be asymptomatic. Continuous epidural anesthetic has been shown to be a significant risk factor for developing peroneal nerve palsy[30].

If a palsy occurs in the face of an expanding hematoma, then urgent exploration may be indicated; otherwise, treatment involves observation, with some clinical series suggesting eventual decompression if the palsy does not resolve in several months[31].

Supracondylar femur fractures remain a significant problem associated with TKAs[32]. They occur most commonly in obese osteoporotic females, and the goal of treatment should be restoration of normal alignment and motion. Surgery is generally needed to attain these goals with options including ORIF with buttress plates, blade plates, dynamic condylar screw/plate designs, or a retrograde intramedullary nail through the intercondylar notch of the prosthesis.

The postoperative weight-bearing regimen varies depending on utilization of a cemented or cementless prosthesis. Generally, with cemented prostheses, the regimen is PWB or WBAT, while with cementless, it is NWB or TDWB for approximately 6 weeks until the patient is cleared to bear weight as tolerated. ROM exercises are usually started on postop day one. Some surgeons use CPM to regain motion, even as early as in the recovery room, with the goal of achieving 90 degrees of flexion sooner than with PROM or AROM exercises. CPM has not demonstrated any increases in the amount of flexion the patient will eventually achieve when fully rehabilitated[33]. One will find that rehab regimens will differ from surgeon to surgeon without any definitive consensus on the most appropriate regimen.

Overall, complications after TKA are relatively rare, but diligent postoperative care is necessary to obtain optimal function and to avoid untoward problems.

TOTAL SHOULDER ARTHROPLASTY[34]

Shoulder arthroplasty whether total (TSA) or hemiarthroplasty is performed less frequently than THA or TKA, but is performed frequently enough to justify gaining familiarity with the basics of the procedure and potential complications.

TSA refers to prosthetic replacement of both the humeral and glenoid surfaces, while hemiarthroplasty refers to replacement of just the humeral surface. Some surgeons routinely perform hemiarthroplasty in degenerative conditions, as TSA has been associated with high rates of radiolucent lines around glenoid components suggesting component loosening. This was especially true with constrained prostheses, which are essentially not used anymore in the United States.

Hemiarthroplasty is also performed in cases with deficient rotator cuffs (cuff-tear arthropathy) and in four-part and some three-part proximal humerus fractures. Shoulder replacement also has excellent results with respect to patient satisfaction. The ultimate functional result is highly dependent on the postoperative rehabilitation to restore motion and strength.

The inpatient perioperative care of these patients is different from that of other arthroplasty patients, as the inpatient course is shorter (1–2 days) and there are generally fewer associated complications. Comorbid conditions still must be managed closely, and complications to be aware of include infection, instability, and neurovascular injury. The long-term complication rate after this procedure is 10%–15%, with instability being the most common complication. Anemia and DVT/PE are rare after shoulder replacements.

Infection after shoulder arthroplasty is rare but devastating if it occurs. Diagnosing it during the hospital stay would be exceedingly rare, given the short postoperative stay. Any prolonged wound drainage in the perioperative period is suggestive of infection and requires further investigation. Late infection can be managed with resection arthroplasty with or without reimplantation.

Instability is perhaps the most common problem in TSA. Any abnormally severe postoperative pain should be investigated with an A-P and axillary radiograph to rule out dislocation. Inpatient instability is rarely diagnosed, as the patient is generally in a sling during this time period. Recurrent instability may require a revision secondary to component malposition or soft-tissue insufficiency (subscapularis tendon tear).

Neurovascular damage is also rare. A thorough postoperative neurologic evaluation of axillary, radial, median, ulnar, and musculocutaneous nerve function is mandatory to assess for palsy. Initial assessment may not provide useful information, as these procedures are now often performed under regional anesthetic, which can block nerve function up to 24 hours after the procedure, depending on the agent used. Once the block wears off, accurate examination is mandatory. Postoperative neurapraxia, although rare, should be followed expectantly for return of function, and if no improvement occurs, then EMG/NCV should be considered to rule out any interruptive lesion.

Postoperatively, these patients are placed in a shoulder immobilizer and generally begin pendulum exercises in 1 to 2 days. Initiation of PROM and AAROM exercises usually under supervision of a therapist begins shortly afterward (discretion of surgeon), and AROM and strengthening generally begin at approximately 6 weeks to 2 months postoperatively.

Overall, this procedure involves less intense inpatient perioperative care than THA and TKA , but the house officer should still be aware of the potential pitfalls associated with this procedure.

TOTAL ELBOW ARTHROPLASTY[35]

Total elbow arthroplasty (TEA) is an excellent treatment option for patients with elbow deformity or pain refractory to nonoperative measures or as a salvage procedure for other failed surgical treatments. Modern prosthetics employ either a semiconstrained design or are resurfacing implants, which have replaced the fully constrained designs secondary to the high loosening rates of the latter. Constrained designs still may play a role in patients with severe instability and associated bone loss.

Indications for TEA include pain or instability that interferes with the ability to use the elbow for activities of daily living. Elbow replacements are most commonly performed in patients with rheumatoid arthritis (RA), with pain being the most common indication. Motion loss is generally not significant in patients with RA except in those with JRA. Other treatment options for the arthritic elbow include distracton or interposition arthroplasty, synovectomy and fusion, but TEA remains the most predictable if used for the proper indications.

Absolute contraindications include active or latent infection of the elbow itself or active systemic infection from any source. Relative contraindications include soft-tissue contracture and muscle paralysis.

Complications include infection, neurapraxia, wound healing problems, triceps insufficiency, fractures, loosening, and instability. These are generally not seen during the short inpatient stay (1–2 days). A thorough neurologic examination of the operated extremity is essential to rule out nerve damage.

Postoperatively, the elbow is immobilized in full extension with range of motion beginning at the discretion of the operating surgeon, since many opinions exist on when to begin motion.

References

1. Kitaoka HB, Patzer GL. Clinical results of the Mayo total ankle arthroplasty. J Bone Joint Surg 1996;78-A:1658–1664.
2. Wynn AH, Wilde AH. Long-term follow-up of the conaxial (Beck-Steffee) total ankle arthroplasty. Foot Ankle 1992;13:303–306.
3. Ranawat CS, Flynn WF Jr, et al. Long-term results of the total condylar knee arthroplasty: a 15-year survivorship study. Clin Orthop 1993; 286:94–102.
4. Rand JA, Ilstrup DM. Survivorship analysis of total knee arthroplasty. Cumulative rates of survival of 9200 total knee arthroplasties. J Bone Joint Surg 1991;73-A:397–408.

5. Rorabeck CH, Bourne RB, et al. A double blind study of 250 cases comparing cemented with cementless total hip arthroplasty. Cost-effectiveness and its impact on health related quality of life. Clin Orthop 1994;298:156–164.

6. Rorabeck CH, Murray P. The cost benefit of total knee arthroplasty. Orthopedics 1996;19(9):777–779.

7. Schulte KR, Callahan JJ, et al. The outcome of Charnley total hip arthroplasty with cement after a minimum 20-year follow-up. J Bone Joint Surg 1993;58-A:961–975.

8. Barnes CL, Scott RD. Unicompartmental knee arthroplasty. Instruct Course Lect 1993;42:309–314.

9. Jacobs JJ, Shanbhag A, et al. Wear debris in total joint replacements. J Am Acad Orthop Surg 1994;2:212–220.

10. Maloney WJ, Smith RL. Periprosthetic osteolysis in total hip arthroplasty: The role of particulate wear debris. Instruct Course Lect 1996;45:171–182.

11. Amstutz HC, Grigoris P. Metal on metal bearings in hip arthroplasty. Clin Orthop 1996;329:11S–34S.

12. Bobyn JD, Tanzer M, Brooks CE. Noncemented total hip arthroplasty in the young patient: considerations for optimizing long term implant survival. Instruct Course Lect 1994;43:299–313.

13. Rorabeck CH, Bourne RB, et al. Cementless fixation of the femur: pros and cons. Instruct Course Lect 1994;43:329–337.

14. Jasty M. Cemented fixation of the femur. Instruct Course Lect 1994;43:373–379.

15. Total Hip Relacement. NIH Consensus Statement 1994;Sep12–14,12(5):1–31.

16. Harris WH. The case for cemented fixation of the femur in every patient. Instruct Course Lect 1994;43:367–371.

17. Fitzgerald RH, Nolan DR, et al. Deep wound sepsis following total hip artroplasty. J Bone Joint Surg 1977;59-A:847–855.

18. Fitzgerald RH. Infected total hip arthroplasty: diagnosis and treatment. J Am Acad Orthop Surg 1995;3:249–262.

19. McCollum DE, Gray WJ. Dislocation after total hip arthroplasty. Causes and prevention. Clin Orthop 1990;262:159–170.

20. Faris P. Use of recombinant human erythropoietin in the perioperative period of orthopaedic surgery. Am J Med 1996;101:28S–32S.

21. Lieberman JR, Huo MM, et al. The prevalence of deep venous thrombosis after total hip arthroplasty with hypotensive epidural anesthesia. J Bone Joint Surg 1994;76-A:341–348.

22. Schmalzried TP, Amstutz HC, Dorey FJ. Nerve palsy associated with total hip replacement. Risk factors and prognosis. J Bone Joint Surg 1991;73-A:1074–1080.

23. Kelley SS. Periprosthetic femoral fractures. J Am Acad Orthop Surg 1994;2:164–172.

24. Ayers DC, Dennis DA, et al. Common complications of total knee arthroplasty. J Bone Joint Surg 1997;79-A:278–311.

25. Pelligrini VD. Management of the patient with an infected knee arthroplasty. Instruct Course Lect 1997;46:215–219.

26. Windsor RE, Bono JV. Infected total knee replacements. J Am Acad Orthop Surg 199;2:44–53.

27. Dennis DA. Wound complications in total knee arthroplasty. Instruct Course Lect 1997;46:165–169.

28. Johanson NA. Neurovascular complications following total knee replacement: causes, treatment and prevention. Instruct Course Lect 1997;46:181–184.

29. Rose HA, Hood R, et al. Peroneal nerve palsy following total knee arthroplasty. A review of the Hospital for Special Surgery experience. J Bone Joint Surg 1982;64-A:347–351.

30. Isdusuy OB, Morrey BF. Peroneal nerve palsy after total knee arthroplasty: Assessment of predisposing and prognostic factors. J Bone Joint Surg 1996;78-A:177–184.

31. Mont MA, Dellon AL, et al. The operative treatment of peroneal nerve palsy. J Bone Joint Surg 1996;78-A:863–869.

32. Chmell MJ, Moran MC, Scott RD. Periarticular fractures after total knee arthroplasty: principles of management. J Am Acad Orthop Surg 1994;4:109–116.

33. Romness DW, Rand JA. The role of continuous passive motion following total knee arthroplasty. Clin Orthop 1988;226:34–37.

34. Wirth MA, Rockwood CA Jr. Complications of shoulder arthroplasty. Clin Orthop 1994;307:47–69.

35. Morrey BF. The elbow. In: Kelley WN, Harris ED, Ruddy S, Sledge CB, eds. Textbook of rheumatology. 5th ed. Philadelphia: WB Saunders, 1997.

Chapter 12

Commonly Used Medications in Orthopaedics

This chapter focuses on medications commonly prescribed by the orthopaedic surgeon including nonsteroidal medications, narcotic analgesics, medications used for deep vein thrombosis, and antibiotics. This chapter also contains dosing guidelines for medications frequently encountered by the orthopaedic surgeon. Sections will be divided into pain medications, DVT prophylaxis, antimicrobial and infectious disease medications, neurological drugs often used by the orthopaedic surgeon, GI medications, osteoporosis medications, medications for diabetes mellitus, and bronchodilators.

PAIN MEDICATIONS

Acetaminophen and NSAIDs[1]

This section focuses on acetaminophen and NSAIDs for controlling mild to moderate pain, including discomfort because of osteoarthritis. **Acetaminophen** is an excellent first-line drug against osteoarthritis. It has an excellent risk-benefit profile and is extremely inexpensive. Regularly dosed acetaminophen is thought to be as effective as NSAIDs in the management of osteoarthritic pain without having nearly the gastric, renal, or hepatic risks. Acetaminophen can be dosed at 650 mg every 4 hours as required for pain, with dosing not to exceed 4 grams per day.

If acetaminophen fails, or if the patient's pain seems to have an inflammatory component, NSAIDs are the next step. Comparative doses of NSAIDs have comparable effectiveness and risks, but prices vary quite drastically. For this reason, **ibuprofen, na-**

proxen, and **ketoprofen** should be utilized first since they are less expensive and have generic options available. Prior to prescribing an NSAID, the surgeon should ask the patient about his or her other medications. Patients should also be asked about peptic ulcer disease, renal insufficiency, chronic anticoagulation, renal hypertension, or aspirin hypersensitivity. One must always remember that many of these patients are older and some have a history of alcoholism, tobacco use, and congestive heart failure or renal failure.

Aspirin causes irreversible dysfunction of platelets, and subsequently is not first-line osteoarthritis therapy in elderly patients who tend to fall. Other carboxylic acids (salicylates) such as Trilisate, Disalcid, and Dolobid have minimal effect on platelets at low doses.

Though the risk profile of most of these medicines is identical, a few exceptions bear mentioning. Relafen (nabumetone) appears to have a lower incidence of peptic ulcers (<1% a year) than other NSAIDs (2%–4% per year). Additionally, Clinoril appears to have a lower renal affect than other NSAIDs. Naprelan (once a day naproxen), Feldene (piroxicam), and Daypro (oxaprozin) have the benefit of once-a-day dosing for those patients who are willing to incur a little expense for the benefit of easier dosing. Other than these previously mentioned exceptions, initial prescriptions should probably be ibuprofen or naproxen in most cases.

Prior to discontinuing a nonsteroidal because of ineffectiveness, one should confirm with the patient that maximum doses have been tried. Additionally, one should always remember that there is no advantage to combining two NSAIDs or combining aspirin use with NSAIDs. The addition of an H2 blocker or Carafate has not been demonstrated to prevent gastric ulcers induced by NSAIDs, and is generally not recommended. Gastric irritation is probably best prevented by instructing patients to take their medications with food. For those patients with a significant risk of gastric ulceration and an obvious indication for antiinflammatory medication, Cytotec (200 mcg orally four times a day) should be administered concurrently with the NSAID.

One should be cautious in patients who have an aspirin sensitivity because cross- reactivity among NSAIDs is extremely high. Patients with aspirin sensitivity have been noted to have increased risk of bronchospasm and anaphylaxis when administered NSAIDs.

Toradol is a relatively new NSAID available in oral, intramuscular, and intravenous form. Postsurgical patients have been extremely satisfied with injectable Toradol in the management of acute pain. Therapy should not exceed 5 days because the risk of adverse side effects is increased with prolonged use.

Patients on ACE inhibitors should not be given NSAIDs if possible, because the combination of the two medications can cause acute renal failure and serious hypercalemia in patients with CHF, preexisting renal disease, or hypovolemic states.

Dosing Instructions—NSAIDs and Acetominophen[2,3]

Tylenol (acetaminophen) 650–925 mg orally every 4–6 hours as needed for pain. Maximum daily dosage 4 grams. Pediatric dosing 10–15 mg/kg/dose every 4–6 hours as needed for pain.

Aspirin (acetylate) 650 to 800 mg orally every 4–6 hours.

Motrin (ibuprofen) 300 to 800 mg orally every 6–8 hours, not to exceed 3200 mg per day. Pediatric dosing 4–10 mg/kg/dose every 6–8 hours.

Naprosyn (naproxen) 250 to 500 mg orally every 8–12 hours, not to exceed 1500 mg per day. Pediatric dosing (>2 years old) 5–7 mg/kg/dose every 8–12 hours.

Meclomen (meclofenamate) 50 to 100 mg orally 4 times a day, not to exceed 400 mg per day.

Anaprox (naproxen sodium) 275 to 550 mg orally 2 times a day, not to exceed 1375 mg per day.

Dolobid (diflunisal) 250 mg orally 2 to 3 times a day, not to exceed 1500 mg per day.

Trilisate (choline magnesium trisalicylate) 750 mg orally 3 times a day to 1500 mg orally 3 times a day.

Orudis (ketoprofen) 50 to 75 mg orally 3 to 4 times a day or 200 mg orally every day, not to exceed 300 mg per day.

Toradol (ketorolac) 10 mg orally 3 times a day or 30 mg intramuscularly or intravenously every 6 hours, not to be dosed for longer than 5 days. Pediatric dosing 0.5 mg/kg every 6 hours intravenously or intramuscularly.

Lodine (etodolac) 400 mg orally 2 to 3 times a day, not to exceed 1200 mg per day.

Indocin (indomethacin) 25 to 50 mg orally 2 to 3 times a day, not to exceed 200 mg per day. Pediatric dosing 1–2 mg/kg/day in 2–4 divided doses, maximum 4 mg/kg/day.

Clinoril (sulindac) 150 mg to 200 mg orally 2 times a day, not to exceed 400 mg per day.

Relafen (nebumatone) 1000 mg orally every day to 2 times a day, not to exceed 2000 mg a day.

Feldene (piroxicam) 20 mg orally every day, not to exceed this dose.

Narcotic Analgesics[1]

Narcotic analgesics are excellent front-line medications for postoperative pain control. Abuse, physical dependence, and tolerance are rare complications that may develop with prolonged use. Patients must be cautioned against this, since many of them are simply not aware. One should also be careful in prescribing oral narcotics because many of these contain aspirin and acetaminophen. Patients should be warned not to exceed 4 grams of aspirin or 4 grams of acetaminophen per day. Patients should be warned not to take these medications with other sedating drugs such as alcohol or antihistamines and muscle relaxants, as they may amplify the effect of the narcotic and make them excessively dizzy or drowsy. Patients should be careful not to operate heavy machinery or automobiles when taking these medications.

Dosing Recommendations—Narcotics[2,3]

Darvon (proxyphene) 65–130 mg orally every 4–6 hours as needed for pain.

Darvon Compound 65 (65 mg propoxyphene, 389 mg aspirin, and 32 mg caffeine) 1 tablet every 4 hours as needed for pain.

Darvocet N-50 (50 mg propoxyphene and 650 mg acetaminophen) 1–2 tablets every 4–6 hours as needed for pain, not to exceed 6 tablets in 1 day.

Darvocet N-100 (100 mg Darvon and 650 mg acetaminophen) 1 tablet every 4–6 hours as needed for pain, not to exceed 6 tablets in one day.

Tylenol #3 (30 mg codeine and 300 mg acetaminophen) 1–2 tablets every 4 hours as needed for pain. Tylenol #2 contains 15 mg codeine per tablet, and Tylenol #4 contains 60 mg of codeine per tablet. Tylenol with Codeine elixir contains 12 mg codeine and 120 mg of acetaminophen per 5 ml of elixir. Pediatric dose 0.5–1 mg codeine/kg every 4–6 hours as needed for pain.

Vicodin (5 mg hydrocodone and 500 mg acetaminophen) 1–2 tablets every 4–6 hours as needed for pain. Pediatric dosing hydrocodone 0.6 mg/kg/day divided in 3–4 doses per day as needed for pain.

Percocet (5 mg oxycodone and 325 mg acetaminophen) 1–2 tablets every 4–6 hours as needed for pain. Pediatric dosing oxycodone 0.05–0.15 mg/kg/dose every 4–6 hours as needed for pain.

Demerol (meperidine) 50–150 mg intramuscularly, subcutaneously, or orally every 3–4 hours as needed. Pediatric dosing 1 to 1.5 mg/kg/dose every 3–4 hours intramuscularly, intravenously or subcutaneously as needed for pain.

MS Contin 15 mg to 200 mg orally every 12 hours. Higher doses to be utilized only in opioid-tolerant patients.

Morphine Sulfate 2–10 mg intravenously or intramuscularly every 4–6 hours as needed for pain. Pediatric dosing 0.1–0.2 mg/kg/dose every 2–4 hours intramuscularly, intravenously or subcutaneously as needed for pain.

Duramorph 5–10 mg in the lumbar region every 24 hours as needed for pain.

Antigout Medications[1]

High doses of NSAIDs are used to treat acute attacks of gout. No one NSAID has been proved to be more effective than any other, although indomethacin is a popular first choice. If the patient has difficulty tolerating NSAIDs, colchicine is an effective alternative, but many patients will refuse to take colchicine because of the GI side effects. It is important to note that aspirin is contraindicated in the treatment of gout. Medications such as allopurinol are typically used in an effort to prevent gouty attacks, but will tend to prolong attacks if started during an acute flare.

Dosing Recommendations for Gout Medications[2,3]

Zyloprim (Allopurinol) dosing ranges from 200 to 800 mg orally every day, depending on renal function and severity of gouty attacks.

Colchichine 2 mg intravenous load followed by 0.5 mg intravenously every 6 hours until a satisfactory response is achieved. Total dosage for the first 24-hour period not to exceed 4 mg. Oral Colchicine may be adminstered at the same dose as intravenous Colchicine.

Indocin (indomethacin). See NSAID section for dosing.

Anturane (sulfinpyrazone) 100–200 mg orally 2 times a day with meals.

Probenecid 1 gram orally 2 times a day.

Deep Vein Thrombosis Prophylaxis[4]

Deep vein thrombosis of the pelvis and lower extremities is a potentially life-threatening complication that frequently occurs following many orthopaedic procedures, particularly total knee arthroplasty and total hip arthroplasty. Virchow's triad of stasis, vessel injury, and coagulopathy is thought to be responsible for the development of this complication. Additional risk factors include advanced age, prolonged immobilization, obesity, CHF, use of oral contraception, and malignancy. In the past, aspirin, dextran, heparin, and warfarin along with mechanical anticoagulation devices have been the cornerstone of DVT prophylaxis. Recently, low molecular weight heparins have become increasingly popular, as they may offer an improved risk-benefit ratio. DVT following THA occurs from 45%–57% without prophylaxis. In 23%–36% of these cases, the thrombosis occurs proximally. Following total knee arthroplasty, the rate of DVT ranges from 40%–84% without prophylaxis, with 9% to 20% of these cases occurring proximally. Without DVT prophylaxis, fatal pulmonary embolism occurs in 3%–6% of the patients.

Aspirin administration renders platelets dysfunctional and, therefore, is thought to decrease the occurrence of thrombi. Aspirin functions by irreversibly binding and deactivating cyclooxygenase in circulating platelets. By inhibiting cyclooxygenase, the production of thromboxane is inhibited and platelet aggregation cannot occur.

Warfarin (Coumadin) has been used for DVT prophylaxis in knee and hip arthroplasty for a long time. This functions by inhibiting vitamin K epoxide leading to limited carboxylation of vitamin K dependent proteins that are necessary in the clotting cascades. Prothrombin, Factor VII, Factor IX, and Factor X, as well as protein C and protein S are impaired. Each of these proteins has a particular half-life, and as warfarin is administered, its effect causes newer dysfunctional, decarboxylated factors to replace the old functional ones. That is why it takes Coumadin 72–96 hours to reach an appropriate level. Proteins C and S are the body's natural anticoagulants, and unfortunately, these tend to have shorter half-lives. Therefore, when Coumadin administration is started, many think that the body passes through a dangerous hypercoagulable phase prior to becoming anticoagulated.

Standard, unfractionated heparin acts by binding to antithrombin III. Antithrombin III is a natural inhibitor of the coagulation cascade and its bond with heparin causes it to become more active. This causes increased inhibition of a number of clotting factors, including 2A and 10A. The ratio of anti-10A activity to anti-2A activity for unfractionated heparin is 1:1 (this is different for low molecular weight heparins). The increased activity of antithrombin III is monitored by following the activated partial thromboplastin time (PTT).

Low molecular weight heparins are derived from standard heparin and have pharmacologic properties that are entirely different from unfractionated heparin. Circulating thrombin (Factor 2A) is needed for local hemostasis following surgery. Meanwhile, factor 10A is considered essential in causing thrombosis. Low molecular weight heparins have an advantage over unfractionated heparin by allowing factor 10A to be inhibited while not affecting factor 2A as significantly. The ratio of anti-2A to anti-10A activity varies among the different low molecular weight heparins. These medications seem to have the advantage of providing a lot of antithrombotic activity while not causing as great a risk of bleeding. They also do not have to be monitored by laboratory tests, unlike both Coumadin and heparin. Additionally, the risk of heparin-induced thrombocytopenia is $\frac{1}{3}$ less with low molecular weight heparins compared with unfractionated heparins.

Current recommendations for total hip arthroplasty, hemiarthroplasty, and hip fracture pinnings include unmonitored LMWH (low molecular weight heparin) subcutaneously or Coumadin (maintaining INR from 2.0 to 3.0). Elastic stockings or intermittent pneumatic compression boots may provide additional protection. The current suggestions for total knee arthroplasty include unmonitored low molecular weight subcutaneously 2 times a day and/or intermittent pneumatic compression boots. Patients with acute spinal cord injury with paralysis should be given adjusted dose heparin or LMWH. Coumadin may be effective as well, though the data is not clear. Multiple trauma patients can be treated with intermittent pneumatic compression devices, Coumadin or LMWH.[5]

The literature is currently unclear as to whether treatment needs to last for 7–10 days or 6 weeks. There are no data suggesting that 7–10 days is insufficient, but Amstutz has reported five late nonfatal PEs from days 24–40 postoperatively in his 3700 THAs.

DVT Prophylaxis Dosing[2]

Aspirin (enteric-coated) 325 mg to 1200 mg orally every day.

Unfractionated heparin 3000 to 5000 units subcutaneously every 6–8 hours or intravenous heparin are utilized in order to maintain a PTT of 50 to 60.

Coumadin 2.5 to 10.0 orally at bedtime in order to maintain an INR of 2.0 to 3.0.

Lovenox 15 to 30 mg subcutaneously every 12–24 hours.

ANTIMICROBIALS IN ORTHOPAEDICS[6]

Antibiotics are most frequently used in orthopaedics for perioperative prophylaxis. Cephalosporins are most typically used in this role. Hypersensivity is the principle side effect of this class of drugs, occurring in approximately 5% of penicillin-sensitive patients. Vancomycin is typically substituted when hypersensitivity to cephalosporins prevents their use. One dose of antibiotics is typically administered during the hour prior to surgery in nearly all orthopaedic procedures, especially those in which metal implants are to be used. In total joint arthroplasty, antibiotics are typically continued for 24–48 hours, though no data exist indicating that this is beneficial. Many practitioners will continue postoperative antibiotics for 24 hours or until drains are removed when hardware has been implanted.

Open fractures are typically treated with cefazolin and an aminoglycoside (usually gentamicin) prophylactically, and their use is often continued for 5–7 days following the injury. The use of these antibiotics is not a substitute for adequate irrigation and debridement, which is the cornerstone of treatment for open fractures. Penicillin is added to the routine prophylaxis for "barn-yard" or heavily soiled, open fractures.

Dog, cat and human bites also require antibiotics, and frequently need open surgical debridement to prevent infection. *Pasteurella multocida* is typically the organism isolated from dog and cat bites, and this is successfully treated with Augmentin or oral penicillin. *Eikenella corrodens* is often isolated from human bites and this is also treated successfully with Augmentin or oral penicillin. Unasyn may need to be used in severe bites requiring intravenous therapy.

Diabetic foot infections are frequently caused by mixed flora, but dominant organisms tend to be staphylococci, streptococci, and *Enterobacter* anaerobes. These infections frequently require surgical debridement. Deep tissue cultures from the operating room are often helpful in defining antibiotic therapy. Superficial cultures are rarely helpful. Empiric therapy should begin with intravenous Unasyn, Cefoxitin, or Timentin.

Necrotizing fasciitis or pyomyositis is often a mixed infection caused by streptococci, enterobacteriaceae, bacteroides species, and clostridium. These can be life-threatening infections, and aggressive surgical debridement can be the difference between life and death. Empiric therapy includes intravenous Unasyn, Cefoxitin, and Timentin. Others recommend Imipenem because of the serious nature of this type of illness. Antibiotic therapy should be tailored according to culture results when they become available.

Acute bronchitis typically does not require antimicrobial treatment in a healthy host. Chronic bronchitis is typically treated by Bactrim, amoxicillin, or erythromycin. Augmentin or a second- or third-generation cephalosporin is utilized for resistant infections.

A community-acquired **pneumonia** can be treated by Cefuroxime intravenously or intravenous Ceftriaxone +/− erythromycin. Oral therapy can include Zithromycin or erythromycin. Nosocomial pneumonias (excluding aspiration) can be treated with intravenous Ceftazidime or Piperacillin and gentamicin. Nosocomial pneumonias owing to aspiration can be treated with Ceftazidime intravenously + Clindamycin intravenously +/− gentamicin intravenously, or Timentin intravenously +/− gentamicin intravenously.

Urinary tract infections (UTIs) should be treated initially with Bactrim or Septra. Ampicillin should be utilized in cases in which the urine Gram stain demonstrates Gram-positive cocci in chains, since these medications are not useful against enterococcal infections. Oral Ciprofloxacin should be used as second-line therapy.

Dosing of Antibiotics[2,6]

Penicillin VK 125 to 500 mg orally every 6–8 hours. Pediatric dose 25–50 mg/kg/day in divided doses orally every 6–8 hours.

Ampicillin 250 to 500 mg orally every 6 hours or 500 mg to 3 grams intravenously or intramuscularly every 4–6 hours. Pediatric doses 50–100 mg/kg/day divided every 6 hours orally and 100 to 200 mg/kg/day divided every 4–6 hours intramuscularly or intravenously.

Amoxicillin 250 to 500 mg orally every 8 hours. Pediatric dose is 20–50 mg/kg/day orally in divided doses every 8 hours.

Augmentin (amoxicillin and clavulanic acid) adult dosing 250 to 500 mg orally every 8 hours. Pediatric dosing 20 to 40 mg/kg/day orally in divided doses every 8 hours.

Keflex (cephalexin) 250 to 500 mg orally every 6 hours. Pediatric dose is 25 to 100 mg/kg/day divided every 6 hours.

Ceclor (cefaclor) 250 to 500 mg orally every 8 hours. Pediatric dose 20 to 40 mg/kg/day orally divided every 8–12 hours.

Ancef (cefazolin) 0.5 to 2 grams every 6–8 hours, with maximum dose 12 grams per day. Pediatric dose 50 to 100 mg/kg/day intravenously divided every 8 hours.

Erythromycin

Erythromycin base: 333 mg orally every 8 hours. Pediatric dose 30–50 mg/kg/day orally divided every 6–8 hours.

Ethyl succinate: 400 to 800 mg orally every 6–12 hours. Pediatric dosing 30–50 mg/kg/day orally divided every 6–8 hours.

Stearate: 20–40 mg/kg/day orally every 6 hours.

NOTE: Abdominal cramping very common. Medication should be taken with food and at least 8 ounces of liquid.

Azithromycin (5-day course) 500 mg orally on first day followed by 250 mg orally every day on days 2–5. Pediatric dosage 10 mg/kg on day 1, followed by 5 mg/kg/day orally every morning on days 2–5. Not currently FDA-approved for use in children. Do not administer with food or antacids. This medication should be used only following failure of erythromycin or clindamycin.

Clindamycin 150 to 450 mg/dose every 6–8 hours orally for maximum of 1.8 g per day. 1.2–1.8 grams per day in 2 to 4 divided doses intravenously or intramuscularly (maximum dose 4.8 g per day). Pediatric dose 10–30 mg/kg/day orally divided every 6–8 hours. 25 to 40 mg/kg/day intravenously or intramuscularly every 6–8 hours.

Septra, Bactrim (TMP/SMX) 1 double-strength tablet every 12 hours for 10 to 14 days for UTI/chronic bronchitis. Pediatric dose 6 to 20 mg/TMP/kg/day in divided doses every 6–8 hours.

NOTE: Patient should avoid prolonged exposure to sunlight for risk of severe sunburn or rash. These drugs have been associated with blood dyscrasias. Blood counts should be monitored for patients on long-term therapy on this antibiotic.

Flagyl (metronidazole) adult dosing 500 mg orally or intravenously every 6–8 hours. Pediatric dose is 15–30 mg/kg/day in divided doses every 8 hours.

Cipro (ciprofloxacin) 250 to 750 mg orally every 12 hours, depending on infection severity. Intravenously, 200 to 400 mg every 12 hours, depending on severity of infection. Pediatric dose 20 to 30 mg/kg/day po in 2 divided doses or 15–20 mg/kg/day intravenously in 2 divided doses.

NOTE: Not recommended in children <18 years of age owing to risk of arthropathy with erosions of weight-bearing cartilage in experimental animals.

Macrodantin (nitrofurantoin) 50 to 100 mg/dose orally every 6 hours. Pediatric dose is 5 to 7 mg/kg/day divided every 6 hours.

Diflucan (fluconazole)Dosing recommendations vary according to indication. Typically, 200 mg orally or intravenously on day 1, then 100 mg every day x 7 to 14 days. Pediatric dose is typically 6 mg/kg orally or intravenously on day 1, followed by 3 mg/kg orally or intravenously for 7–14 days.

Unasyn (ampicillin/sulbactam) 1–2 g every 6–8 hours intramuscularly or intravenously. Pediatric dose 100 to 200 mg ampicillin/kg/day every 6 hours.

Mefoxin (cefoxitin sodium) 1–2 g every 6–8 hours intramuscularly or intravenously. Pediatric dose 80–160 mg/kg/day divided every 4–8 hours, depending on severity of infection.

Timentin (ticarcillin/clavulanate potassium) Adults 3.1 g intravenously every 4–6 hours. Pediatric dosing 240 mg Ticarcillin component/kg/day divided in doses every 8 hours.

Gentamicin Adults 3–6 mg/kg/day intramuscularly or intravenously in divided doses every 8 hours. Pediatric dose is 2 to 2.5 mg/kg every 8 hours. Levels should be carefully monitored to prevent toxicity.

Vibramycin (doxycycline) 100 to 200 mg per day in 1 to 2 divided doses, orally or intravenously. Pediatric dose (>9 years old) 2–5 mg/kg/day in 1–2 divided doses.

Cefuroxime 750 mg to 1.5 grams per dose every 8 hours intravenously or intramuscularly. Pediatric dose is 75 to 150 mg/kg/day divided every 8 hours intravenously or intramuscularly.

Ceftriaxone sodium 1–2 g intravenously every 12–24 hours, depending on severity of infection. Pediatric doses vary on indication.

Fortaz (ceftazidime) 1–2 g every 8–12 hours intravenously or intramuscularly. Pediatric dose is 100 to 150 mg/kg/day divided every 8 hours.

Piperacillin sodium 2–4 g/dose every 4–8 hours. Pediatric dose is 200 to 300 mg/kg/day in divided doses, every 4–6 hours intravenously.

Nafcillin sodium 500 to 2000 mg every 4–6 hours intravenously. Pediatric dose is 50 to 200 mg/kg/day in divided doses every 4–6 hours intravenously, depending on severity of infection.

Primaxin (imipenem) 2–4 g/day in 3 to 4 divided doses. Pediatric dose is 60 to 100 mg/kg/day divided every 6–8 hours.

MUSCLE RELAXANTS[1,2]

Skeletal muscle relaxants are frequently used by the orthopaedic surgeon for patients with muscle spasms. These medications are also recommended with NSAIDs following some acute injuries. Some of these medications may cause sedation, so patients should be cautioned. Some of these may also be habit forming.

Valium (diazepam) 2 to 10 mg orally 2 to 4 times a day or 5 to 10 mg intramuscularly or intravenously every 2–4 hours as needed for spasm.

Flexeril (cyclobenzaprine hyperchloride) 20 to 40 mg/day orally in 2 to 4 divided doses.

Parafon Forte (chlorzoxazone) 250 to 500 mg 3 to 4 times a day orally. Pediatric dose is 20 mg/kg/day in 3 to 4 divided doses.

DIARRHEA AND EMESIS[1,2]

The initial treatment of **acute diarrhea** should focus on the prevention of fluid and electrolyte loss. This is especially important in the elderly and the very young. Acute diarrhea must be evaluated so the proper treatment can be administered. Patients should be questioned about travel and drinking water sources. Pseudomembranous colitis is a frequent cause of diarrhea in the hospital because of antibiotic alteration of the gut flora. Oral metronidazole and vancomycin are both effective agents. Metronidazole is cheaper. Only after infectious etiologies of diarrhea have been ruled out may antidiarrheal drugs be utilized. Some of these antidiarrheal drugs may cause pain if used for chronic diarrhea. Antispasmodics may relieve this discomfort.

Imodium (lopermamide hydrochloride) 4 mg initially followed by 2 mg after each loose stool up to 16 mg a day.

Lomotil (diphenoxylate/atropine) 15–20 mg/day in 3–4 divided doses.

Promethazine is typically the front-line medication for postoperative **emesis**. *Zofran* (ondansetron) is a back-up medication that is FDA-approved for nausea caused by chemotherapy, radiotherapy, or postop medications. Postop nausea owing to delayed gastric emptying should initially be treated with Metoclopramide or Cisapride.

Phenergan (promethazine hydrochloride) 12.5–25 mg intramuscularly, intravenously, or orally every 4 hours as needed for nausea. Pediatric dose is 0.25–1 mg/kg every 4–6 hours as needed for nausea.

Zofran (ondansetron) 0.15 mg/kg/dose intravenously every 4 hours as needed for nausea, in both adults and children.

Reglan (metoclopramide hydrocloride) 10–15 mg orally 4 times a day. Pediatric dose 0.1 mg/kg/dose 3 to 4 times a day.

Propulsid (cisapride) 10 mg orally 4 times a day 15 minutes before meals and at bedtime.

ANTIULCER MEDICATIONS[1,2]

Over-the-counter antacids are typically effective against minor dyspepsia. For patients with dyspepsia or ulcerlike symptoms not responsive to antacids, H2 antagonists are indicated. All H2 antagonists are similar in efficacy when prescribed at equipotent dosages. Cimetidine is a generic alternative and ought to be used preferentially. However, cimetidine can interact with theophylline, warfarin, phenytoin, propranolol, diazepam, lidocaine, and other medications. Patients who take one of these medicines should likely be treated with another alternative medication (e.g., Zantac or Pepcid).

Cytotec (misoprospol) is the only FDA-approved agent for use in the prevention of NSAID-induced gastric ulcers. This probably should be used only in high-risk patients when an NSAID is being taken. This medicine is contraindicated during pregnancy and should not be taken by women of child-bearing potential unless on birth control.

Patients who are infected with *Helicobacter pylori* should be treated with an antibiotic such as metronidazole, amoxicillin, or doxycycline and Pepto-Bismol or an antisecretory agent (H2 blocker or Prilosec). If the presence of this bacteria is confirmed, the antibiotic regimen may, in fact, be able to eradicate the bacteria and the ulcer problem. Prilosec (omeprazole) and Prevacid (lansoprazole) are both documented to heal active duodenal ulcers within 4 weeks. Treatment for this condition should last at least 4–8 weeks. Omeprazole has demonstrated drug interactions with diazepam, phenytoin, and warfarin.

Dosing and Medications[2]

Tagamet (cimetidine) 300 mg orally, intramuscularly, or intravenously every 6 hours or 800 mg orally at bedtime or 400 mg orally 2 times a day for short-term treatment of active ulcers. Pediatric doses are 20 to 40 mg/kg/day orally intramuscularly or intravenously in divided doses, every 6 hours.

Carafate (sucralfate) 1 gram orally every 6–12 hours. Pediatric doses are not established, though doses of 40 mg/kg/day divided every 6 hours have been used.

Zantac (ranitidine) 150 mg orally 2 times a day or 300 mg orally at bedtime, 50 mg intravenously or intramuscularly every 6–8 hours. Pediatric dose is 4–5 mg/kg/day orally divided every 8–12 hours. Intravenous or intramuscular dosing is 2–4 mg/kg/day divided every 6–8 hours.

Pepcid (famotidine) 40 mg orally at bedtime or 20 mg orally 2 times a day. Intravenous dosing is 20 mg every 12 hours. Pediatric dosing is 1–2 mg/kg/day given once or twice daily in oral and intravenous form.

Prilosec (omeprazole) 20 mg orally every day for 4–6 weeks. Pediatric dosing not established, but the effective dosing range is 0.7 to 3.3 mg/kg/day.

Cytotec (misoprostol) 200 mg orally 4 times a day.

References

1. Duke Outpatient Clinical Formulary, 1996–1997. A focus on quality. Copyright 1995 by PCS Health Systems, Inc.
2. Arky R, ed. Physician's desk reference. Montvale, NJ: Medical Economics Data Production Co., 1995.
3. Taketomo C, Hodding JH, Krous DM. The pediatric dosage handbook. Lexi-Comp, Inc., 1996.
4. Zimlich, et al. Current status of anti-coagulation therapy after total hip and total knee arthroplasty. J Am Acad Orthop Surg 1996;4:54–62.
5. Clagett GP, et al. Prevention of venous thromboembolism. Chest 1995;108:312S–334S.
6. Drew R, Dukes C, Hayward S. Guide to antimicrobial therapy 1996–1997. Antimicrobial Decision Support Team.

Index

Page numbers in *italics* refer to figures; those followed by the letter "t" refer to tables.

Titles to Make the Most of Your Clerkship Experience

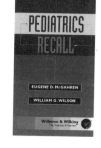